ESSENTIALS OF NEUROLOGY

ESSENTIALS OF
NEUROLOGY

by

JOHN N. WALTON, T.D. M.D. F.R.C.P.

*Neurologist, Newcastle General Hospital
and Newcastle Regional Hospital Board.
Physician in Neurology, Royal Victoria
Infirmary, Newcastle upon Tyne. Clinical
Teacher in Neurology, University of
Newcastle upon Tyne*

SECOND EDITION

LONDON

Pitman Medical Publishing Company Ltd

First published 1961
Second edition 1966

PITMAN MEDICAL PUBLISHING COMPANY, LTD.
46 CHARLOTTE STREET, LONDON, W.1

ASSOCIATED COMPANIES
SIR ISAAC PITMAN & SONS, LTD.
PITMAN HOUSE, PARKER STREET, KINGSWAY, LONDON, W.C.2
THE PITMAN PRESS, BATH
PITMAN HOUSE, BOUVERIE STREET, CARLTON, MELBOURNE
22-25 BECKETT'S BUILDINGS, PRESIDENT STREET, JOHANNESBURG

PITMAN PUBLISHING CORPORATION
20, EAST 46TH STREET, NEW YORK, N.Y. 10017

SIR ISAAC PITMAN (CANADA), LTD.
PITMAN HOUSE, 381–383 CHURCH STREET, TORONTO

PRINTED IN GREAT BRITAIN BY C. TINLING AND CO LTD
LIVERPOOL, LONDON AND PRESCOT

PREFACE TO THE SECOND EDITION

DEVELOPMENTS in the field of neurology during the last four years, together with the comments and advice of those who read and reviewed the first edition, have necessitated substantial changes in the text, although the general structure of the book remains the same. Each chapter has been carefully revised, some sections have been rewritten and there have been numerous additions which have inevitably resulted in some increase in length. For example, sections on the examination of individual muscles, reproductions of some representative radiographs, brief comments on echo-encephalography and gamma-encephalography and a new illustration of electro-encephalographic appearances have been added, and the chapter on treatment has been revised extensively, bearing in mind advances in pharmacology which have occurred in recent years. The references at the end of each chapter have also been brought up to date but, as in the first edition, those given have been selected in order to bring to the attention of the reader other books which he may consult in order to widen his knowledge of neurology and related disciplines and in which he will find references to original sources of information. In a text-book of this size and scope, it is still my view that references to scientific papers would be inappropriate; it would be difficult to select a suitable short list which would cover adequately all of the topics which are discussed, while comprehensive lists of references to journals would be too weighty in a short commentary of this nature.

I am grateful to Dr E. R. Bickerstaff and to Blackwell Scientific Publications Ltd. for permission to reproduce illustrations from *Neurological Examination in Clinical Practice*, to Dr G. L. Gryspeerdt for the reproductions of radiographs and to Dr D. D. Barwick and Miss B. P. Longley for the composite illustration of the electroencephalogram; photographic reproductions have been made in the Department of Photography, the University of Newcastle upon Tyne. As always I am deeply indebted to my secretary, Miss Rosemary Allan, for her invaluable assistance in the preparation of this second edition, and to Mr Michael Jackson and the staff of the Pitman Medical Publishing Co. Ltd. for all their help and co-operation.

JOHN N. WALTON

Newcastle upon Tyne
March 1965

PREFACE TO THE FIRST EDITION

ALTHOUGH there can be no absolute distinction between diseases of the nervous system and those which affect other organs or systems of the human body, by convention the clinical science of neurology embraces those many disorders which affect the functioning of the central and peripheral nervous system. This book has been written in order to help the undergraduate or postgraduate student to learn the principles of neurological diagnosis and treatment. It is hoped that it will also assist the practising physician in his management of patients suffering from this variety of illness.

The first ten chapters of the book are devoted to a consideration of the cardinal symptoms and signs of neurological disease, to the mechanism of their production and the various pathological changes which may produce these clinical manifestations. In this review of the principles of neurological diagnosis, brief mention is made of investigative methods, some simple and others highly specialised, but only in sufficient detail to indicate to the student or practitioner the indications for employing these methods, their failings and their dangers, and the information which they are likely to divulge. The ensuing chapters contain brief descriptions of specific syndromes of nervous disease, taking into account the general principles previously stressed. Exhaustive descriptions of pathological changes and of differential diagnosis are omitted and the reader will look in vain for lists and tables of diseases and syndromes. Nor will he find detailed analyses of the physiological mechanisms by which symptoms and signs are produced, since this work is based upon clinical methodology, and scientific premises are only mentioned when absolutely necessary for an understanding of clinical principles. The intention has been to make this a book which can be read by the student who wishes to obtain a composite picture of neurological illness, but can also be used for reference if need be. Each chapter is concluded with a list of references to other volumes in which more detailed information can be found and from which the reader can obtain further references to original sources of information, should he wish to consult them.

The book ends with a general review of therapeutic measures which are of value in the field of neurological medicine, but only those appropriate to general practice are considered fully, while more specialised techniques receive mention sufficient only to indicate which patients should be referred to a specialist for these measures to be undertaken.

In preparing this book, I am conscious of the debt I owe to those from whom I learned the principles of neurological diagnosis and management and I wish particularly to thank Professor F. J. Nattrass, Sir Charles Symonds, Dr E. A. Carmichael, Dr Raymond D. Adams and Dr H. G. Miller for the help and encouragement they have given me in the past. No textbook is written without reference to other volumes. I have obtained help particularly from *An Introduction to Clinical Neurology* by Sir Gordon Holmes, Sir Russell Brain's *Diseases of the Nervous System* and the chapters by Dr R. D. Adams in Harrison's *Principles of Internal Medicine,* and wish to express my indebtedness to the authors and publishers concerned. I must also thank the many authors and publishers who have given permission for the reproduction of stated illustrations. I am also grateful to Dr A. E. Clark-Kennedy for his helpful advice and to Dr Peter Nathan, Dr J. B. Foster and Dr David Poskanzer for their valuable criticisms of the manuscript. The work of preparing the typescript was performed by Miss Shirley Whillis and Miss Rosemary Allan, and many of the illustrations were prepared by Miss M. Mustart of the Department of Photography, King's College, Newcastle upon Tyne. I also wish to thank Mr D. K. C. Dickens and the staff of the Pitman Medical Publishing Company Ltd. for their enthusiastic and willing co-operation in the production of this volume.

JOHN N. WALTON

Newcastle upon Tyne
July 1959

CONTENTS

LIST OF PLATES

CHAPTER 1

SOME GENERAL PRINCIPLES IN NEUROLOGY

THE nervous system of the individual cannot be considered in isolation, for without an adequate supply of oxygen and of nutrients, which depend in turn upon efficient circulatory and respiratory activity, the nervous system cannot survive. The converse is also true, for the activity of the autonomic portion of the nervous system in particular exercises a profound and continuing influence upon the behaviour of the heart and circulation, upon respiratory activity, upon the gastrointestinal system, and upon the function of the endocrine glands. The mysteries of these complex and important interrelationships, upon which the normal functioning of the human body depends, are being elucidated to an increasing extent by anatomical and physiological studies; their understanding requires an appreciation of certain homeostatic mechanisms which are already familiar to readers of this volume. But there are still a great many problems which defy comprehension. Upon what, for instance, does the ability of the brain to control thought processes depend? It is well recognised that disordered activity of the mind is commonly present when modern techniques fail to demonstrate any abnormality in the structure or function of the brain; and the influence of the mind upon the behaviour of the organs of the body can be profound. Disorders of the mind can sometimes initiate and sometimes accentuate the symptoms of physical disease, while conversely certain organic diseases are regularly accompanied by psychological manifestations. The mechanisms underlying these relationships are still obscure but their importance must be recognised by the physician who deals with sick people. Diseases do not exist as independent entities; it is the patient who suffers from the disease who is real and who shows a personal and individual reaction to it. The pattern of his illness depends upon many factors, for the pathological process is influenced by his genetic constitution, by the condition of other organs of his body apart from that which is primarily affected, and by his state of mind.

There are many physical disorders of the nervous system which regularly produce a consistent series of symptoms and physical signs independent of the personality and constitution of the individual. The clinical syndrome resulting from division of one median nerve, for instance, is not significantly modified by the mental state of the

1

patient. But if the lesion of the nerve is incomplete, due perhaps to transient compression, the severity of the resultant symptoms and the rate of the recovery can be influenced by factors which are independent of the physical process concerned with the restoration of normal conduction in the damaged nerve fibres. Much may depend, for instance, upon the nature of the lesion responsible; if it was an industrial injury, involving a claim for financial compensation, the patient's disability may be excessive and his recovery unduly delayed.

Many functions of the nervous system, such as those concerned with speech, with seeing and hearing, with the control of movement and with the appreciation of sensation, are subserved by the passage of nervous impulses along pathways which have been clearly delineated by anatomists and physiologists. These functions can be disordered if there is a fault in development (a congenital defect). They may also be rendered abnormal by a pathological process, whether it is the result of inherited factors (genetically-determined illness) or whether it is acquired. The lesions so produced will give rise to certain symptoms and physical signs depending upon their situation and character and the functions of the pathways which they involve; many of the subsequent chapters of this book are devoted to a detailed consideration of these functions, to the means by which abnormalities can be recognised, the lesions responsible localised and their nature determined. The purpose of this introductory commentary is to indicate that the clinical effects of these pathological processes are not immutable, and that the resultant disease can be greatly influenced by the personality and constitution of the individual and by his state of mind. Some patients are born physically and mentally less perfect than others and yet show no obvious defect; but constitutionally they are less capable of resistance to stress, both mental and physical, and are seriously disturbed by environmental influences which would leave others unaffected. The possible effects of fatigue, of ageing processes, and of other contributory influences which cannot easily be measured by scientific parameters, must also be stressed. Are the headaches of which the patient complains due to emotional tension or to an intracranial tumour? Are his suspicions that he is suffering from malignant disease well-founded or is he suffering from cancerophobia? Do his insomnia and his symptoms of anxiety neurosis depend upon constitutional inadequacy and a low resistance to stress, or are they the result of some underlying physical disease? These are some of the common questions which the doctor is called upon to answer, questions which require, for their elucidation, all his reserves of experience and understanding.

It is also important at this stage to consider the use of the term 'functional' as commonly utilised in medicine to identify the nature and cause of a patient's illness, since the use of this word is a common cause of misconception. It would in fact be correct to regard as functional disorders, those diseases in which there is an important disorder of the function of some organ of the body, but which do not depend upon any recognisable pathological change in the organ concerned, whether structural or biochemical. In neurology, so-called 'idiopathic' epilepsy would be a good example, though it is of course possible that in this and many other states of altered function, some biochemical or structural abnormality is present which cannot be recognised with the techniques at present available. But, in fact, the term 'functional disorder', as conventionally used, is not generally applied to disease of this kind, but rather to symptoms and signs which result from a disordered state of mind. Thus when a physician says that a particular symptom is functional, he usually means that it has no physical cause and, by implication, that its origin is psychological. For instance, headaches due to anxiety or nervous tension are 'functional', and so too is loss of the voice (hysterical aphonia) in the young singer about to face her first professional engagement. In other words, anxiety reactions, symptoms resulting from mental or emotional fatigue, and those which are due to a subconscious desire to escape from stress (hysteria) are usually included in this category. It would, on the other hand, be incorrect to classify under this heading deterioration of intellectual function (dementia) which generally results from physical disease of the brain. Functional disorders, therefore, are those conditions in which symptoms and signs result not from any primary physical disease, but from mental processes, whether conscious or subconscious. These mental processes may in turn influence profoundly the physical functioning of the body; the increased heart rate, perspiration and insomnia which commonly accompany anxiety will serve as examples. Hence, the clinical use of the term 'functional', if not strictly correct in a semantic sense, is hallowed through common usage and can usefully be employed by the student, provided he appreciates its meaning, and does not regard this as a final diagnosis. For if a disorder is accepted as being 'functional' it is then necessary to decide whether the patient's disability is due to conscious anxiety, whether it is hysterical, or whether it could even be psychotic. In other words, its nature, and if possible its cause, must be determined if treatment is to be effective. Disorders of the mind will be considered and some of the terms mentioned above will be defined in a subsequent chapter, but it is well to appreciate at the outset that the distinction between organic and functional disease is often one of the most difficult diagnoses to make in medicine. And even when there is clear evidence of a primary physical abnormality it is common for the symptoms and signs to be accentuated or distorted by concurrent psychological factors. The doctor must always strive not only to recognise and interpret the symptoms and signs of physical disease which he observes in his patient, but also to understand the workings of his mind and to appreciate the influence which the one may have upon the other. Having accepted these facts it will now be convenient to consider some general principles which help in the recognition of diseases of the nervous system.

THE FOUNDATIONS OF NEUROLOGICAL DIAGNOSIS

In order to forecast accurately the outcome of a patient's illness and to advise upon appropriate treatment, accurate diagnosis is usually necessary. In disorders of the nervous system, more perhaps than in disease of other systems, the physical signs will indicate the anatomical localisation of the lesion or lesions responsible for the abnormalities of function which are present, while it is the history of the illness, revealing the detailed evolution of the patient's symptoms, which generally indicates the nature of the pathological process. Hence the intelligent interpretation of the significance of physical signs demands an adequate knowledge, first, of neuroanatomy. This does not imply that the student must be familiar with intricate details of the anatomical organisation of the nervous system, though he should be aware of the reference sources to which he may turn in order to find the anatomical information required in a particular case which presents a difficult problem in localisation. He should, however, be able to identify the areas of the cerebral cortex which control certain major functions, such as those of speech, the control of movement, and the appreciation of visual and somatic sensation. He must also be familiar with the general topography of the cerebral hemispheres, brain stem and spinal cord and with the organisation of the autonomic nervous system, at least in so far as the situation of the more important cranial nerve nuclei and the pathways traversed by the main motor and sensory pathways are concerned. Knowledge of anatomy alone, however, is clearly not enough, for one must understand the normal activities of these anatomical structures before it is possible to decide that their function or functions are disturbed. In subsequent chapters we shall deal with disorders in functioning of the motor, sensory and other systems and we shall consider how these may be recognised, how they may be brought about, and how the responsible lesion may be localised and identified. Certain general principles may, however, be usefully stated here.

Most symptoms and signs resulting from nervous disease can be referred to as positive or negative. **Positive symptoms** are those produced by irritation or stimulation of a part of the nervous system, causing it to behave in an abnormal manner; focal epilepsy resulting from irritation of or pressure upon the motor area of the cerebral cortex is an example. **Negative symptoms,** by contrast, are those produced by a temporary or permanent depression in function, so that some activity or ability, normally present, is lost; paralysis of a limb is a typical negative symptom. The law of **dissolution,** first propounded by Hughlings Jackson, should also be remembered. Those functions and skills most recently acquired during the processes of evolution and training are the first to be lost in disease of the brain, while primitive activities and instincts survive longer. A similar principle applies to temporary disturbances of cerebral function produced, say, by anaesthetics or other drugs. For instance, a naturalised foreigner may revert to using his native tongue during recovery from anaesthesia, and only when recovery is more complete will he be able to utilise the language of his adopted country. To take another example, man differs from the higher primates in his ability to move individual fingers and to use opposition of the thumb to the other fingers for the purpose of carrying out fine and deliberate movements. The latter can be called the 'precision grip'; the primate possesses only the 'power grip', produced by flexion of all the fingers. In an early lesion of the appropriate area of the motor cortex or of its efferent corticospinal or pyramidal fibres in man the 'precision grip' is impaired as is discrete movement of the individual fingers, at a time when the 'power grip' appears normal. Similarly, in the leg, movement of the toes is affected by such a lesion at an early stage.

Disordered function depends not only upon the localisation of pathological change, but upon its severity, its extent and the effects it has upon contiguous nervous tissue and upon interconnected though anatomically remote structures in the nervous system. Thus an acute and extensive lesion may affect a greater area of the brain than its anatomical extent would lead one to expect, for around the edge of the lesion itself the activity of the surrounding nervous tissue is disturbed by oedema, vascular changes and other ill-defined abnormalities. Furthermore, an acute lesion can produce a state of 'shock' or temporary dissolution of function in connected areas of the brain or spinal cord. This is seen in the patient with a hemiplegia which is initially flaccid, later spastic, or in one with an acute spinal lesion; the limbs below the level of the lesion are initially flaccid and totally paralysed but later, as the shock wears off, spasticity resulting from bilateral lesions of the corticospinal (pyramidal) tracts develops. By contrast, lesions of equal extent which are slow to develop, produce far fewer symptoms and physical signs, as it is only the structures which are actively invaded or destroyed by the lesion whose function is disturbed; the surrounding tissues have more time to adapt themselves to the presence of the lesion. Other forms of adaptation also occur, particularly in the cerebral cortex, for here it is sometimes possible for a function which has been lost through a cortical lesion to be 'adopted', though usually much less efficiently, by another area of the brain. This type of adaptation occurs more readily in children than in adults, for the younger the patient the greater the flexibility of cerebral organisation. In the spinal cord, there is much less opportunity for this type of reorganisation than in the brain, for the pathways followed here by nervous activity are more stereotyped and less complex. In the peripheral nerves opportunities for adoption of functions in this way are almost non-existent, but it should be remembered that the peripheral nerves are able to regenerate effectively following injury, while effective regeneration does not occur within the spinal cord or brain.

PATHOLOGICAL REACTIONS IN THE NERVOUS SYSTEM

A detailed consideration of neuropathology is beyond the scope of this volume, but certain general principles which are necessary for an informed approach to neurological diagnosis may be stated. Pathological changes in the nervous system can first be classified into three broad groups, namely, **focal lesions,** which cause a disturbance in function of a strictly localised area; **diffuse or generalised disorders,** whether of metabolic, toxic, vascular or other aetiology, which affect nervous and supporting elements throughout the nervous system; and **systemic nervous diseases,** in which the pathological process shows a predilection for a particular neuronal structure or group of structures, such as the anterior horn cells, the cerebellum and its connexions, or the pyramidal tracts. The focal lesions and diffuse disorders affect nervous tissue more or less by accident and many of these are not primarily neurological diseases. Thus cerebral vascular disease, which may produce a focal cerebral lesion, say, an infarct, is usually a complication of generalised atherosclerosis, while the diffuse pathological changes which occur in the brain in syphilis, for instance, form only one part of the changes resulting from infection of the entire human organism. In the systemic nervous diseases, by contrast, as in motor neurone disease, there is clearly some biochemical or other factor which causes the pathological process to be confined to a particular group of nerve cells or fibre pathways. In this context it is important to note that the tissues of the nervous system vary considerably in their response to a variety of different noxious influences. Thus ischaemia tends to affect nerve cells more severely than fibres, while plaques of demyelination, as in disseminated sclerosis, have a more profound influence upon the nerve fibres of the white matter. There are also considerable differences in the effects of ischaemia, compression and various toxins upon nerve fibres, depending upon whether they conduct motor or sensory impulses.

Having accepted the above outline of pathological changes which affect the functioning of the nervous system it is then necessary to subdivide these groups, and particularly the local lesions, on an aetiological basis. Virtually every pathological lesion of the nervous system will be embraced by one of the following headings—

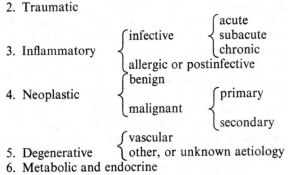

1. Congenital
2. Traumatic
3. Inflammatory
   - infective
     - acute
     - subacute
     - chronic
   - allergic or postinfective
4. Neoplastic
   - benign
   - malignant
     - primary
     - secondary
5. Degenerative
   - vascular
   - other, or unknown aetiology
6. Metabolic and endocrine

For detailed consideration of the pathological changes characterising lesions of these different types, the student is referred to textbooks of neuropathology. Most of the important central nervous lesions of **congenital** origin are clearly apparent as gross disorders of anatomical development and configuration; examples are anencephaly, hydrocephalus due to stenosis of the aqueduct of Sylvius, and meningomyelocele. Arteriovenous malformations or angiomas, which are commonly found in the substance of the brain, are also of congenital origin. **Trauma** to the nervous system, as elsewhere, produces the familiar effects of necrosis, haemorrhage and subsequent scar formation, the scar consisting of proliferated neuroglial cells and fibrils (gliosis) and of mesenchymal fibrous tissue derived from fibroblasts in the supporting tissue of the blood vessels. Among the **acute inflammatory disorders** we have first the meningitides which produce the typical pathological changes of inflammation and exudation in the meninges. Meningitis may give rise to superficial degenerative changes in the underlying nervous tissue or to more extensive ischaemic changes in the nervous parenchyma resulting from an obliterative endarteritis of blood vessels which traverse the subarachnoid space. **Pyogenic infection** of the substance of the brain and spinal cord begins as a diffuse suppuration, but localisation and abscess formation generally follows with the formation of a capsule through gliosis and fibrosis, as in a scar following trauma.

Most of the neurotropic **viruses,** such as those which give rise to virus encephalitis and anterior poliomyelitis, are polioclastic, that is, they show an affinity for nerve cells; inflammatory changes, with perivascular cellular infiltration and degeneration of nerve cells, are therefore seen in the grey matter of the brain and spinal cord in this group of diseases. Sometimes inclusion bodies are found within the nucleus or cytoplasm of infected nerve cells. The virus of herpes zoster shows a particular affinity for the cells of the posterior root ganglia. **Syphilis,** despite its decreasing incidence, is still the most important chronic infection of the central nervous system. The meningovascular form of the disease produces meningeal inflamma- tion and endarteritis of cerebral and spinal arteries; in general paresis there are degeneration of nerve cells, gliosis and minimal inflammatory changes in the cerebral cortex; while in tabes dorsalis the most prominent pathological change is gliosis and meningeal fibrosis at the entry zone of the posterior spinal nerve roots with secondary ascending degeneration of the posterior columns of the spinal cord. In **allergic or postinfective encephalomyelitis,** by contrast to the virus infections, inflammatory changes are largely confined to the white matter, where perivascular collections of inflammatory cells and loss of myelin are seen. The pathological changes in this group of diseases show some resemblance to those observed in the **demyelinating diseases** of unknown aetiology, such as disseminated sclerosis, in which there is patchy loss of myelin throughout the white matter of the brain and spinal cord. This primary lesion, in which the axis cylinders of the nerve fibres may initially be preserved, is eventually replaced by a glial scar.

Most of the **benign tumours** which affect the functioning of the central nervous system are extracerebral and extramedullary, that is they lie outside the brain or spinal cord, though within their bony encasements. The two most common are the meningioma, which probably arises from cells of the arachnoidal membrane, and the neurofibroma or neurilemmoma, which grows from the sheath of Schwann of the cranial nerves, spinal roots or peripheral nerves. These neoplasms compress and distort but do not invade nervous tissue. The gliomas constitute the major group of **malignant tumours** of the central nervous system; these are infiltrating and invasive tumours whose relative malignancy depends upon whether the principal constituent cell of the tumour is a relatively mature astrocyte or one of its more rapidly multiplying primitive precursors. Metastatic malignant neoplasms are also common in the nervous system; cancer of the lung, breast and kidney and the malignant melanoma are among those which most often metastasise to the brain. Secondary deposits, which are often seen at the junction of the white and grey matter of the brain, are sometimes single but much more often multiple. Less commonly these deposits, or plaques of lymphadenoma, may be laid down in the meninges; if this occurs in the spinal canal, or if a vertebral body has collapsed following malignant infiltration, spinal cord compression may result.

Vascular disorders of the nervous system are a common cause of pathological change. Bleeding into the subarachnoid space produces a meningeal inflammation comparable to meningitis and in some few cases a degree of meningeal organisation or so-called arachnoiditis may result. Chronic bleeding into the subarachnoid space can give rise to a state of haemosiderosis of the meninges. Haemorrhage in the nervous parenchyma produces an area of total necrosis which is eventually walled off by gliosis and fibrosis; if it is small the necrotic area is absorbed and a scar results, but more often a cavity is left which is filled with a clear straw-coloured fluid containing bilirubin. An infarct, too, will show an area of central ischaemic necrosis. Within twenty-four hours, activated microglial cells (the histiocytes or scavengers of the nervous system) invade the necrotic area and some become distended with the fatty remnants of the necrotic myelin which they have ingested. A minute infarct, produced by embolic occlusion of a tiny cortical vessel, may consist of nothing more histologically than a small cluster of activated microglial cells, whereas a large one will show an extensive central area of necrosis surrounded by distended phagocytes ('gitter' cells) and proliferating astrocytes. A large area of infarction may eventually be represented by a contracted glial scar or by a cavity, while multifocal infarction sometimes leads to the formation of multiple small cavities ('status lacunosus').

There remain a large group of **degenerative disorders** of the nervous system whose aetiology is at present unknown, but in some of which specific neuropathological changes are seen. In motor neurone disease, for instance, the cells of the motor nuclei of the brain stem, the anterior horn cells of the spinal cord, and the pyramidal tracts show a progressive degeneration; in Huntington's chorea there is a selective degeneration of the caudate nucleus and of the nerve cells of the frontal cortex. But in these and in many other disorders, although the anatomical distribution of the pathological lesions has been well-defined, their nature is little understood. Nor do we know why anoxia should affect particularly the cells of the deepest layer of the cerebral cortex, the Ammon's horn area of the hippocampus and the Purkinje cells of the cerebellum, nor even why deficiency of vitamin B_{12}, as in subacute combined degeneration of the spinal cord, should damage so selectively the posterior columns and pyramidal tracts. Many **metabolic disorders** which seriously disturb nervous functions produce relatively little pathological change, although in hypoglycaemia the changes are similar to those of anoxia, while in hepatic failure there is astrocytic proliferation, particularly in the basal ganglia. The pathological changes in many different forms of polyneuropathy are also non-specific, consisting of a swelling and fragmentation of axis cylinders in the peripheral nerves. Since the purpose of this section is to describe briefly some of the basic pathological reactions which may occur in the diseased nervous system and not to give comprehensive descriptions of the detailed changes which occur in individual disease entities, these histopathological changes whose significance is not understood will not be considered further.

CONSTITUTION AND HEREDITY

In considering the aetiological factors which may be responsible for a patient's illness it is only too easy to overlook the important influences which may be derived from inherited characteristics. Many neurological disorders, and particularly some of those which were referred to above as 'degenerative' in character, are clearly inherited in a strictly Mendelian manner. A disease resulting from a dominant gene situated on one of the autosomes, a so-called autosomal dominant character, is passed on by an affected individual to half his or her children of either sex if penetrance or expressivity of the gene is complete. Examples of neurological disorders which are often inherited in this way are migraine, Huntington's chorea, peroneal muscular atrophy and facio-scapulo-humeral muscular dystrophy. A recessive gene, carried on the autosome, however, can only produce its effect if it is paired with a similar gene lying on the other chromosome of the pair. A character of this type, known as an autosomal recessive, can only come to light, therefore, when two unaffected carriers marry, and hence there is usually no previous history of the disease in the family, unless there has been intermarriage between relatives (consanguinity). In families of this type, the likelihood is that the disease will affect one in four of a series of brothers and sisters (a sibship); Friedreich's ataxia, hepatolenticular degeneration and limb-girdle muscular dystrophy are usually inherited in this way.

A recessive gene can produce an effect, however, if it is situated on the unpaired portion of the X-chromosome; hence this type of condition occurs in males and is carried by unaffected females. It is then known as a sex-linked recessive character; the disease may have affected maternal uncles and now appears in half the male children of an apparently unaffected female carrier. Diseases inherited in this manner include colour-blindness, haemophilia and pseudohypertrophic (Duchenne type) muscular dystrophy. It is, of course, true that any inherited disease can appear anew in a family if a previously normal gene has undergone a process of spontaneous change or mutation.

Apart from the diseases mentioned above which are clearly inherited by recognisable genetic mechanisms, there are many other disorders of the nervous system in which genetic influences are of importance, though these factors are difficult to define. In epilepsy and in disseminated sclerosis, for example, the disease affects more than one member of a family far more often than could be accounted for by chance, though no clear pattern of inheritance emerges. From time to time, too, one may find families in which several individuals have died from cerebral tumour or subarachnoid haemorrhage. Furthermore, there is some evidence that an individual's emotional and constitutional make-up may influence his susceptibility to certain infections or neurological disorders; thus many patients with migraine are intense, hard-working and obsessional. It is therefore of the greatest importance to consider not only the environmental, but also the constitutional influences which may have a bearing upon each patient's disease.

CONCLUSIONS

The purpose of the foregoing commentary has been to indicate that a systematic approach to each patient with symptoms suggesting disease of the nervous system is an essential preliminary to accurate diagnosis. The question should first be asked, in what situation may be the lesion responsible for these symptoms and physical signs? Is it extracerebral, in the skull or meninges, in the cerebral cortex, in the white matter, in the brain stem or cerebellum? Or if the clinical picture indicates, say, a disorder of the spinal cord or of the lower motor neurone, is the lesion in the spinal column, the meninges, the spinal cord, the spinal roots, plexuses, peripheral nerves, motor end-plates or muscles? And in each of these situations, could it be congenital, traumatic, inflammatory, neoplastic, degenerative or metabolic? What influences are constitutional factors playing in its genesis? Is there disease in the heart, great vessels, lungs or other organs which could be primarily responsible for these neurological symptoms and signs? Are emotional or psychological factors responsible for any part of the patient's disability? While it is true that in many cases the answers to some of these questions are self-evident it is well that they should be asked, since it is only through such a comprehensive approach to patients with neurological disease that the student will eventually acquire the skill and experience which will allow him to discard the irrelevant and to concentrate upon those salient facts which will lead to accurate diagnosis.

REFERENCES

BIGGART, J. H., *Pathology of the Nervous System*, 3rd ed. (Edinburgh, Livingstone, 1961).

BLACKWOOD, W., MCMENEMY, W. H., MEYER, A., NORMAN, R. M. and RUSSELL, D. S., *Greenfield's Neuropathology*, 2nd ed. (London, Arnold, 1963).

HOLMES, G., *An Introduction to Clinical Neurology*, 2nd ed. (Edinburgh, Livingstone, 1952).

MATTHEWS, W. B., *Practical Neurology* (Oxford, Blackwell, 1963).

STERN, C., *Principles of Human Genetics* (San Francisco, Freeman, 1955).

CHAPTER 2

THE SYMPTOMS AND SIGNS OF DISEASE IN THE NERVOUS SYSTEM

IN neurology, as in any branch of medicine, prognosis and treatment will usually depend upon accurate diagnosis, while diagnosis, in turn, stems from an elucidation of symptoms and signs, combined with information obtained from the appropriate ancillary investigations. In certain nervous disorders, of which epilepsy and migraine are good examples, a careful appraisal of the patient's symptoms is all-important if the correct diagnosis is to be reached, and in such cases physical examination is essentially negative. Conversely in many other diseases, the history can be singularly uninformative and all will depend upon a meticulous neurological examination. In most cases, however, the history and examination are mutually inter-dependent, one throwing light upon the significance of the other. In general it is the physical signs which identify the anatomical situation of a lesion responsible for a patient's illness, while the evolutionary pattern of its symptomatology will indicate the nature of the patho-logical process. So many are the individual symptoms and signs which may be the result of a nervous disease that it is essential to have a planned approach to each individual patient, an approach so designed that major manifestations of illness which may at first seem irrelevant are not overlooked, but are fitted into place so that the patient and his disease may be viewed as a whole. In this chapter, bearing in mind the principles previously outlined, an attempt will be made to construct the framework upon which the edifice of neurological diagnosis and management can be erected.

Diagnosis is not, however, an end in itself, not even for the purpose of obtaining medical qualifications, and any examination which fails to take into account the candidate's ability to treat patients as people is failing in its object. The doctor will be assessed by his patients, who justify his professional existence, not upon his flair for diagnosing rare diseases, but upon his understanding of their needs, of their hopes and fears and of the intensely personal problem which their illness presents. Sometimes fears of cancer or of insanity may be playing a considerable part in the genesis of the patient's symptoms, and it may be difficult to uncover these or other significant anxieties, which are being consciously suppressed, but are nevertheless of great aetiological importance. Furthermore, the correct management of

B
13

two identical cases of disabling disease of the nervous system will be totally different if the sufferers differ widely in attitude, emotional constitution and domestic environment. There are a great many chronic and crippling progressive disorders of the nervous system which continually pose serious problems of management to patient and doctor. These conditions present a challenge which require from the doctor tact, sympathy and understanding, as well as diagnostic skill and ingenuity in changing circumstances. These qualities cannot be learned from any textbook but must be derived from continuing contact with patients and their relatives, not only in hospital, but in their homes. In cases of this type, diagnosis is only the beginning, and need not necessarily be strictly accurate for management to be correct, provided the broad pattern of the patient's disease is recognised. On the other hand, there are many other conditions, such as meningitis, subdural haematoma and spinal tumour, in which diagnosis must be made early and accurately if death or severe disability is to be avoided.

TAKING THE HISTORY

The principles of history-taking in neurological disease do not differ in general from those applicable to any branch of medicine. It is usual to begin by listing the **principal symptoms** of which the patient complains and then to give, in chronological order, a detailed description in the patient's own words of the way in which they developed. Judicious questions may be needed at this stage to restrain the garrulous and cut short irrelevancies, as well as to expand and clarify individual points in the history. It is easy to forget that patients have not usually been trained in anatomy and physiology; to them, opinions previously expressed by Dr X, or the fall downstairs five years ago may seem much more important than the transient blurring of vision, say, apparently unconnected with the present complaint, which occurred three months ago. Hence it is always important, once the patient has given his story, amplified by judicious guidance and prompting, to ask a number of **leading questions,** questions which have been avoided assiduously at an earlier stage so as not to present the suggestible patient with additional symptoms which he may profess. These questions should relate to some of the principal symptoms of nervous disease, symptoms which will be considered individually in succeeding chapters. Has there been, for instance, any pain or headache, any loss or impairment of consciousness, either brief or prolonged? Have there been any visual disorders, such as impairment of sight or diplopia, or has the patient noticed any alteration in his speech or swallowing?

Are memory, behaviour and concentration unimpaired, have deafness, tinnitus, giddiness or unsteadiness been experienced, or any involuntary movements of the head, trunk or limbs? Usually, too, it is wise to enquire specifically about weakness or paralysis or clumsiness of the limbs (though few patients would overlook such striking symptoms) and about numbness, tingling, pins and needles or other unusual sensations. Finally, enquiry should be made as to whether control of the vesical or anal sphincters has been impaired and whether there have any other more general symptoms such as breathlessness, weight loss (or gain), anxiety, depression, sleeplessness, anorexia or vomiting.

Having elicited the fact that a particular patient has one or more symptoms, it is usually apparent that this knowledge alone is insufficient. If the complaint is of a headache, for instance, much more must be known. Where in the head is it situated, and does it spread? What is its character? When does it or did it begin? How long does it last and how often does it occur? Is there any warning of its onset? Does anything seem to precipitate it or make it worse once it has begun, and does anything relieve it? This kind of enquiry may be applied, with minor modifications, to almost any symptom of nervous disease, but should not be learned by rule. It is far better to cultivate an inquisitive approach in which each symptom is scrutinised and analysed in detail, being viewed, as it were, from every possible angle. Such a spirit of critical enquiry and appraisal is more revealing and profitable to both doctor and patient than a carefully ordered routine which has been learned by heart. On the other hand, the enquiry must be comprehensive. While the experienced physician may reach the heart of the problem with a few well-chosen questions, there are no short cuts for the beginner. This is one of the most important lessons for the student to learn. If history-taking is at first slow and laborious, growing experience, and experience alone, will teach which symptoms may safely be discarded as irrelevant and which are of crucial importance.

In taking the history it should also be remembered that sometimes the patient's own testimony is unreliable. In the unconscious patient it is manifestly necessary to interview relatives and others who may possess the essential information, while it is equally important to have independent evidence concerning individuals who have experienced lapses of consciousness or mental and behaviour disorders. Few epileptics, for instance, are capable of describing their own seizures, while the history given by demented or psychotic patients, though revealing, will often be lacking in essential details.

Having dealt with the history of the patient's present illness it is then necessary to enquire as to his **previous health.** Have there been any serious accidents or illnesses in the past, or any unusual sequelae of the common childish ailments? Social and occupational details may also be of considerable importance. What was the patient's educational standard at school or university and what occupations has he followed? Is he married, with a family, or does he live alone? Are his domestic circumstances satisfactory or are there financial and/or personal difficulties? And what evidence is available as to the patient's physical and emotional constitution? Has he been physically active, athletic and extraverted, or studious, retiring and introspective? Was he excessively nervous or over-protected as a child, did he wet the bed or walk in his sleep, and has he changed his employment frequently? What are his interests and hobbies, and have these changed of late? Questions of this nature can be very rewarding, indicating perhaps deterioration in intellect, change in personality, or life-long psychopathy and failure of adjustment to the demands of society. The information so obtained about the patient as an individual may throw important light upon the nature and significance of his symptoms. Clearly, too, in this connexion, the consumption of alcohol, of tobacco and of drugs should be recorded.

Finally, the **family history** can be very important, as some neurological disorders are clearly inherited, while in certain other conditions it is apparent that an inherited predisposition plays some part in the development of the disease. Hence enquiry should be made as to the existence of nervous or mental disease in the sibs, parents and more distant relatives of the patient; if further cases of disease come to light, then a pedigree should be drawn. Important diseases of other systems should also be noted if they have affected other members of the family; for instance, a strong family history of coronary artery disease may suggest that atherosclerosis of the cerebral, rather than of the coronary arteries, is responsible for the patient's symptoms.

Clearly, in so brief a compass, this guide to history-taking in nervous diseases is perforce incomplete, but if these general principles are followed, few mistakes will be made and the amplified descriptions of symptoms and symptom-complexes which appear in subsequent chapters should assist in stressing those interrelationships between individual symptoms which must always be borne in mind.

THE NEUROLOGICAL EXAMINATION

Whereas in taking the history of a patient with nervous disease, an inspired virtuosity born of experience may yield results superior to those achieved by means of a didactic and methodical approach, a comprehensive neurological examination depends much more upon a carefully itemised routine. Many schemes for examining the nervous system have been recommended and most are satisfactory, provided they are complete. The outline given below is of a method for examining the nervous system which the author has found to be satisfactory in practice. A full examination performed in this way is admittedly time-consuming, but once it has been learned and practised assiduously, experience will teach which parts of the examination may be discarded or abridged in any individual case. However, when experience is inadequate, attempts to abbreviate the examination of the nervous system will lead to inevitable and important oversights.

The Mental State

Disease of the brain may have a profound effect upon the patient's behaviour and awareness, so that an accurate assessment of the mental state can be of great importance. Individual symptoms and signs will be considered at length in subsequent chapters; it is therefore unnecessary at this stage to define terms but brief outlines will be given of certain common abnormalities which may be looked for.

First, the patient's state of awareness must be assessed. Is he comatose or semicomatose, confused or disorientated, or is he perfectly alert and well orientated in time and in place? Secondly, is his mood normal, or is he euphoric or elated, depressed, anxious or agitated? Thirdly, is his behaviour and social adjustment normal or is he antisocial and amoral, or dirty in his habits and blandly unconcerned? Does he show disordered thought processes with ideas of persecution (paranoia) or other delusions, or are there visual or auditory hallucinations? While questions of this nature can be answered by means of careful observation and by questioning the patient, simple tests of a more formal nature may be required in order to assess the present state of the memory and intellect and the powers of abstract thought. To assess the powers of attention and concentration it is usual to ask the patient to repeat a series of numbers forwards and then backwards; the normal individual can easily remember seven figures forwards and five backwards. Similarly, the patient is asked to subtract serial sevens from 100 and the number of mistakes made as well as the time taken are recorded. It is generally possible to tell whether memory for the remote past is intact when the history is being taken. In assessing the recent memory and the ability to record and retain new impressions it may be necessary to ask the patient for details of his last meal or to give him a name, address and the name of a flower to remember; he should be asked to repeat these several minutes later. It may be useful to ask him to repeat a standard sentence such as the Babcock sentence, viz. 'One thing a nation must have to be rich and great is a large, secure supply of wood'. Most normal individuals can repeat this correctly by the third attempt. In testing the patient's ability to think in an abstract manner, it is usual to ask him for an interpretation of common proverbs or of a fable. A defect of abstract thinking will be apparent, for instance, in the individual who suggests that people who live in glass houses should not throw stones as they would break the glass. Finally, in assessing the patient's intellectual state, it is usual to ask for the names of recent monarchs and Prime Ministers, the names of six large cities in Britain, or of European capitals. For accurate assessment of minor degrees of change, detailed psychometric testing by a psychologist may be required, but these simple tests will often reveal important disorders of cerebral function.

Praxis and Gnosis and the Body Image

Praxis is the ability to perform purposive skilled movements; if this function is impaired, those skills most recently acquired may be the first to be lost. In testing this function it is usual to ask the patient to perform movements of moderate complexity, such as those involved in dressing, in shaving, in opening a box of matches and striking one and in constructing a model with toy bricks. Inability to perform these movements in a patient without obvious motor weakness or sensory impairment may indicate a disorder of praxis, known as apraxia.

Gnosis is the ability, based upon the reception of sensory stimuli, either visual or tactile, to recognise the nature and significance of objects. This may relate to articles in the patient's environment, but may also be concerned with the parts of his own body. In testing this function the patient may be asked to interpret humorous drawings or pictures which tell a story, or to identify objects, such as coins placed in the hands. He should also be asked to identify parts of his body, for example, one ear, a knee or individual fingers. The patient's awareness of his own body and of its relationship to external space is known as the body image and a loss of awareness of a part of the body image is a form of agnosia or impairment of gnosis. This may also involve an inability to distinguish right from left, a possibility which should be borne in mind when testing.

Speech

The function of speech may conveniently be subdivided into first, the higher or cortical control of speech, and secondly the lower or peripheral mechanism which is responsible for phonation and articulation. Reading (understanding of the written word) and writing (expression by means of the written, rather than the spoken word) are closely related to the function of speech, as is the ability to calculate. An inability to express one's thoughts in words when the peripheral mechanisms of articulation are intact, and understanding of the spoken word is preserved, is known as motor or expressive aphasia; while a failure to understand the spoken word is called sensory or receptive aphasia. These and related functions are most easily tested by asking the patient to name a series of common objects of progressive difficulty (hand, mouth, pen, radiator, spectacles, stethoscope, etc.) and by giving a series of simple commands, or by asking simple questions. A patient with slight motor aphasia may be accurate in his speech but yet at a loss for simple words, while one with sensory aphasia may fail to obey commands or name simple objects or he may use totally inappropriate words in his reply to questions, since words to him, as symbols, have lost their meaning and significance. When the exact answers to these questions have been recorded the patient should then be asked to read, interpret and perhaps paraphrase a short passage from a book and to write down his name and address and some of his outstanding symptoms. The ability to do a number of simple sums should also be tested.

A patient with complete paralysis of the muscles of articulation may be well able to understand and interpret the spoken and written word and to express himself fluently in writing. If he cannot make a sound (phonation) this is called aphonia, but if the sound is uttered and cannot be moulded into words, this sign is entitled anarthria. Complete anarthria is rare, but slurring or indistinctness of speech due to disease of the peripheral neuromuscular mechanisms is much more common and is called dysarthria. The patient should be asked to repeat a number of set phrases which may reveal clearly that he is dysarthric; 'British constitution' and 'Methodist episcopal' are good examples of phrases in common use.

The Skull and Skeleton

Inspection and palpation of the skull is an essential part of the neurological examination. The size and shape of the skull and any asymmetry should be noted, as should the presence of any abnormal bony protuberances or points of tenderness. Auscultation in the temporal fossae and over the globes of both eyes should also be carried out and the patient should be asked to stop breathing, so that the presence or absence of a **cranial bruit** or murmur may be recorded. The presence or absence of a bruit over the carotid arteries in the neck should also be recorded; very rarely a significant bruit can be heard over the vertebral column (a spinal bruit). So far as the remainder of the skeleton is concerned, any bony deformities (abnormal spinal curvature, pes cavus, etc.) should be noted as should any limitation of movement in the spine (cervical, dorsal or lumbar) or in limb joints. Limitation of straight leg raising with pain down the back of the thigh may be due to meningeal irritation (Kernig's sign) or to a compression of one of the nerve roots which form the sciatic nerve, as by a prolapsed intervertebral disk (Lasègue's sign).

The Special Senses

The sense of **smell** (the olfactory nerves) should be tested in each nostril independently with the other occluded. Camphor, coffee, peppermint and oil of cloves are convenient test substances.

Taste should be tested on either side of the tongue, first on the anterior two-thirds, then on the posterior third, where accurate assessment is often very difficult. The four modalities of taste which can be recognised are sweet (sugar), salt (salt), bitter (quinine) and sour or acid (vinegar). It is usual to have the tongue protruded and dried and held with a piece of gauze while a fine brush dipped in a solution of one of the test agents is applied to the surface. The patient should then be asked to point to one of four cards on which these four modalities of taste sensation are given. Taste sensation from the anterior two-thirds of the tongue is carried in the chorda tympani (facial nerve) and from the posterior one-third in the glossopharyngeal nerve.

VISION (The Optic Nerves)

In testing vision it is customary to begin by testing the **visual acuity** in each eye independently, the other being covered. Usually, Snellen's test types are used, and the patient is asked to read, at a distance of 6 m, the letters on the card. Each line of type is numbered and the acuity is recorded as 6 over the number of the lowest line of type which can be read accurately; for instance, 6/6 is normal. If the patient normally needs spectacles it is then reasonable to record the acuity when they are worn, the so-called corrected acuity. This test is appropriate to distance vision, while near vision may be tested with Jaeger's reading card, in which case acuity is expressed as from J1 to J6, J1 being normal, J6 severely impaired acuity. There are, of course, cases in which vision in one or both eyes is so severely impaired that none of the test types can be seen. Here it is usual to record that sight is limited to 'counting fingers', 'hand movements' or 'light perception only', whichever is the case. In patients who claim to be blind and in whom hysteria is suspected, it may be of value to see whether blinking occurs at the threat of a blow.

Colour vision is rarely impaired as a result of disease, but colour-blindness is present from birth in about 8 per cent of males and in occasional females, being inherited as a sex-linked recessive character. This function is tested most satisfactorily with the Ishihara charts with which full instructions are supplied.

The **visual fields** must next be tested, and it is usual to begin by testing on confrontation. The patient and the examiner sit face to face and the patient is instructed to gaze steadily at the bridge of the examiner's nose. One eye is then covered and a convenient test object (the examiner's finger, or preferably a hat-pin with a white head) is brought into the patient's field of vision from all angles, the patient being instructed to say 'now' whenever it first comes into view. The procedure is then repeated with the other eye. In this way, gross defects in the peripheral visual fields may be detected and must then be confirmed by means of accurate charting on the perimeter. Even the perimeter, however, is not sufficiently accurate to plot in full the important area of central vision, the area around the fixation point, which is subserved by the macular area of the retina. To examine this area fully, and particularly if small scotomas (small areas of visual loss) are to be detected, central vision should be charted on the Bjerrum screen. Patients with central scotomas, due to disease of the macula or of the nerve fibres from this area, may have a greatly reduced visual acuity and may for instance be quite unable to read, though the peripheral fields as charted on the perimeter are full. Details of technique belong to the ophthalmologist rather than the neurologist and are outside the scope of this volume, but it may be mentioned that the visual field for large objects is larger than that for small, and for white objects it is more extensive than for red; a scotoma for red may sometimes be detected before one for white can be found.

The **optic disks and fundi** should next be inspected, after dilatation of the pupils with homatropine if necessary. The optic disk is normally faintly pink in colour, but the temporal half is usually somewhat paler than the nasal. A deep physiological cup into which the vessels enter may give a mistaken impression of pallor of the central and temporal areas of the disk until a pink rim of normal-appearing disk is seen to the temporal side of the cup. Furthermore, some blurring of the nasal margin of the disk is common in many normal individuals and sometimes only the extreme temporal margin is clearcut. In papilloedema, or swelling of the optic nerve head, not only are the margins of the disk blurred and sometimes impossible to define, but the vessels may be seen to be 'heaped up' in the centre of the disk, no physiological cup is present, the veins are distended, and there may even be haemorrhages and exudates in the surrounding retina. In optic atrophy, by contrast, the disk is flat and dead-white in colour with clearly-defined and often irregular margins. In the type of optic atrophy which may occur in disseminated sclerosis, the temporal half of the disk is strikingly pale. In examining the fundus, abnormal pigmentation, white patches of retinal degeneration, haemorrhage, hard white exudates and vascular changes (arterial narrowing, 'nipping' of veins at arteriovenous crossings, micro-aneurysms) as well as any other abnormality should all be noted and described if present.

Any abnormal position of the globe of one or other eye, such as proptosis (asymmetrical protrusion), exophthalmos (uniform protrusion), or enophthalmos (sunken eye) must also be recorded, as must the state of the **eyelids and pupils.** Drooping of the eyelids, or ptosis, may be observed, or alternatively lid-lag, revealing white sclera above the cornea on downward ocular movement. The size, equality or otherwise, and regularity of the pupils should now be examined, along with the changes in them which occur on shining a bright light into the eye; when this is done the effect upon the other pupil (the consensual reaction) as well as the direct light reaction should be observed. Changes occurring on accommodation-convergence, when transferring the gaze rapidly from a distant to a near object, such as a finger placed a few inches from the eyes, should also be tested. The afferent pathway for the pupillary reflex to light is in the optic nerve, the efferent pathway in the parasympathetic constrictor fibres of the oculomotor nerve or in the dilator fibres of the ocular sympathetic.

Ocular movements (the oculomotor, trochlear and abducent nerves) must now be examined. It is customary to ask the patient to follow with both eyes an object, such as a finger or hat-pin, which is moved quickly from right to left and then up and down in front of the eyes. If diplopia (double vision) occurs in any direction of gaze, this should be noted, as well as the position of the two images in relation to one another. Any deviation of the ocular axes during movement should be recorded as well as the occurrence of nystagmus, an oscillatory or rotatory movement which may be a most important physical sign. If nystagmus occurs, its character and direction should also be carefully observed, as well as the ocular movements which produce it. In certain cases, it is not the movement of one or other eye which is defective, but movement of the two eyes together, either laterally, upwards or downwards, is impaired. These are movements which are necessary for the maintenance of binocular vision. Such defects of conjugate ocular movement have considerable localising value and should, if present, be carefully defined. Similarly, the ability to converge the ocular axes when watching an object approach the bridge of the nose, may be lost in disease and should be tested.

HEARING AND LABYRINTHINE FUNCTION (The Auditory and Vestibular Nerves)

An approximate assessment of the efficiency of a patient's **hearing** can be obtained by recording the distance at which a whispered voice or the ticking of a watch can be heard by each ear, with the other temporarily occluded. If comparison with a normal subject suggests that one or both ears is deaf, then it is necessary to decide whether the deafness is due to disease in the middle ear (middle-ear or conduction deafness) or to disease of the cochlear or auditory nerve (nerve or perceptive deafness). This may be done with a 256-frequency tuning fork. Normally air conduction is better than bone conduction and in nerve deafness this principle is still true though the hearing by either means may be greatly diminished; in middle-ear deafness on the other hand, bone conduction is better. In **Rinne's test,** a vibrating tuning fork is applied to the mastoid process and when the sound is no longer heard the fork is held at the external auditory meatus; the normal and those with nerve deafness will still hear it, while those with middle-ear deafness will not. In **Weber's test** the vibrating fork is applied to the vertex; normal individuals will hear the sound equally in the two ears, while patients with nerve deafness will hear it louder in the normal ear, in contrast to those with middle-ear deafness to whom it will seem louder in the affected ear. Accurate assessment of hearing must, of course, depend upon audiometry.

Clinical assessment of **labyrinthine** function may be difficult, but in patients with vertigo it is reasonable to make sudden alterations in the position of the head to see whether this produces nystagmus or vertigo. For instance, a patient may be asked to lie down suddenly and to turn the head sharply to one or other side. This test is particularly useful in patients who complain of giddiness brought on by change in posture. Caloric tests, which are mentioned in Chapter 3, constitute an important means of testing the function of the labyrinths.

The Motor System

Foremost in examination of the motor system in the patient who is able to walk, is observation of the **gait.** Certain neurological diseases produce striking abnormalities in the gait and many of these are distinctive. The hemiplegic patient tends to drag or to circumduct his weak and spastic leg, while the arm is commonly flexed at the elbow and lies across the abdomen when he walks; the patient with a spastic paraparesis, by constrast, shows a stiff and clumsy mode of progression, in which both feet seem to drag along the ground. The festinant gait of Parkinsonism is even more striking; the patient shuffles along with short hurried steps, the head bowed and the back bent, as if he were having continually to press forwards to prevent himself from falling on his face. By contrast, the individual with cerebellar ataxia walks on a wide base, the feet unusually far apart; he staggers occasionally from side to side and if asked to stop suddenly or to turn round he may be very unsteady and may even fall. Equally characteristic is the 'clopping' or slapping gait of the individual with unilateral or bilateral foot-drop resulting from weakness of the dorsiflexors of the feet, while the waddle, protuberant abdomen and accentuated lumbar lordosis of the patient with pelvic girdle weakness due to muscular dystrophy is also virtually diagnostic. Another important abnormality of gait is the high-stepping unsteady demeanour of the patient with sensory ataxia, as in tabes dorsalis, who slaps his feet down hard as if he is not sure where they are in space.

Having observed the gait it is then necessary to note any **abnormalities of posture** or **involuntary movements.** These are abnormalities which cannot be corrected, and movements which cannot be prevented, by willed effort on the part of the patient. If involuntary movements are present, their situation, nature, amplitude, rhythmicity and frequency should be assessed and it is also important to observe whether changes in posture are permanent or temporary and whether they are influenced by volitional activity.

One must next turn to detailed examination of the **neuromuscular system.** It is customary first to inspect the muscles of the cranium, trunk and limbs, for the presence or absence of **atrophy** (a reduction in muscular bulk), **hypertrophy** (muscular enlargement) or **fasciculation** (involuntary twitching of isolated bundles of muscle fibres). Next, contractures or irreversible shortening of muscles and tendons, possibly resulting in skeletal atrophy or deformity, should be looked for and then one will proceed to an examination of muscular **power.**

Beginning with the **motor cranial nerves,** the muscles of mastication (temporals, masseters and pterygoids), supplied by the motor division of the fifth or trigeminal nerve, are tested by asking the patient to clench the teeth or to move the jaw from side to side against resistance while the bulk and firmness of the muscles on the two sides are compared. The function of the seventh or facial nerve is first assessed by inspection of the face and then by asking the patient to close the eyes tightly and to show the teeth. Inability to bury the eyelashes adequately on one side may be a significant physical sign, while differences in power between the upper and lower facial muscles should be noted. Similarly the fact that emotional movement of the face, as in smiling, is normal, while volitional movement on command is impaired, may be important. Movement of the palate on saying 'ah' may reveal a disorder of one or other vagus nerve, and if the uvula moves to one side this implies weakness of the opposite side of the palate, possibly resulting from a lesion of the nerve. Similarly, atrophy and weakness of one trapezius and sternomastoid may imply disease of the homolateral spinal accessory nerve, while atrophy and fasciculation of the tongue and a deviation to one side when it is protruded indicates a lesion of the twelfth or hypoglossal nerve on the side to which the tongue protrudes.

In testing the **power of the trunk and limb muscles,** most of these may be tested individually if necessary. Rational application of simple anatomical knowledge will indicate how these individual muscles may be tested, but unless there is striking atrophy of single muscles or muscle groups, so detailed an examination is rarely necessary. In a routine examination it is usual to test representative groups, which are contracted against resistance from the examiner; such muscles are those concerned in abduction of the shoulder, flexion and extension of the elbow, extension and flexion of the fingers (the grip) in the upper limbs. The upper and lower abdominal muscles may be compared in the recumbent patient by noting whether the umbilicus deviates upwards or downwards on lifting the head. In the lower limbs it is usual to test hip flexion, flexion at the knee, and dorsi- and plantar-flexion of the feet.

No single method of assessing the power of individual muscles is perfect in view of subjective variations from one examiner to the next, but that given in the Medical Research Council's pamphlet *Aids to the Investigation of Peripheral Nerve Injuries* (H.M.S.O. 1943) is most widely used and gives numerical gradings from 5 to 0 to identify degrees of power as given below:

5 = Normal power.
4 = The muscle, though able to make its full normal movement, is overcome by resistance.
3 = The muscle is able to make its normal movement against gravity but not against additional resistance.
2 = The muscle can only make its full normal movement when the opposing force of gravity is eliminated by appropriate positioning.
1 = There is a visible or palpable flicker of contraction, but no resultant movement of a limb or joint.
0 = Total paralysis.

If examination reveals weakness of one or more major muscle groups it may then sometimes be necessary to examine in detail the power of individual muscles in order to determine whether the pattern of weakness indicates, for instance, disordered function of a single peripheral nerve or nerve root. Details of methods of examination of all of the limb and trunk muscles are outside the scope of this volume and for more comprehensive descriptions the reader is referred to texts on the neurological examination which are listed at the end of this chapter. However, methods of testing a number of representative muscles are illustrated in Plate 1.

The **tone** of the limb muscles should next be tested by noting and comparing the resistance which the muscles show to passive movement at the shoulder, elbow, knee and ankle joints. This may be a most difficult examination as some patients find it almost impossible to relax the limb being tested and try to help by carrying out the movements themselves. If tone is reduced (hypotonia) the limbs are limp and 'floppy' and excessively mobile with little resistance, while if it is increased (hypertonia) the limbs may be spastic in which case there is a severe initial resistance which suddenly 'gives' (clasp-knife rigidity); alternatively the tone may be increased throughout the entire range of movement (plastic or lead-pipe rigidity) or intermittently normal and increased (cog-wheel rigidity). In spastic limbs, a muscle which is being stretched may show the phenomenon of **clonus** (rapid intermittent involuntary contraction and relaxation); this may be seen best at the ankle on sudden dorsiflexion of the foot, at the knee on pushing sharply against the upper border of the patella, and occasionally on sudden extension of the fingers.

Tests for **co-ordination** are next carried out with the intention of eliciting signs of cerebellar disease. The patient should be asked to touch his nose and the examiner's finger alternately, with the tip of his index finger, and any tremor or past-pointing should be noted. In the lower limbs, the heel–knee test, in which the heel of one foot is placed on the opposite knee and then moved smoothly down the shin, is commonly used. Other valuable tests which may reveal the clumsy inco-ordinate movements of cerebellar disease include rapid tapping with the fingers or toes on a convenient surface, 'playing the piano' on a table top, or rapid alternating pronation and supination of the hands and forearms; clumsiness in performance of the latter test, which is one of the least useful, is called dysdiadochokinesis.

Finally, the **deep and superficial reflexes** should be tested. First the jaw jerk should be elicited by placing a finger across the patient's chin, with the mouth slightly open and then tapping sharply downwards on the finger. A brisk contraction of the masseters is a positive jaw jerk, which is present in about 10 per cent of normal individuals but is exaggerated when there is bilateral corticospinal tract disease in the upper brain stem. In the upper limbs, the biceps jerk is elicited by a blow on a finger which is placed across the biceps tendon with the elbow flexed; the radial jerk by a brisk stimulus to the tendon of the brachioradialis as it traverses the lateral aspect of the lower end of the radius; and the triceps jerk by tapping the tendon of the triceps just above its insertion into the olecranon, again with the elbow flexed. To produce a finger jerk the examiner's fingers are tapped as they lie in contact with the palmar aspect of the tips of the patient's fingers; these should be partially flexed. Like the jaw jerk, the finger jerk is present in some normal individuals and in those who are tense; if it is present only on one side, however, this may be very significant. A concomitant flexion of the terminal phalanx of the thumb when the finger jerk is elicited, usually indicates that this reflex is exaggerated. Similar flexion of the terminal phalanx of the thumb occurring when the terminal phalanx of the middle finger is flicked sharply downwards between the examiner's finger and thumb (Hoffman's sign) may also indicate corticospinal tract dysfunction, particularly if present on one side only. In the lower limbs, the knee jerk is elicited by a blow on the patellar tendon with the knee in a semiflexed position, while the ankle jerk is obtained by tapping the tendo Achilles while the foot is dorsiflexed passively. Sometimes reinforcement (Jendrassik's manœuvre) is necessary to bring out these reflexes. The patient is asked to grip an object or to clasp the hands firmly when any tendon is about to be tapped, as this generally has the effect of producing a state of partial tension in his muscles so that all stretch reflexes are increased.

So far as the superficial reflexes are concerned, the first to be tested are usually the abdominals; to elicit these, brisk strokes are made downwards and inwards in each quadrant of the abdomen with a sharp instrument such as the point of a pin, when the umbilicus should move towards the area of application of stimulus. The cremasteric reflex is less valuable clinically; it consists in an upward movement of the ipsilateral testis on stroking the inside of the thigh. Finally, a most important reflex is the plantar response. A firm stroke is made along the sole from the heel to the base of the fifth toe, along the outer side of the foot. Plantar-flexion of all the toes is a flexor or normal response, while dorsiflexion of the great toe with plantar-flexion and 'fanning' of the other toes is the extensor or Babinski response.

It is essential in recording each of these reflexes that the patient should be resting comfortably and that the muscles being tested should be relaxed. Furthermore it is best to compare each reflex on one side of the body with the corresponding one on the opposite side, observing any asymmetry of response. Conventionally, each reflex is recorded as −, +, ++ or +++ depending upon its activity, while the plantar responses are recorded as ↓ (flexor), ⇂ (equivocal) or ↑ (extensor).

The Sensory System

It is usual to test the different modalities of sensation independently, as they follow different pathways in the spinal cord and brain. The perception of pain may conveniently be tested by pinprick and that of touch with a fine wisp of cotton wool. Each of these forms of sensation may be tested quantitatively by applying painful stimuli of graduated weight (algesiometers) or hairs which are calibrated so that a particular force is required to bend them (von Frey hairs). Such refinements are, however, unnecessary in clinical practice. Abnormalities in sensory perception should be sought for on the face, trunk and limbs, by exploring representative areas with the two types of stimuli mentioned above; the corneal reflexes, evoked by touching each cornea with a fine wisp of cotton wool, should also be compared. If an area of diminished pain sensation (hypalgesia) or touch sensation (hypaesthesia) is discovered, or even one of heightened sensation (hyperaesthesia), this should be defined and outlined by applying repetitive stimuli from within to without the area and vice versa, asking the patient to say when any change occurs. The area of sensory change should then be charted on a drawing of the human body, each modality of sensation being recorded separately. If pain loss is found, then temperature perception should be tested within the same area, using test-tubes filled with hot and cold water.

The finer and more discriminative aspects of sensibility should also be tested. Thus the patient may be asked to identify objects placed in the hands when his eyes are closed, or figures drawn on the skin. He is also requested to mention the direction of movement each time a finger or the great toe is moved passively upwards or downwards and any defects in position and joint sense, so elicited, must be recorded. The appreciation of vibration should also be tested with a 128-frequency tuning fork over bony prominences such as the sternum, elbow, knuckle, anterior superior iliac spine, patella and external malleolus. The ability to perceive whether the tips of the fingers or the soles of the feet are being touched with one or two points may also be noted. The normal threshold for two-point discrimination on the tips of the fingers is 3-4 mm, while on the sole of the foot it is 2-3 cm. Another useful test for eliciting very minor alterations in sensation is to touch similar points on opposite limbs, sometimes

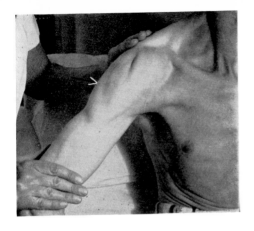

A. Deltoid muscle (C5, circumflex nerve); the patient abducts the arm to 60° against the examiner's resistance.

B. Pectoralis major (C6, 7 and 8, lateral and medial pectoral nerves); this illustration shows both the sternocostal and clavicular portions of the muscle; with the arms raised to 60° and the elbows flexed, the patient is trying to bring the hands together against the examiner's resistance.

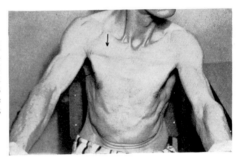

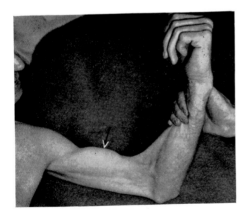

C. Biceps brachii (C5, musculo-cutaneous nerve); the patient flexes his elbow against resistance with the forearm supinated; brachio-radialis is also well shown in this illustration.

Plate I. Methods of examination of the power of certain individual skeletal muscles. (From 'Neurological Examination in Clinical Practice' by E. R. Bickerstaff.)

D. Extensor digitorum communis (C7, radial nerve); the examiner attempts to flex the patient's extended fingers at the metacarpal-phalangeal joints.

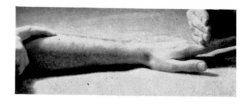

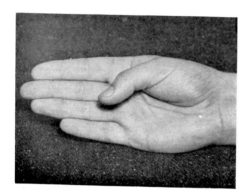

E. Opponens pollicis (T1, median nerve); the patient attempts to touch the little finger with the thumb.

F. Adductor pollicis (T1, ulnar nerve); the patient attempts to hold a piece of paper between the thumb and the palmar aspect of the forefinger.

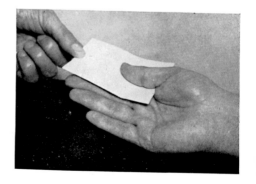

Plate I

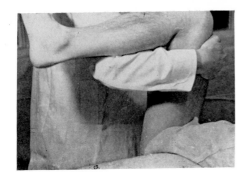

G. Iliopsoas (L1, 2, 3, femoral nerve); the patient lies on his back and attempts to flex his thigh against resistance.

H. Gluteus maximus (L5, S1, inferior gluteal nerve); the patient lies on his face, tightens the buttocks and attempts to raise the thigh against resistance.

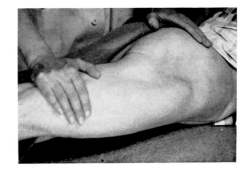

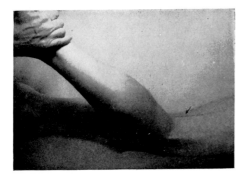

J. Hamstrings (L4 and 5, S1 and 2, sciatic nerve); the patient attempts to flex the knee against resistance; the biceps is seen laterally, the semitendinosus medially.

Plate I

K. Quadriceps femoris (L3, 4, femoral nerve); the patient attempts to extend the knee against resistance.

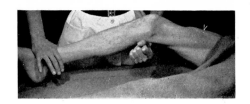

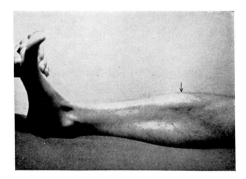

L. Tibialis anterior (L4, 5, anterior tibial nerve); the patient dorsiflexes his foot against resistance.

M. Peronei (L5, S1, musculo-cutaneous nerve); the patient everts the foot against resistance.

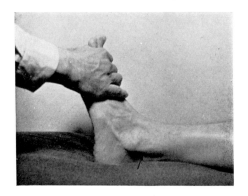

Plate I

independently and sometimes together, while asking the patient to say which has been touched. A patient who can feel perfectly stimuli applied independently to the two limbs may only feel the stimulus on one side when both are touched together. This phenomenon is known as tactile inattention.

Testing of sensory function carries many pitfalls for the unwary and needs considerable practice and experience before it can be accurately performed. One reason for this is that many suggestible individuals may easily produce spurious areas of cutaneous sensory loss, and hypalgesia is one of the commonest neurological signs of hysterical origin. Furthermore, many less intelligent patients find it difficult to understand what is being required of them, while the more intelligent may find sensory changes which are more dependent upon unintentional variation in intensity of stimulus rather than upon organic disease. A circumspect approach free from suggestion and combined with a dispassionate objectivity is therefore required.

Signs of Disease in Other Systems

It is well to remember that no body can function as an isolated nervous system and that neurological symptoms and signs may depend upon primary disorders of other systems. Cerebral infarction, for instance, can be a sequel of cardiac infarction, a brain abscess may be the result of bronchiectasis or paranasal sinusitis, or a confusional state can result from uraemia due to renal disease, from pernicious anaemia or from liver failure. Hence even though the patient's symptoms and physical signs may indicate that the nervous system is diseased, examination of the patient as a whole must be no less assiduous, for the essential clue to the nature of the patient's illness may lie in some other system.

DISCUSSION AND DIFFERENTIAL DIAGNOSIS

A detailed clinical history and a physical examination recorded in meticulous detail can be of no value unless it can be interpreted and it is upon this interpretation that treatment may depend. It is at this stage particularly that experience plays the greatest part, but experience can only be acquired if the student or young doctor learns to sift the accumulated data, discarding the irrelevant and tabulating the significant. He must therefore at this stage apply his powers of inductive and deductive reasoning in order to decide first the situation and secondly the nature of the pathological changes responsible for the patient's disease. He must be expected to tabulate in order of likelihood the possible diagnoses which he is considering, and must then decide which ancillary investigations, if any, are required in order to establish whichever is correct. For the history and examination are but a means to an end, the end being diagnosis, upon which management of the patient must depend.

REFERENCES

BICKERSTAFF, E. R., *Neurological Examination in Clinical Practice* (Oxford, Blackwell, 1963).

HOLMES, G., *An Introduction to Clinical Neurology*, 2nd ed. (Edinburgh, Livingstone, 1952).

DE JONG, R., *The Neurologic Examination*, 2nd ed. (New York, Hoeber, 1960).

KLEIN, R. and MAYER-GROSS, W., *The Clinical Examination of Patients with Organic Cerebral Disease* (London, Cassell, 1957).

MAYO CLINIC, SECTION OF NEUROLOGY, *Clinical Examinations in Neurology* (Philadelphia, Saunders, 1956).

MEDICAL RESEARCH COUNCIL, *Aids to the Investigation of Peripheral Nerve Injuries*, War Memorandum (London, H.M.S.O., 1943).

CHAPTER 3

INVESTIGATION OF THE PATIENT WITH NEUROLOGICAL DISEASE

WHEN we come to consider the ancillary investigations which are used as aids to diagnosis in a patient whose symptoms and signs suggest a disorder of the nervous system it is of the greatest importance to appreciate that symptoms of neurological dysfunction may result from disease in some other part of the body. The patient must therefore be viewed as a whole if he is not to be subjected to a series of prolonged and unpleasant tests designed to demonstrate a primarily nervous disease, when the lesion responsible may be in some other organ far removed from the brain and spinal cord. A second principle which is too often forgotten is that investigations should always be planned to give the maximum required information about the patient's illness with the least possible discomfort and risk. There is an unfortunate tendency in some centres to submit all patients to a routine series of disturbing and often expensive laboratory or radiological studies, some of which may have no relevance to the primary complaint. Such a rigid and mechanistic approach to medicine, as observed in certain modern 'diagnostic' hospitals and clinics, must be mentioned only to be deplored. A system of this type takes little account of the patient as an individual and of his comforts and discomforts. Whereas a thousand routine barium enema studies may perhaps reveal one unsuspected early carcinoma of the large bowel, one must ask whether the other nine hundred and ninety-nine could reasonably be justified on this score, taking into account the time spent by skilled radiologists, the patient's discomfort and the cost to him or to the community.

In many patients with neurological disorders there is in fact no need for investigations either for diagnosis or to give guidance in management. Migraine, for instance, is a condition in which the diagnosis can usually be made on the clinical history alone and in which ancillary tests are rarely indicated. In other cases, investigations should be carefully designed in order to establish or exclude the diagnoses which are brought to mind by the patient's symptoms and signs. It is also reasonable to begin by carrying out the simpler tests which the doctor is capable of doing himself, before proceeding, if the diagnosis remains in doubt, to the more difficult investigations which require specialised apparatus and skilled technical help.

31

GENERAL MEDICAL INVESTIGATIONS

The central and autonomic nervous systems play an important role in the regulation of the body **temperature**. Hence in a febrile patient with neurological symptoms and signs it is important to determine whether the pyrexia is due to inflammatory changes in the nervous system or elsewhere, or whether it is due to a lesion of the neuraxis giving rise to a disorder of temperature regulation. Pyrexia and fever are of course seen in patients with meningitis and encephalitis, whether infective or postinfective, and a remittent fever characteristic of suppuration is seen in those with an intracranial or spinal abscess. An aseptic or chemical meningitis, resulting from bleeding in the subarachnoid space, will also give fever. Lesions of the pons and hypothalamic region, however, may give hyperpyrexia, with temperatures of 105° F or more; this typically results from pontine haemorrhage, brain-stem injury or massive haemorrhage into the third ventricle with consequent compression of the hypothalamic centres in its floor. It should, however, be remembered that drowsiness, headache and neck stiffness (meningism) sometimes occur in patients with pneumonia, especially in childhood, while a stuporose or delirious febrile patient who is at first thought to have a primarily neurological illness may possibly be suffering from enteric or some other specific fever.

Examination of the **pulse** is of considerable value in neurology. A slow pulse in a patient with neurological symptoms and signs will often indicate increased intracranial pressure, giving rise to compression of medullary centres, but when this is so, there is usually some impairment of consciousness. Bradycardia in the alert and conscious patient is more probably constitutional, or rarely due to heart block. A rapid pulse, on the other hand, is a terminal feature in certain fatal diseases of the brain (e.g. cerebral haemorrhage or tumour), but in the conscious patient, tachycardia will often be the result of anxiety (when there will usually be other evidence of nervousness), or of systemic disease such as infection or thyrotoxicosis. Irregularity of the pulse is also important; sinus arrhythmia and extrasystoles have little pathological significance, but auricular fibrillation occurring in a patient with a hemiplegia may indicate that the hemiplegia was the result of cerebral embolism from a thrombus in the left auricle. Similarly a full, bounding pulse will suggest hypertension and a tendency towards cerebral haemorrhage, while a collapsing pulse, resulting from aortic valve incompetence, may suggest that the patient's neurological symptoms are due to neurosyphilis. Recording of the **blood pressure** is also an essential part of any physical examination. If the sphygmomanometer reading, combined with the presence of haemorrhage, exudates and vascular changes in the retina, indicate a diagnosis of malignant hypertension, this may well be the explanation of neurological signs and symptoms such as headaches, drowsiness, convulsions or even coma. Hypertension is almost invariably severe, too, in patients with cerebral haemorrhage, while in cases of so-called cerebral thrombosis it is atheroma rather than hypertension which is the primary offender and in these individuals the blood pressure is sometimes normal. However, atheromatous changes can be seen in the retinal arteries of such patients on **ophthalmoscopy,** and **electrocardiography** may indicate that there is also atherosclerosis of the coronary arteries, with cardiac ischaemia; irregularities of the pulse, and abnormalities of the serum potassium which can be the cause of neurological symptoms, will also be defined by this investigation. Very occasionally intracranial disease and subarachnoid haemorrhage in particular can produce transient abnormalities in the ECG.

Examination of the **urine** is also of value. The presence of *glycosuria* may suggest that the patient has diabetes mellitus and will in turn explain why he shows signs of peripheral neuropathy. *Polyuria* is occasionally a functional or psychiatric symptom, but if much urine of low specific gravity is passed, it may indicate diabetes insipidus due to a disorder of the hypothalamus–pituitary axis. *Albuminuria* and the presence of *abnormal cells* and *casts* in the urine may be evidence of the primary renal disease which is causing uraemia and making the patient drowsy, or producing hypertension and consequent cerebral symptoms. Alternatively, minimal albuminuria with some red cells may indicate embolism (as in subacute bacterial endocarditis) or diffuse arterial disease (as in polyarteritis nodosa) and these conditions also give neurological manifestations. A number of biochemical tests also give useful information. Thus *bilirubin* in the urine may be an expression of liver disease, in which episodes of confusion and disturbed behaviour may occur, while a dark port-wine coloured urine which goes darker on standing is sometimes indicative of *porphyria*, a condition in which confusion, abdominal pain and peripheral neuropathy occur. Furthermore, there may be a diminished urinary output of *17-ketosteroids* in patients with hypopituitarism resulting from a chromophobe adenoma which is destroying the pituitary gland. Alternatively, in Cushing's syndrome, a condition which is usually of adrenal origin but occasionally results from a basophil adenoma of the pituitary gland, the ketosteroid output is raised. Estimation of *sodium and potassium output* is also occasionally of value in patients suffering from intermittent attacks of flaccid muscular paralysis, for some have a nephritis causing excessive loss of salt and consequent hypokalaemia, while others, in whom there is a diminished output of sodium, may have attacks of periodic paralysis caused perhaps by excessive aldosterone secretion by the adrenal gland. Estimation of *heavy metals* in the urine is also useful; thus in a painter or battery-maker with unilateral wrist drop, or in a child with convulsions due to lead encephalopathy, there is an excessive output of lead, while in Wilson's disease (hepatolenti-cular degeneration) the urinary copper content is increased. It has also been found that in some cases of chronic degenerative neuro-logical disease the urinary excretion of *amino acids*, determined by paper chromatography, is abnormal.

Examination of the **blood** often gives important clues as to the significance of certain neurological symptoms and signs. One most valuable test is estimation of the *erythrocyte sedimentation rate* (E.S.R.). Primary disorders of the nervous system, save for the suppurative infections, rarely influence this reading, though it is occasionally slightly raised in patients with intracranial haemorrhage and primary intracranial neoplasms. A moderate rise in the E.S.R., however, to above 10 mm/hr (Westergren) in men, or above 15 mm/hr in women, may indicate an infective or inflammatory disorder or malignant disease, while an excessively high reading in the region of 50-100 mm/hr is often indicative of one of the 'collagen-vascular' group of disorders such as rheumatism, polyarteritis nodosa, lupus erythematosus or dermatomyositis.

Haematological studies also shed important light on certain manifestations of nervous disease. Thus dysphagia, at first suggesting a paresis of swallowing, may be found to be associated with hypo-chromic anaemia. In addition to microcytosis and a low colour index, the *serum iron* is low in this condition. More frequent are the neuro-logical complications (subacute combined degeneration of the spinal cord with variable confusion or even dementia) of pernicious anaemia. Most such cases have a macrocytic anaemia with a colour index of greater than unity and an increased mean cell volume, while megaloblasts are found in profusion in the bone marrow. Occasion-ally, however, typical neurological signs are found before any of these haematological findings develop, and the diagnosis must then rest upon the finding of histamine-fast achlorhydria in the **gastric juice** and an abnormally low value of *serum B_{12}* (less than 100 $\mu\mu g/100$ ml). It should also be remembered that a number of systemic diseases which may have neurological manifestations (malignant disease and 'collagen' disease are examples) can produce an anaemia which is normocytic and orthochromic in type. By contrast there are often neurological symptoms (headache, giddiness and minor 'strokes') in patients with polycythaemia vera, in whom the *red and white cell components of the blood* are greatly increased.

A *differential white cell count* is also a valuable aid in neurological diagnosis. A polymorphonuclear leucocytosis is found in many infective disorders, while leucopenia or eosinophilia may occur in 'collagen' diseases involving the nervous system, such as lupus erythematosus or polyarteritis nodosa. Certain primary disorders of the reticuloendothelial system also have important neurological complications; thus meningoencephalitis is an occasional complication of infective mononucleosis (glandular fever). Furthermore, leukaemic deposits in the central nervous system sometimes give focal neurological symptoms and signs of which facial palsy is one of the commonest; leukaemia will of course be identified by blood and marrow examinations. Neurological signs, and particularly those of cord compression, can also result from reticulosis, particularly Hodgkin's disease, but here blood examination is usually uninformative and diagnosis will generally rest upon the result of **lymph node biopsy.** Similarly, multiple myeloma may cause compression of the brain, optic nerves or spinal cord, and in this condition diagnosis depends upon marrow biopsy and radiological changes in the bones. Haemorrhagic disorders, such as haemophilia or thrombocytopenic purpura, can also give rise to neurological complications of which subdural, intracerebral and subarachnoid haemorrhage are the most frequent and these conditions will usually be identified by estimation of the *bleeding and clotting time* and of the *platelet count.*

Many more neurological diagnoses can be established by the determination of the absolute values of various **biochemical substances** in the serum. Thus in some individuals with long-standing respiratory insufficiency a syndrome of chronic cerebral anoxia and carbon dioxide narcosis gives rise to a severe confusional state, and this is identified first by the clinical evidence of chronic lung disease (usually emphysema and chronic bronchitis) and by the estimation of the *arterial oxygen* and *carbon dioxide tension.* The coma or drowsiness of uraemia will be recognised by the clinical evidence of acidosis and by the finding of a high blood urea, while diabetic ketosis is confirmed by *blood-sugar estimation* and by finding acetone in the breath and urine. Another important cause of coma which also gives rise to focal neurological signs is hypoglycaemia, which is identified by a blood-sugar estimation carried out during an attack. A five-hour *glucose tolerance curve*, repeated blood-sugar estimations during prolonged fasting, and insulin or tolbutamide tolerance tests will often be necessary in patients with frequent fainting spells or epileptic seizures in whom there is reason to suspect either reactive or organic hyperinsulinism. Examination of the *serum electrolytes* is also of considerable value, as muscular asthenia and drowsiness are common features of Addison's disease, in which condition the serum sodium is usually low, while hypokalaemia or hyperkalaemia are important causes of periodic attacks of generalised flaccid muscular paralysis. In mentally-defective patients with epilepsy it is impor·tant to estimate the *serum calcium and phosphorus* as some such patients have idiopathic hypoparathyroidism and may be helped by calciferol or similar therapy which raises their abnormally low serum calcium. Furthermore, fainting attacks and muscular weakness sometimes occur in patients with hypercalcaemia whether due to hyperparathyroidism or to renal disease.

Neurological complications of liver disease often take the form of intermittent confusion and abnormal behaviour, associated with a curious flapping, or wing-beating, tremor of the hands. In any patient presenting with symptoms of this nature, it is often necessary to carry out a battery of *liver function tests*, including the serum bilirubin, alkaline phosphatase and various flocculation tests; one of the most valuable estimations is that of the blood ammonia, which is usually greatly raised in cases of this syndrome of 'hepatic encephalopathy'. In such individuals, there is often an abnormal pattern of serum proteins, and this may be confirmed by electrophoretic separation of the proteins on paper. Identification in this way of a rise in *serum Y-globulin* is also a valuable aid in the diagnosis of 'collagen' disease.

A rise in the *serum cholesterol* may be a guide to the diagnosis of myxoedema, a condition which occasionally presents with mental symptoms or with stiffness, aching and sluggishness of the skeletal muscles. In such cases, confirmation of the diagnosis is obtained from the *basal metabolic rate, serum protein-bound iodine* and *radio-iodine uptake* studies, or by the detection of anti-thyroid antibodies in the serum. Another test which is sometimes of value in neurological diagnosis, particularly in patients with a polyneuropathy, is a *pyruvate tolerance curve*, in which the serum pyruvate is estimated half-hourly after giving 50 g of glucose. An abnormal pyruvate tolerance indicates a deficiency of vitamin B_1, either primary (nutritional), or resulting from heavy-metal poisoning. Estimation of the *serum copper*, copper oxidase and caeruloplasmin content are also valuable on occasions, as these values are low in patients with Wilson's disease.

A number of **bacteriological** studies are also applicable in neurological diagnosis. In addition to the *culture of organisms* from the cerebrospinal fluid or from abscesses in or near nervous tissue, blood culture is indicated if there is any clinical evidence to suggest a bacteraemia. *Agglutination reactions* are also important, not only in the diagnosis of enteric, abortus and glandular fever, but also in suspected cases of leptospirosis (Weil's disease and canicola fever) in which the nervous system is often involved. *Virological studies* are of increasing importance, not only in the diagnosis of recognised viral infections such as poliomyelitis, but also in the investigation of cases of lymphocytic meningitis and encephalomyelitis of unknown aetiology. In addition to the well-known *Wasserman and Kahn reactions* utilised in the diagnosis of syphilis as well as the more specific *treponema-immobilisation test*, there are also available a number of other complement-fixation and agglutination reactions which aid in the recognition of less common infective and parasitic disorders of the nervous system, such as toxoplasmosis.

Biopsy techniques, other than lymph-node biopsy which was previously mentioned, are of great value in the investigation of suspected nervous disease; in certain cases, skin, liver or renal biopsy and other methods commonly used in general medicine may be applicable. *Muscle biopsy* has, however, a more immediate relevance to neurological medicine as this method can be very useful in deciding whether muscular weakness and wasting is due to a disease of the motor nerves (neuropathy) or of the muscles (myopathy), while it often assists in the diagnosis of 'collagen' disease and particularly of polyarteritis nodosa. Digital *nerve biopsy* is occasionally of use in the investigation of cases of peripheral neuropathy, while *brain biopsy* is utilised in the diagnosis of cerebral tumour or of diffuse degenerative cerebral disease; these techniques have relatively restricted clinical applications.

THE CEREBROSPINAL FLUID

Formation and Composition

From experimental work carried out in the early part of this century it became apparent that the choroid plexuses of the cerebral ventricles play an important part in the formation of the cerebrospinal fluid. Blockage of the aqueduct of Sylvius was found to give rise to a striking dilatation of the lateral and third ventricles, a dilatation which is consequent upon the continued production of cerebrospinal fluid for which there is no longer an outlet. From these early observations and from the fact that hydrocephalus could follow blockage of the superior longitudinal sinus and was then presumed to be the result of impaired re-absorption of the fluid, the classical view of C.S.F. formation and circulation has evolved. According to this view, the fluid is formed in the choroid plexuses, not by simple diffusion or dialysis but by a process of active secretion; that secreted in the lateral ventricles then passes through the foramina of Monro, the third ventricle, the aqueduct and fourth ventricle, to enter the basal cisterns of the subarachnoid space through the foramina of Magendie and Luschka. It then flows upwards over the surface of the cerebral hemispheres, while some flows down into the spinal subarachnoid space; reabsorption into the blood stream then occurs through the arachnoidal villi which protrude into the superior longitudinal and other venous sinuses. Recent work on the passage of radioactive substances into the cerebrospinal fluid has confirmed that this mechanism of secretion and reabsorption does in fact operate but that in addition there is a constant process of dialysis, with exchange of chemical constituents between the C.S.F. and blood, occurring across the arachnoid membrane at all levels. The composition of the ventricular fluid is very different from that in the lumbar subarachnoid space and it seems that many of the consti- tuents in the lumbar fluid have been added to it by diffusion across the spinal arachnoid membrane.

The total volume of cerebrospinal fluid in the normal adult is between 120 and 130 ml. The fluid is quite clear and colourless; it contains less than five white blood cells per cubic millimetre and all of these are lymphocytes. The protein content of the lumbar fluid is 15-40 mg/100 ml, the respective values for ventricular and cisternal fluid being 5-15 mg and 15-25 mg/100 ml; most of the protein present is albumin. Normally, too, the fluid contains 50-80 mg glucose and 725-750 mg chloride (expressed as NaCl) per 100 ml. Thus the protein content of the fluid is very low when compared with that of the blood serum, the sugar level is also lower than that in the serum, while the chloride is higher. Sodium, potassium, urea and certain drugs such as the sulphonamides, pass freely into the fluid and are there found in concentrations equal to that in the serum, whereas other substances such as antibodies, salicylates, penicillin and streptomycin pass into the fluid in relatively minute quantities even if the serum concentration is high. Bromide, too, is found in the lumbar C.S.F. in only about one-third the concentration in which it is present in the blood. Clearly, therefore, the entry of many chemicals into the cerebrospinal fluid is a highly selective matter and does not depend upon a simple process of diffusion across a semipermeable membrane. Disease, and particularly inflammation of the arachnoid, may influence this process and in some cases of meningitis, peni- cillin, say, and bromide enter the fluid more easily.

Lumbar Puncture

Cytological and chemical examination of the cerebrospinal fluid is of great value in neurological diagnosis and specimens of fluid are most readily obtained by lumbar puncture, which is usually a com- paratively simple and safe procedure though never to be undertaken lightly. In this technique the exploring needle is inserted into the lumbar subarachnoid space below the temination of the spinal cord, and since the roots of the cauda equina are pushed aside by the needle, the risks of damage to nervous tissue by the needle puncture are negligible. The investigation can, however, be dangerous if the intracranial pressure is high, and particularly if an intracranial tumour is present, since reduction in the pressure of fluid in the lumbar subarachnoid space can result in impaction of the cerebellar tonsils in the foramen magnum or of the medial aspects of one or both temporal lobes between the brain stem and the edge of the tentorium cerebelli, with fatal results. Hence papilloedema is usually a contra-indication to lumbar puncture and the examination should be very cautiously performed if the patient's symptoms suggest that the intracranial pressure is raised; should manometry reveal, in such a case, that the pressure is high, it is wise to remove only a few drops of fluid. Even this precaution, however, will not always avoid cerebellar or tentorial herniation, as a persistent leakage of fluid may occur though the hole in the spinal dura mater left by the exploring needle. The latter mechanism, with consequent reduction of the intracranial pressure below the normal level, is probably the cause of the common post-lumbar-puncture headache.

In carrying out lumbar puncture, positioning of the patient is all-important. He should lie horizontally on the left side with his neck firmly flexed, the knees drawn up to the chin and the trunk flexed. The skin of the back is then cleaned with ether and a suitable anti-septic; a line is then drawn down the spinous processes of the vertebrae and another joining the highest points of the iliac crests. This line usually crosses the spine of the fourth lumbar vertebra and the needle may be inserted either in the intervertebral space above or in the one below this line. Full precautions regarding asepsis are of course essential; it is usual for the operator to wear a mask and sterile gloves and the lumbar puncture outfit, including needles, stylets and manometer should have been autoclaved. Harris's or similar needles are the most satisfactory. After infiltration of the skin and subcutaneous tissue with local anaesthetic (e.g. 1 per cent procaine hydrochloride solution) the lumbar puncture needle is then inserted with its stylet in position and is passed horizontally inwards in a slightly cephalad direction. It passes through the interspinous ligaments and soon afterwards encounters the resistant ligamentum flavum. After penetrating this firm ligament resistance suddenly lessens and the needle enters the subarachnoid space. The stylet is now removed from the needle and the fluid will drip out slowly. Care must be taken not to insert the needle too far, as a vertebral vein may then be punctured or an intervertebral disk can be damaged.

It is next customary to measure the pressure of the fluid by attaching a manometer to the needle and the level of the column of fluid in millimetres of C.S.F. is measured when it ceases to rise in the upright tube. The normal pressure in the recumbent adult patient is 60-180 mm of fluid; when he is sitting upright the pressure in the lumbar subarachnoid space is about 200 to 250 mm. It is most important that the patient should be lying comfortably relaxed during this procedure. Coughing or straining causes an increased pressure in abdominal veins and consequently in the vertebral veins; this displaces cerebrospinal fluid from the spinal canal and its pressure therefore rises. Similarly, if there is a free communication between the cerebral and lumbar subarachnoid spaces, a temporary increase in the intracranial pressure will be reflected in the manometer. Such an increase may be produced by compressing one or both internal jugular veins in the neck, thus reducing venous outflow from the cranium. In carrying out this procedure, which is known as Queckenstedt's test, there is usually a sharp rise in pressure to 300 mm or more, with an equally rapid fall to the normal level when the pressure is released. If there is a block to the free passage of fluid in the subarachnoid space, then no rise in pressure occurs during the manœuvre, while if the block is partial the rise and fall are both abnormally slow.

After pressure readings have been taken it is then usual to collect fluid in two separate sterile and chemically clean test-tubes or other appropriate containers. One specimen is used for bacteriological, the other for cytological and chemical studies. When the examination is complete, the stylet is reinserted into the needle, it is withdrawn and the track is sealed by the application of a piece of cotton wool or lint which has been dipped in collodion or by a simple dry dressing.

Cisternal Puncture

Cisternal puncture is a more difficult and dangerous procedure than lumbar puncture, since if the needle is inserted too far into the cisterna magna, the lower part of the medulla oblongata is pierced. Hence this method is only used if lumbar puncture is technically impossible owing to spinal deformity, if an opaque substance must be injected to define the upper level of a spinal lesion causing a block, if it is necessary to compare the chemical constitution of the lumbar and cisternal fluids, or if intrathecal injections of therapeutic agents are to be given and there is a block in the spinal subarachnoid space.

In preparation, the neck is shaved to the level of the external occipital protuberance and the head is flexed. After skin preparation and local anaesthesia as for lumbar puncture, the needle is inserted about 1 cm above the highest palpable spinous process and is passed upwards and inwards until it strikes the posterior atlanto-occipital ligament. It is then passed through the ligament and advanced cautiously for another 0·5 cm; the stylet is now withdrawn, as the tip should be lying in the cisterna magna. Sometimes the fluid fails to flow out from the cistern, as the pressure here is considerably lower than in the lumbar subarachnoid space, and gentle suction with a syringe is often necessary in order to obtain a specimen of fluid. This technique is one which, unlike lumbar puncture, should only be performed as a rule by a skilled operator working in a specialised unit.

Ventricular Puncture

Direct needle puncture of the lateral cerebral ventricles is sometimes necessary in order to relieve symptoms of increased intracranial pressure prior to an operation for intracranial tumour, or in order to inject air for ventriculography. Rarely, when there is much inflammatory exudate in the subarachnoid space and lumbar or cisternal puncture fails to produce a free flow of cerebrospinal fluid, this route is used for the administration of drugs such as penicillin or streptomycin. In infants the ventricles can be entered directly by a needle which is inserted in the lateral angle of the fontanelle and is then passed through the cerebral substance. In older children and in adults, cranial burr-holes must first be made. In view of the hazards which may result from the passage of a needle through brain tissue, this technique is one which must be left to the specialist.

Examination of the Cerebrospinal Fluid and Some Common Abnormalities

PRESSURE

An increase in the pressure of the cerebrospinal fluid above 200 mm in a relaxed, recumbent patient usually implies a raised pressure inside the cranium. This is usually due to an increase in the volume of the brain produced by oedema or by a lesion such as a tumour or abscess or haematoma. A moderate rise occurs in patients with severe arterial hypertension. An unusually low pressure is much less significant if Queckenstedt's test gives a normal response, and is generally of no diagnostic value, although patients in whom the pressure is low to begin with seem more liable to develop headache as a sequel of lumbar puncture; a syndrome of intracranial hypotension has been postulated as an explanation of this finding, but the evidence that such a condition exists is inconclusive.

NAKED-EYE APPEARANCE

Turbidity of the fluid usually indicates a polymorphonnclear pleocytosis; excessive lymphocytes, even in large number, rarely give changes visible to the naked eye. Some specimens of fluid which contain an excessive quantity of protein may clot on standing; a fine cobweb-like **fibrin deposit** appearing after a few hours also implies an increased protein content; it is seen in tuberculous meningitis and less commonly in poliomyelitis and meningovascular syphilis. Frank **blood** in the C.S.F. may be present owing to puncture of a vertebral vein by the exploring needle, in which case the contamination of the fluid becomes less as it flows; if two test-tubes are filled, the second is less stained than the first, and if the specimen is centrifuged the supernatant fluid is clear. Uniform blood-staining is, however, seen in subarachnoid haemorrhage or if a primary cerebral haemorrhage has extended to the subarachnoid space; in such a case, the supernatant fluid, after centrifuging, generally shows a yellow coloration or **xanthochroma.** A faint colour, generally orange, appears within four hours of a subarachnoid haemorrhage and is then due to the presence of oxyhaemoglobin; within forty-eight hours the deep yellow colour of bilirubin also develops. This colour may persist for six weeks after a haemorrhage but usually disappears in from two to three weeks. Xanthochromia is also seen in C.S.F. with a very high protein content (as in spinal tumour cases) in some patients with subdural bleeding, and in others who are deeply jaundiced.

CYTOLOGY

Numerous techniques of counting the white cells in the C.S.F. are in common use. That most commonly used is to draw up 0·1 ml of methyl green diluting fluid in a white-cell-counting pipette and to fill the pipette with C.S.F. After mixing, the number of cells seen in the entire lined area of a Neubauer counting chamber are counted; this gives the number per cubic millimetre of fluid. Staining is usually good enough for red cells, lymphocytes and polymorphonuclear leucocytes to be identified. Tumour cells, yeasts and other abnormal cells are occasionally found but require specialised cytological techniques and skilled scrutiny for their recognition and interpretation.

A small number of **red cells** may be present owing to the trauma of the puncture but if they persist in several specimens they usually indicate a cerebral infarct, a haemorrhage approaching the surface of the brain, or bleeding into the subdural, as distinct from the subarachnoid space; the possibility of minor leakage from an intracranial aneurysm must also be borne in mind. An increase in **white cells** generally implies inflammatory changes in the meninges and these can be primary, as in meningitis, or secondary to diffuse cerebral disease, as in encephalitis. In general, polymorphonuclear leucocytes are predominant in pyogenic infections such as coccal or influenzal meningitis and many thousands of cells may be present per cubic millimetre of fluid. As the condition resolves, so the polymorphs are gradually replaced by lymphocytes in decreasing numbers. In a case of cerebral abscess, but without obvious meningitis, it is usual to find between twenty and 200 cells/mm^3 of which most are polymorphs. In tuberculous meningitis there is a polymorphonuclear reaction at the beginning of the illness but within a few days the pleocytosis is generally entirely mononuclear (lymphocytes and histiocytes) and usually of the order of from 200 to 1,000 cells/mm^3. Meningovascular syphilis generally gives a mononuclear pleocytosis of up to 200 cells/mm^3, but some polymorphonuclears are present in the more acute cases; patients with tabes dorsalis rarely shown an excess of cells in the fluid, but in patients with general paresis counts of from five to fifty lymphocytes/mm^3 are usual.

In virus infections of the nervous system such as encephalitis, lymphocytic meningitis and poliomyelitis, a moderate lymphocytic reaction, up to 1,000 cells/mm^3 is general, but in poliomyelitis a number of polymorphs, and even a predominance, may be observed in the first one or two days of the illness.

A slight pleocytosis, nearly always of lymphocytes, is also sometimes found in a number of other miscellaneous conditions, including cerebral tumour (primary or secondary), cerebral infarction, venous sinus thrombosis and disseminated sclerosis. Only rarely in these conditions does the count exceed from forty to fifty cells/mm^3. In subarachnoid haemorrhage, too, the aseptic meningitis produced by the blood in the C.S.F. excites a moderate lymphocytic pleocytosis, and the number of white cells present is proportionately greater than would be expected from the number of red cells which are seen. In occasional cases of intracranial tumour, particularly medulloblastomas in childhood, neoplastic cells, which look very like lymphocytes, are present in the fluid in comparative profusion.

CHEMICAL ABNORMALITIES

PROTEIN. An increase in the protein content of the C.S.F. is one of the commonest of abnormalities discovered in neurological practice and also one of the most difficult to interpret. A rise to several hundred milligrammes per 100 ml is usual in inflammatory disorders of the meninges such as meningitis and persists for some time after the pleocytosis is no longer present; this is also true of poliomyelitis, in which disease a rise in protein without an increase in cells is sometimes noted only four or five days after the onset. A moderate increase, usually to about 100 mg/100 or less may be found in encephalitis, cerebral abscess, cerebral infarction, neurosyphilis (excluding tabes dorsalis), intracranial venous sinus thrombosis and disseminated sclerosis. A similar moderate rise is common in patients with intracranial gliomas and metastases but extracerebral neoplasms such as meningiomas often give a somewhat higher reading and the protein content of the fluid is usually well over 100 mg/100 ml in a patient with an acoustic neuroma. Particularly high values for C.S.F. protein, often of several hundred milligrammes and sometimes as much as 1 g/100 ml are found in patients with post-infective polyneuropathy (the Guillain–Barré syndrome), and in these cases there is typically no pleocytosis ('dissociation cyto-albuminologique'). Virtually the only other circumstance in which similarly high readings are found in the lumbar C.S.F. is in cases of spinal block, usually due to a neoplasm in the spinal canal, but occasionally resulting from vertebral collapse and angulation, extradural abscess formation, or inflammatory adhesions following tuberculous meningitis. Not uncommonly this fluid with a high-protein content is somewhat xanthochromic, and these signs, combined with a Queckenstedt test indicating a block, constitute Froin's syndrome, which can clearly result from a variety of causes. Minor degrees of spinal cord compression without a complete block, as in cervical spondylosis, show less striking rises in the protein content of the fluid, rarely to above 100 mg/100 ml. A moderate rise to a figure which is usually below this level is also found sometimes in patients suffering from a recent prolapse of an intervertebral disk, either lumbar or cervical.

Albumin–globulin ratio. In the normal C.S.F. the albumin–globulin ratio is approximately 8:1 but in many of the inflammatory conditions referred to above there is a selective rise in globulin; this is identified by Pandy's test, using a solution of carbolic acid with which a turbidity appears if excess globulin is present. More accurate is electrophoresis which has revealed that in some conditions, such as disseminated sclerosis, there is a particular rise in γ-globulin and in other immunoglobulins. If the total protein content of the fluid is normal and yet more than 28 per cent of the protein is γ-globulin, this finding is strongly suggestive of disseminated sclerosis.

Gold colloidal (Lange) curve. It is probably selective changes in the protein content of the C.S.F. which are responsible for variations observed in the gold colloidal curve. This is charted by noting the numbered colour reactions produced when various dilutions of fluid are added to Lange's colloidal gold solution.

The normal Lange curve is 0000000000, but slight rises to 1 or even 2 in any of the tubes are not necessarily significant. The *paretic* or 'first-zone' curve (e.g. 5544322110) is characteristic of general paresis but also occurs occasionally in meningovascular syphilis, tabes dorsalis, disseminated sclerosis (about 30 per cent of cases) and following a subarachnoid haemorrhage. The *luetic* or tabetic curve (e.g. 0123322100) is usually found in tabes dorsalis or meningovascular syphilis, while the *meningitic* curve (e.g. 0001223210) is found in meningitis of various types.

SUGAR. Sugar disappears completely from the C.S.F. in patients with pyogenic meningitis, but in tuberculous meningitis, unlike lymphocytic meningitis, a moderate fall in glucose level to about 20-45 mg/100 ml is often found and is a valuable aid in diagnosis.

CHLORIDES. The chlorides in the C.S.F. generally run in a fairly parallel manner to those in the blood and are therefore reduced in patients who have been vomiting frequently. Perhaps for this reason they are usually low in patients with tuberculous meningitis, but this finding has no certain diagnostic value.

BROMIDE. The C.S.F. bromide level in the normal human is negligible, but if a patient is given a dose of bromide by mouth or by injection, the drug soon appears in the C.S.F. in one-third the concentration it is present in the blood. In tuberculous meningitis, more than in any other condition, this serum–C.S.F. bromide ratio after a dose of the drug is reduced from 3 to about unity and this is sometimes a most important diagnostic test in suspected cases of tuberculous meningitis. A similar finding is sometimes obtained in cases of carcinomatosis of the meninges.

BACTERIOLOGICAL EXAMINATION

If turbid C.S.F. is removed, a smear should be stained with Gram's stain and examined for micro-organisms and another specimen cultured. In pneumococcal, staphylococcal, streptococcal and influenzal meningitis the causal organisms are usually quite profuse in a direct smear, but meningococci may be extremely difficult to find and culture. Tubercle bacilli should also be looked for in preparations stained by the Ziehl–Neelsen technique and are usually found in cases of tuberculous meningitis after an assiduous search, particularly if a fibrin 'web' can be examined. If no bacilli are found, confirmation of the diagnosis depends upon finding the organisms on culture or guinea-pig inoculation, but these measures take about six weeks. In some cases of chronic meningitis, special culture media (e.g. Sabouraud's medium) are required for the identification of rare infections such as torulosis. Virological studies also tend to give results only when the illness is over but are very useful

C

even at this stage in establishing the nature of the organism responsible for a number of obscure infections of the nervous system.
Serological tests for syphilis, such as the Wasserman and Kahn, are
sometimes positive in the C.S.F. but negative in the serum of cases
of neurosyphilis.

ELECTROENCEPHALOGRAPHY

Electroencephalography is a technique of recording the electrical
activity of the brain through the intact skull. Electrodes are applied
to the scalp and the potential changes so recorded are amplified and
presented for interpretation as an inked tracing on moving paper.
Machines in common use today have eight or more channels so that
it is possible to record the activity from many different areas of the
head simultaneously. The technique is relatively simple and entirely
harmless and may give information which is of great value in neurological diagnosis.

In the normal adult the dominant electrical activity in the EEG
from the post-central areas is usually a sinusoidal wave form with a
frequency of 8-13 cycles per second. This is the alpha rhythm; it
commonly disappears on attention, as when the eyes open. Normally
there is often some faster or so-called beta activity (14-22 c/s) in the
frontal regions; this is greatly accentuated by the administration of
barbiturates and sometimes by anxiety. In young infants the EEG
is dominated by generalised slow activity of so-called delta frequency (up to 3·5 c/s); gradually during the processes of maturation
this is replaced by theta activity (4-7 c/s) and subsequently by the
alpha rhythm. Theta activity disappears last from the posterior
temporal regions, particularly on the right side, and the record is
usually completely mature, showing no theta activity, by the age of
from twelve to fourteen years. During drowsiness and sleep in the
normal individual theta activity and later delta activity reappear.
Some common appearances in the EEG are illustrated in Fig. 1.

The EEG may be of great value in the diagnosis of **epilepsy.** In
cases of **petit mal** it often shows regular, rhythmical, generalised outbursts of repetitive complexes, each consisting of a spike and a delta
wave (spike-and-wave), and recurring at a frequency of about 3 c/s.
In idiopathic or 'centrencephalic' **major epilepsy,** the record may
show brief generalised outbursts of spikes or sharp waves, or of
mixed spikes and slow activity (an irregular spike-and-wave discharge). In patients suffering from **focal epilepsy,** including **temporal
lobe or 'psychomotor' attacks,** there are often spikes, sharp waves or
rhythmical outbursts of slow (delta or theta) activity arising in the
epileptogenic area of cortex. Unfortunately, a single record taken in

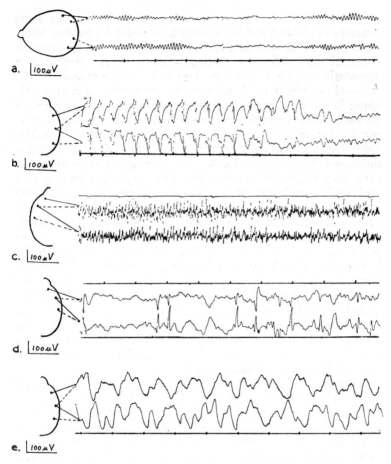

FIG. 1. Some common appearances in electroencephalographic (EEG) recordings.

a. A normal alpha rhythm recorded from both occipital regions and disappearing (in the centre of the recording) when the eyes are closed.

b. A 3 c/sec. spike and wave discharge of petit mal epilepsy, recorded in this illustration from the right temporal region.

c. High frequency discharges (mainly muscle artefact) recorded from the left fronto-temporal region during a major epileptic seizure.

d. A right anterior temporal focus of spike discharge in a patient suffering from temporal lobe epilepsy.

e. A focus of high-amplitude delta activity seen in the right mid-temporal region in a patient suffering from a cerebral abscess in this situation.

an epileptic patient is often normal; positive findings are more common in children and less common the older the patient. Many other patients show non-specific abnormalities, such as excessive temporal theta activity, a finding which is usually attributed to immaturity in the broadest sense. Hence, it may be necessary to take repeated recordings or alternatively to use various **activation techniques** in order to uncover epileptic discharges. Overbreathing for a period of from two to three minutes is particularly effective in evoking the discharges of petit mal, while photic stimulation (repetitive light flashes of variable frequency) can also bring out epileptic discharges. Since temporal spikes or sharp waves often appear in early sleep it has become conventional to carry out recordings after oral (quinalbarbitone) or intravenous (thiopentone) barbiturate sedation in cases of suspected temporal lobe epilepsy. In some such cases, and particularly when the patient's symptoms are sufficiently severe for surgical treatment to be contemplated, recordings are made from underneath the medial surface of the temporal lobe by inserting a needle electrode to lie in contact with the basi-sphenoid. Occasionally, when other techniques have failed, epileptic discharges can be provoked by the intravenous injection of metrazol or megimide (bemigride), but these substances commonly produce clinical convulsions and may do so even in the non-epileptic if given in adequate dosage. The interpretation of results obtained with these drugs is therefore difficult, and this technique should only be applied as a rule in highly specialised centres.

It can be concluded that a single routine EEG is of limited value, but should generally be performed, using the simple activation techniques if necessary, in most patients who are suspected to be suffering from epilepsy. If epileptic discharges are found in the record this will confirm the diagnosis and the nature of the discharge may help in deciding upon appropriate treatment. Negative findings, however, cannot be taken to exclude this diagnosis. The more difficult techniques should be reserved for use in intractable or problem cases or those in which confirmation of the diagnosis is particularly important, say, for, medicolegal reasons.

The EEG is also of value in the diagnosis of **focal cerebral lesions.** A relatively acute lesion of one cerebral hemisphere usually gives a focus of delta activity in or around the area of the lesion. It is not the lesion itself which produces this abnormal discharge, but the changes which it has produced in the surrounding brain. A **cerebral abscess** usually produces a very slow discharge of high amplitude, and similar though less striking abnormalities result from **tumour, haemorrhage, local injury** or **infarction.** Thus the EEG can give valuable aid in localisation, but is of little help in pathological diagnosis, and this must depend upon clinical and other information, or upon progressive changes occurring in a series of records. An abnormality due to a tumour will usually become worse, while that due to an infarct will tend to improve. In the case of lesions which are more chronic or more deeply situated in the cerebral hemisphere, focal theta activity of low amplitude or even an absence of the alpha rhythm or of beta activity which is present on the other side, may be the only abnormality. Indeed in some patients with very chronic, slowly growing tumours, such as a meningioma, the record is entirely normal. However, some localised abnormality is generally found in upwards of 70 per cent of patients with cerebral neoplasms, and although, as in epilepsy, a negative record has no real value in excluding tumour, the investigation is often a simple and harmless method of localisation.

A **subdural haematoma** is another condition which may be revealed by the EEG, as cases of this type often show a unilateral suppression of the alpha rhythm and some irregular slow activity on the affected side. Certain rare conditions such as **subacute encephalitis** also show characteristic findings, but in many chronic neurological disorders such as **Parkinsonism** and **disseminated sclerosis** the EEG is usually normal. Tumours in the posterior fossa or deeply situated lesions near the midline often give paroxysmal outbursts of theta or delta activity at the surface, but these changes are by no means specific as they occur in patients with many diffuse cerebral disorders including **meningitis, subarachnoid haemorrhage** and **encephalitis** or conditions giving a generalised **disorder of cerebral metabolism** such as anoxia, uraemia, hypoglycaemia, hepatic coma or pernicious anaemia. Similar non-specific abnormalities are found in patients who are confused or comatose from any cause.

The EEG is of comparatively little value in **psychiatric diagnosis** although anxious and obsessional patients often show excessive frontal fast activity, while **psychopaths** and children with **behaviour disorders** have typically immature records with excessive temporal slow activity, particularly on the right side posteriorly. Patients with **organic dementia** often show a dominant rhythm of theta rather than alpha frequency; this is in a sense a reversion to the childhood pattern and may even occur naturally as a result of an ageing process; it is certainly not specific.

Hence it will be seen that the EEG has considerable value in the diagnosis of epilepsy and in the investigation of patients with suspected subdural haematoma or intracranial tumour. Repeated studies are often of value in assessing the response to treatment of certain diffuse metabolic disturbances. The method has also considerable applications as a research tool.

ECHO-ENCEPHALOGRAPHY

A comparatively recent development has been the introduction of ultrasonics into neurological diagnosis. A number of simple and relatively inexpensive machines are now available commercially and are being used to an increasing extent in neurological departments. With apparatus of this type an ultrasonic beam is passed horizontally through the intact skull and an 'echo' can be recorded from mid-line structures. A 'shift' of the mid-line can readily be demonstrated and this method, which carries no risk to the patient, is thus of considerable value in confirming the presence of a space-occupying lesion in or overlying one cerebral hemisphere. With increasing precision it is likely that 'echoes' arising from other parts of the brain will be identified so that eventually this technique may prove to have an increasing application in the localisation of intracranial lesions.

GAMMA-ENCEPHALOGRAPHY

Until recently a research technique, the use of radioactive isotopes in the localisation of intracranial neoplasms is being increasingly applied in many neurological and neurosurgical units. The blood vessels and very possibly the cells of a number of types of tumour show a selective affinity for certain isotopes which emit gamma radiation, and in some instances a 'scan' of the external surface of the skull using radioactive counting equipment gives remarkably accurate localisation of a tumour within the brain. This method too is likely to be utilised increasingly as its accuracy improves.

STUDIES OF PERIPHERAL NERVE AND MUSCLE FUNCTION

A number of methods of electrodiagnosis are in common use in studying the function of peripheral nerves. It has long been known that motor nerves will respond to an applied electrical current of brief duration (faradism) and that muscle, even when it has lost its motor nerve supply, will contract, though sluggishly, in response to a long-duration current (galvanism). In Erb's **reaction of degeneration** (R.D.) there is loss of the response to faradism and retention of the response to galvanism, a finding which implies loss of nerve supply to the muscle concerned. Unfortunately this classical method does not indicate whether the denervation is partial or complete; to overcome this difficulty, the method has now been replaced in most centres by the charting of **strength-duration** or **intensity-duration** (I.D.) curves which are more quantitative.

To chart an I.D. curve, a square-wave electrical stimulator is used, so designed as to give a current (or voltage) which remains constant independently of varying resistance in the patient's tissues. An electrode is applied to the motor point of the muscle under test, and an earthing electrode is placed in contact with the skin elsewhere. A square wave of long duration is then applied repetitively and the current (or voltage) is gradually increased until a muscular contraction is just produced. The procedure is then repeated with square waves of increasingly brief duration and the current (or voltage) required on each occasion is charted. Characteristic curves are obtained for normally innervated muscle, for totally denervated muscle and for partially denervated muscle. Since many muscles can be tested it is therefore possible to determine which muscles have lost their nerve supply, and approximately to what extent.

This technique is of considerable value in studying patients with **peripheral nerve lesions** and in some cases of **neuromuscular disease.** It also has a prognostic value, as characteristic changes occur when a muscle is regaining its nerve supply. It is also possible sometimes to confirm a diagnosis of **myasthenia gravis** in this way, since in some cases of this disease, muscular contractions become progressively more feeble during repeated nerve stimulation. In **myotonia,** by contrast, there is a prolonged after-contraction with delayed relaxation.

Electromyography

Electromyography is a technique of recording the electrical activity produced by muscle at rest and during contraction. Surface electrodes can be used but are only of value for physiological studies, in determining, for instance, which muscles or muscle groups contribute to a particular movement, or for recording the frequency of involuntary movements (e.g. tremor). For diagnostic work, bipolar needle electrodes are inserted into the muscle being tested; the electrical activity is then passed through a high-gain amplifier and is presented for interpretation both on a cathode-ray screen and in a loudspeaker. Sometimes the visual trace is more valuable, sometimes the auditory pattern, but the combination is more valuable than either alone. **Normal voluntary muscle** is electrically silent at rest, but on contraction motor-unit potentials are seen and appear in increasing number and frequency as contraction increases, to give a continuous trace across the cathode-ray screen and a low-pitched rumble in the loudspeaker. These potentials are smooth monophasic, diphasic or triphasic waves, each about 5-7 msec in duration and about 1 mV in amplitude; each is produced by the contraction of all the muscle fibres supplied by one anterior horn cell and its motor neurone.

When a muscle **loses its nerve supply,** spontaneous **fibrillation** or contraction of individual muscle fibres begins within fourteen to twenty-one days and can be recorded from the relaxed and resting muscle; this takes the form of a series of repetitive small spikes on the cathode-ray screen and a ticking noise in the loudspeaker. If the muscle has lost only a part of its nerve supply, some motor unit potentials will still appear on attempted contraction, but the pattern of voluntary effort will be much reduced. During re-innervation following nerve regeneration complex polyphasic potentials of long duration appear, so-called **recovery potentials.** Hence in patients with disease of the motor neurone at any point from the anterior horn cell to the motor end-plate the EMG will show spontaneous fibrillation and a **reduced pattern** of motor units on voluntary effort. Sometimes there will also be spontaneous **fasciculation potentials** which look like normal motor unit potentials but are recorded from the resting muscle, while if there is nerve or nerve root irritation, groups of two or three motor unit potentials may be recorded, again from a muscle which is apparently at rest.

In **primary diseases of muscle,** such as muscular dystrophy, the pattern is different. Here there is no spontaneous activity, but on volition the motor unit potentials are seen to be broken-up, **polyphasic** and of **short duration.** Hence the pattern is complex and spiky and the noise in the loudspeaker is a crackling sound, like hail on a tin roof. The phenomenon of **myotonia** also gives a characteristic EMG; chains of oscillations of high frequency are seen which give a typical 'snarling' or 'dive-bomber' sound in the loudspeaker.

The electromyogram has a definite, though limited, value in neurological diagnosis. It is of particular use in the investigation of peripheral nerve injuries and in the study of difficult cases of muscular wasting and weakness in which it may be used with confidence to distinguish disease of the muscle from that of the motor nerves.

Nerve Conduction Velocity

By stimulating a motor nerve at two separate points along its course and by recording the motor unit potentials so produced, it is possible to measure the stimulus–contraction delay interval in each case and hence to calculate the rate of conduction of the impulse along the nerve. Nerve conduction has been found to be greatly slowed in some cases of polyneuropathy and the technique can also be utilised to localise focal lesions in the peripheral nerves, such as compression of the median nerve in the carpal tunnel, compression of the ulnar nerve at the elbow or of the lateral popliteal nerve at the neck of the fibula. Measurement of the conduction velocity in sensory fibres, stimulated by ring electrodes on a finger and picking up the sensory volley by an electrode over the trunk of the nerve, is also being used increasingly for diagnostic purposes.

Studies of Sensory Nerve Function

If a nerve is rendered ischaemic, by the inflation of a sphygmo-manometer cuff around a limb to above the systolic arterial blood pressure, ischaemic paraesthesiae develop in the skin areas supplied by the nerve concerned within five to ten minutes. On release of the cuff a series of post-ischaemic paraesthesiae are experienced. If the blood supply of the nerve concerned is already reduced due to pressure, ischaemic paraesthesiae appear much earlier, perhaps within one to two minutes and post-ischaemic paraesthesiae are more severe. This technique is of considerable value in diagnosing pressure lesions of peripheral nerves, of which median nerve compression in the carpal tunnel is a good example. It has also been found that ischaemic paraesthesiae are generally absent in patients with motor neurone disease, even though this condition is one in which sensory abnormalities are not discovered clinically.

Motor End-plate Dysfunction

It has been found that patients with myasthenia gravis show certain abnormal responses to muscular relaxant drugs and these may be of diagnostic value. Patients with true myasthenia are abnormally sensitive to curare and resistant to decamethonium iodide; this is not, however, the case as a rule in patients with a myasthenic syndrome associated with bronchial carcinoma.

RADIOLOGY

Radiological methods are among the most helpful and widely-used of all the ancillary techniques used in neurological diagnosis. Often final diagnosis must depend upon highly specialised methods involving the use of air or other contrast media, but each of these techniques, which will be considered below, is time-consuming, expensive and often disturbing to the patient. It must therefore be remembered that valuable and sometimes even conclusive information can be obtained from plain radiographs of the skull and/or spine and even of other parts of the body. Thus in patients with a clinical picture suggestive of intracranial tumour, or in others with a subacute meningitic illness, it will be important to X-ray the chest, as in one case a bronchogenic carcinoma may be revealed indicating that the intracranial lesion is probably metastatic, while in the other the appearances of pulmonary tuberculosis may be discovered. In

C*

certain other cases changes in the skeleton will cast light upon the significance of neurological symptoms and signs as, for instance, in cases of prostatic carcinoma or multiple myelomatosis.

Straight Radiography of the Skull

It is usual to take routine anteroposterior and lateral views of the skull, while in most specialised centres an anteroposterior view is also taken with the brow depressed some 35° so that the petrous temporal bones become visible (Towne's view), and another of the skull base. Stenver's view is also utilised to examine the petrous temporal bone. Usually the **skull vault** is first examined to see if there is reasonable uniformity of bony thickness or whether there is any **erosion** or **bony overgrowth** (as may result from a meningioma) or **abnormal vascular markings** due to dilatation of the middle meningeal artery which is supplying a meningeal tumour or vascular malformation. Sometimes, as in carcinomatosis or myelomatosis, there are multiple areas of **bony rarefaction** in the skull vault or there is a general thickening or 'woolliness' of the bone as in Paget's disease. In young children, hydrocephalus due to any cause gives **separation of the cranial sutures** and a characteristic **'beaten copper'** **mottling** of the bone. However, the latter appearance is so often seen in normal individuals, even in adult life, that in itself it is not diagnostic. Fractures of the vault are, of course, noted if present, and in passing it is wise to examine the frontal, maxillary and sphenoidal paranasal sinuses for opacities which would suggest infection or neoplasia. **Hyperostosis** of the inner table of the frontal bone is a not uncommon finding but has no definite pathological significance.

The **base of the skull** is next examined, first in the lateral projection. Here the relationship of the upper **cervical spine** to the **foramen magnum** is observed and it is noted whether there is any protrusion of the odontoid process of the axis above a line joining the posterior margin of the hard palate to the posterior lip of the foramen magnum (Chamberlain's line). If the odontoid does show above this line, or if there is an abnormal tilt of the body of the atlas implying invagination of the basi-occiput, then **basilar impression,** which may give important neurological symptoms and signs, is present. However, the most important structure at the base of the skull which is visible on the lateral projection is the **sella turcica.** The size and shape of the sella and the integrity and density of the anterior and posterior clinoid processes which form its lips are noted. In patients with primary pituitary neoplasms the sella is expanded or ballooned and partially decalcified. In patients with suprasellar lesions the sella is also expanded, but tends to be shallower and flattened and there is often erosion of the clinoid processes. A moderate degree of flattening and expansion of the sella with decalcification of the posterior clinoid processes may occur in any patient with increased intracranial pressure whether there is a lesion near the sella or not.

Also to be noted on the lateral projection is the presence or absence of **intracranial calcification.** If present, such calcification can then be more accurately localised by means of anteroposterior views, or sometimes by stereoscopic lateral projections. In about 50 per cent of adults, and even in a proportion of normal children, the **pineal gland,** which lies some distance above and behind the sella, is calcified and sometimes even measures up to 0·5 cm in diameter. If the gland is calcified it is most important to measure its distance from the inner table of the skull at either side on anteroposterior radiographs, as displacement of the gland to one or other side may indicate the presence of a space-occupying lesion in one cerebral hemisphere. Other intracranial structures which occasionally calcify in the normal individual are the choroid plexuses, the falx cerebri and the petro-clinoid ligaments. **Pathological intracranial calcification,** if mottled in type and suprasellar in situation, usually indicates a craniopharyngioma, but many other intracranial tumours, including meningiomas, gliomas and oligodendrogliomas, occasionally show a fine spidery pattern of calcification. Fine curvilinear lines of calcification are rarely seen in the wall of a large aneurysm, while calcific stippling or even dense calcification may occur within a haematoma or in an arteriovenous angioma. Rare causes of intracranial calcification include cysticercosis (calcified cysts), toxoplasmosis (mottling in the basal ganglia) and hypoparathyroidism (also in the basal ganglia). A form of widespread calcification outlining clearly the gyri of one occipital and/or parietal lobe is seen in diffuse cortical angiomatosis associated with a portwine naevus of the face (the Sturge–Weber syndrome).

In anteroposterior, Towne's, Stenver's and the basal views, the most important feature to look for is **enlargement or erosion of cranial exit foramina. Sclerosis and overgrowth of bone** may also occur, particularly in the wings of the sphenoid, in patients who have a meningioma in this situation. Otherwise it is usual to examine the optic foramina, superior orbital fissures, and internal auditory meati particularly. A funnel-shaped erosion of the internal auditory meati, revealed by Towne's and Stenver's views, is characteristic of acoustic neuroma. The basal view is valuable in revealing bony erosion due to malignant infiltration of the bony base of the skull and may also reveal enlargement of one foramen spinosum in a patient with a meningioma producing dilatation of one middle meningeal artery.

Radiology of the Spinal Column

In examining radiographs of the spine we are concerned first with changes in the **vertebrae** themselves, secondly with the **intervertebral disks** and thirdly with the **intervertebral foramina.** It is usual to carry out anteroposterior and lateral views to study the vertebrae and disks, but for examination of the intervertebral foramina, oblique views are necessary. In the vertebrae themselves one may first observe **congenital abnormalities** such as **fusion** of several vertebral bodies (if in the cervical region this may be called the Klippel–Feil syndrome) or **spina bifida,** either of which may be responsible for or associated with, neurological signs. Fracture, fracture-dislocation, Paget's disease, osteomyelitis, neoplasia, either benign or malignant, of vertebral bodies, any one of which might give vertebral collapse and spinal cord compression, will generally be revealed by routine X-rays. **Bony erosion** and, in particular, enlargement of the relevant intervertebral foramen is typically seen, often with the extraspinal soft tissue shadow of a dumb-bell tumour, in cases of spinal neurofibroma. Less striking but of equal diagnostic importance is a **variation in interpedicular distance.** The distance between the vertebral pedicles is large in the cervical region, gradually diminishes to a minimum in the mid-dorsal region, and then expands again in the lumbar region, corresponding to the cervical and lumbar enlargements of the spinal cord. If successive interpedicular distances are measured and one or more measurement falls outside the expected arithmetical progression, this indicates the presence of an expanding lesion within the spinal cord or spinal canal in this region. Dorsal meningiomas may produce no more radiological change than this, whereas neurofibromas commonly give bony erosion as well. Measurement of the **anteroposterior diameter** of the spinal canal is also of value, particularly in the cervical region; an unduly wide canal is seen, for instance, in some cases of syringomyelia.

In a patient with an acute **prolapse of an intervertebral disk,** radiographs of the spine are often normal or reveal simply a narrowing of the disk space concerned. The prolapsed disk is not itself radio-opaque. If one or more disk protrusions have been present for some months or years, the margins of the prolapsed tissue gradually become calcified, giving posterior (and often anterior) **osteophyte formation** at the upper and lower borders of the contiguous vertebrae. As the prolapsed tissue often projects laterally as well, osteophytes also tend to encroach upon the intervertebral foramina and this change is shown on oblique views. A combination of changes of this type, which are most commonly observed in the cervical and lumbar regions, is referred to as **spondylosis.**

Contrast Methods

The contrast methods most often used in neurological diagnosis are air encephalography, ventriculography with air or myodil, carotid, vertebral and aortic arch angiography and myelography (Plate II). Each of these methods carries certain possible hazards to the patient and all involve some degree of pain or discomfort. Hence they are by no means to be regarded as routine methods of investigation but should only be utilised when an accurate diagnosis can be reached in no other way. When this is the case, it should then be decided which method is likely to give the most helpful information and whether the method chosen is likely to be safe or whether there are contra-indications. Sometimes it is necessary to carry out a number of these studies successively, but they should always be kept to the minimum necessary to give adequate information concerning the patient's disease. In general it can be said that **air encephalography** is indicated in patients in whom cerebral tumour or cortical atrophy, either focal or generalised, are suspected and in whom there are no clinical localising signs and no features to suggest raised intracranial pressure. When an intracranial aneurysm or angioma is believed to be present or else a tumour which is shown by clinical findings, the EEG or the echo-encephalogram to be in one cerebral hemisphere, then **carotid arteriography** is usually the next step. In patients with papilloedema and other evidence of increased intracranial pressure but without localising signs, air **ventriculography** is generally indicated in order to localise the tumour or other lesion responsible. This must sometimes be followed after an interval by myodil ventriculography if the outline of the lateral ventricles is uninformative or if the third and fourth ventricles are not adequately outlined by air. It cannot be stressed too strongly that these are highly-specialised investigations which require immaculate radiographic technique and skilled neuroradiological interpretation. They should only be carried out in units where neurosurgical help is readily available should unforeseen complications arise. Often ventriculography must be followed by immediate craniotomy.

In the investigation of suspected spinal cord compression, **myelography** is the technique of choice and is usually performed by the lumbar route, though rarely cisternal injection of contrast medium is required in order to define the upper limit of a spinal lesion prior to surgical exploration.

AIR ENCEPHALOGRAPHY

Air encephalography, like lumbar puncture, is generally contra-indicated in patients with papilloedema or other evidence of increased intracranial pressure, in view of the dangers of cerebellar or tentorial herniation. It should be performed with utmost caution, and then only if skilled neurosurgical aid is at hand, in patients suspected of having a posterior fossa neoplasm, even if the C.S.F. pressure in the lumbar region is normal.

To perform an air encephalogram a lumbar puncture is performed with the patient sitting upright. After a few drops of C.S.F. have been allowed to flow, sufficient only to determine that the needle is in postion, 5 ml of air is injected slowly and radiographs are taken as the bubble of air passes through the basal cisterns and fourth ventricle. Then 5 ml of C.S.F. is removed, 10 ml of air is injected and subsequently 10 ml of fluid is withdrawn. The procedure is continued until a total of 25-30 ml of air has been injected and adequate filling of the ventricular system has been obtained. Usually this amount of air is adequate and can be manipulated in order to give a complete demonstration of the entire ventricular system and of the basal cisterns. It was once the custom to inject a considerably larger quantity of air, but the procedure in any event produces a severe headache and sometimes even prostration and vomiting; the severity of these symptoms is usually in direct proportion to the amount of air injected. It is usual to give pethidine or a similar analgesic both as a premedication and subsequently, and chlorpromazine may be required in order to relieve vomiting, though it should not as a rule be given beforehand as it may promote syncope during the procedure. Despite its unpleasant side-effects, encephalography is a remarkably safe investigation if used in appropriate cases.

Much valuable information may be obtained by this procedure. Thus the upper limits of a **pituitary neoplasm** can be defined by distortion of the basal cisterns or a **posterior fossa neoplasm** by displacement of or encroachment upon the fourth ventricle. Similarly, **neoplasms of the cerebral hemispheres** are localised by signs of distortion and displacement of the lateral and third ventricles (Pl. IIA). A localised dilatation of some part of the ventricular system may indicate a localised area of **cerebral atrophy** in this situation, while a general enlargement of the cerebral ventricles results from diffuse cortical atrophy, as in presenile dementia (Pl. IIB). The accurate interpretation of encephalographic findings demands much skill and experience; detailed descriptions are beyond the scope of this volume, but it is nevertheless important to appreciate the type of information which this investigation can give.

VENTRICULOGRAPHY

To perform ventriculography, air is injected into one lateral ventricle through a needle which has been inserted through a burr-hole in the skull and then passed through brain tissue. Hence to carry out this investigation the scalp must be shaved and bilateral posterior burr-holes in the skull must first be made. The procedure is not without risk as the needle may pierce a vessel during its passage through brain tissue, while a sudden release of pressure in one lateral ventricle may sometimes result in herniation of the contralateral cerebral hemisphere across the midline beneath the falx cerebri. Immediate puncture of the other lateral ventricle or even operative decompression will then be necessary. Hence this investigation should only be carried out when it is possible to proceed with the appropriate neurosurgical operation without delay.

The information obtainable by this method is comparable to that derived from encephalography and hence it is usually performed in patients with suspected **cerebral tumour** in whom the intracranial pressure is high. A **stenosis of the aqueduct of Sylvius,** giving internal hydrocephalus, is also demonstrated by this method, as the air will fail to pass through the aqueduct into the fourth ventricle. Sometimes, when despite manipulation it is impossible to demonstrate the fourth ventricle adequately, it is necessary to inject 1-2 ml of oily contrast medium such as myodil into the lateral ventricle and to observe its flow downwards through the third and fourth ventricles. This technique must only be used in carefully selected cases as the myodil acts as a cerebral irritant unless it is able to flow down into the spinal theca when the examination has been completed.

CEREBRAL ANGIOGRAPHY

Three techniques of cerebral angiography are in common use. In the first, **carotid arteriography,** the common carotid artery is injected with an iodine-containing contrast medium such as diodone, in a 35-40 per cent watery solution. With this technique, which is carried out by percutaneous injection under either local or general anaesthesia, the internal carotid artery and its branches (middle and anterior cerebral and their radicals) are demonstrated. The second technique, **vertebral arteriography,** can also be performed by percutaneous injection of the vertebral artery in the neck, and the vertebral, basilar and posterior cerebral arteries are then filled; this method is, however, difficult and is much less often used than carotid injection. In skilled hands, complications are few, but undue trauma to the wall of the injected artery may cause it to go into spasm, and in the elderly, hypertensive or atherosclerotic individual this can lead to cerebral ischaemia or infarction with a transient or even occasionally a permanent hemiplegia. Many radiologists now prefer to inject contrast medium into the vertebral arteries through a catheter inserted into a limb artery such as the femoral or radial; a similar

Plate II. Some important radiological abnormalities seen in patients with neurological disease.

A. A ventriculogram demonstrating the presence of a right temporal glioma which is causing elevation of the right temporal horn and is also infiltrating the basal ganglia to give distortion and displacement of the lateral ventricles. A = right temporal horn, B = left temporal horn, C = displaced and distorted right lateral ventricle.

B. A lumbar air encephalogram demonstrating diffuse ventricular dilatation with pooling of air in the sulci in a case of pre-senile dementia.

C. Right carotid arteriogram demonstrating a supraclinoid aneurysm of the internal carotid artery arising at the origin of the posterior communicating artery.

D. Left carotid arteriogram demonstrating an arteriovenous malformation in the posterior occipital region in a man of 29 years.

E. Left carotid arteriogram demonstrating stenosis at the origin of the internal carotid artery.

F. Right carotid arteriogram (late arterial phase) demonstrating the sinusoidal pathological circulation of a highly malignant glioma in the parietal region.

G. Left carotid arteriogram demonstrating a frontal meningioma (arterial phase).

H. Left carotid arteriogram demonstrating a frontal meningioma (the same as that seen in G—venous phase showing a 'blush').

J. A myelogram (antero-posterior view) demonstrating a smoothly rounded extramedullary but intrathecal space-occupying lesion in the dorsal region which is displacing and compressing the spinal cord. The spinal cord is seen outlined as an area of decreased density running down the centre of the myodil column.

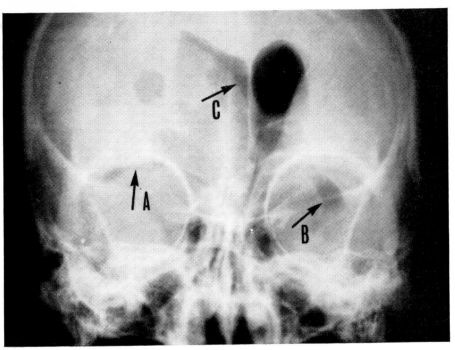

A

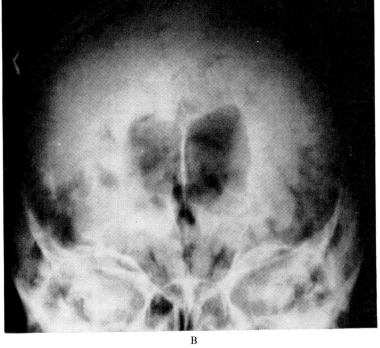

B

Plate II

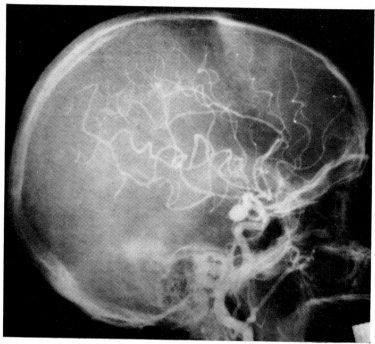

C

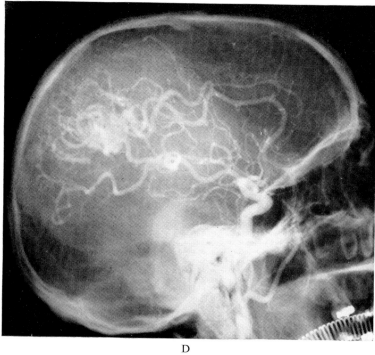

D

Plate II

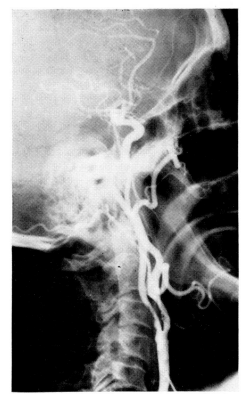

E

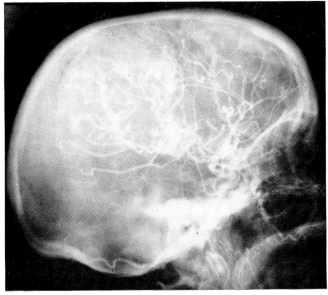

F

Plate II

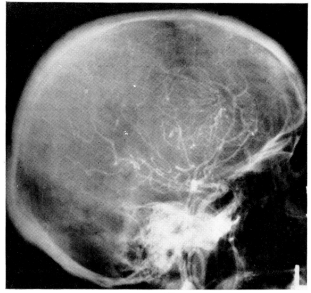

G

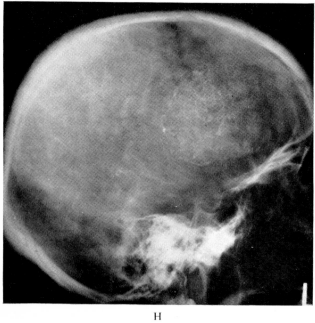

H

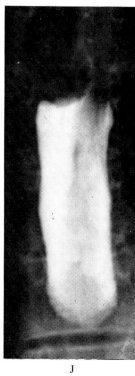

J

technique can be utilised when it is necessary to demonstrate the **aortic arch** and its main branches in cases of cerebral vascular disease. This third technique of angiography is being used increasingly.

Normally at least three lateral, anteroposterior and oblique views are taken at one- or two-second intervals to give early and late arterial and venous filling, but machines are now available to take much more frequent pictures, giving a more comprehensive demonstration of the vascular tree (rapid serial angiography).

Angiography is particularly valuable in the diagnosis of **vascular lesions.** Thus **intracranial aneurysms** and **arteriovenous angiomas** (Pl. IIc and D) are demonstrated and localised with a high degree of success; the technique must be used with caution in cases of presumed cerebral infarction, because of the danger of complications, but in some such cases obstruction or **stenosis of the internal carotid artery** (Pl. IIE), or of other major vessels in the neck or cranium are clearly demonstrated. **Subdural haematoma,** too, can be diagnosed with confidence, by the finding of an avascular area beneath the vault of the skull in the anteroposterior view.

Carotid arteriography also assists in the diagnosis and localisation of **space-occupying lesions** of the cerebral hemispheres. Distortion and displacement of vessels will localise the lesion whether it be tumour, abscess or haemorrhage, while many tumours show a characteristic pattern of vascularisation. **Astrocytomas** are relatively avascular, while **glioblastomas** commonly show a tangle of small abnormal blood vessels (Pl. IIF); **meningiomas** often give a characteristic 'blush' in the venous phase of the angiogram (Pl. IIG and H), owing to retention of contrast medium in the tiny vessels of the tumour. Vertebral arteriography may help in the diagnosis of tumours in the posterior fossa and is of great value in patients suspected of having vascular anomalies of the hind-brain circulation.

CONCLUSIONS

It may be concluded that in patients in whom the symptoms and physical signs indicate a space-occupying lesion of one cerebral hemisphere, carotid arteriography is probably the investigation of choice. Where an intracranial tumour or cortical atrophy are suspected but there are no localising signs and no evidence of increased pressure, air encephalography is indicated; when, however, the intracranial pressure is clearly raised, ventriculography is required.

MYELOGRAPHY

Myelography is a most valuable means of localising lesions which are compressing the spinal cord. It is usual to inject 5-6 ml of oily contrast medium into the lumbar subarachnoid space and then to observe under the screen (fluoroscope) the flow of contrast medium up and down the spinal canal on tilting the patient. Anteroposterior and lateral radiographs are also taken at intervals. It is only necessary to inject myodil cisternally when there is a block beyond which contrast medium injected in the lumbar region will not pass and information is required concerning the upper limit of the lesion. The investigation has few complications, though some pain and paraesthesiae in the lower back and legs, along with mild fever, may persist for a few days afterwards. Very rarely a transient 'cauda equina syndrome' occurs, or else lumbar or sacral root pain, presumably due to irritation, persists for some weeks or months. It is probably unnecessary to attempt to remove the myodil after the examination has been completed, but this is done in some centres.

An **extramedullary neoplasm** will almost always be localised accurately on myelography, either by the presence of a block or by a characteristic filling defect in the column of contrast medium (Pl. IIj). Expansion of the spinal cord, indicative of an **intramedullary neoplasm**, or of **syringomyelia** can also be demonstrated, while an outline of abnormal vessels in patients with **spinal vascular malformations** may also be seen. **Prolapsed intervertebral disks** and spondylotic changes are demonstrated best in lateral views, when indentations in the myodil column are seen opposite the disk space or spaces concerned; lateral protrusions may result in a failure of certain root sleeves to fill with contrast medium, and this is seen best in the anteroposterior view. Myelography is thus an essential preliminary to any operation performed for the relief of spinal cord compression, as clinical signs in themselves are never sufficiently accurate for exact localisation of the lesion.

THE SPECIAL SENSES

Visual and Oculomotor Functions

Methods of examination of the visual apparatus which form a part of the routine neurological examination have already been described in Chapter 1. These include testing of the visual acuity, charting of the peripheral and central visual fields, examination of the pupils, of the ocular movements and ophthalmoscopy.

Slit-lamp examination is occasionally helpful in neurological diagnosis, either for the detection of early degrees of cataract, or in looking for the pigmentation of the periphery of the cornea which occurs in Wilson's disease (the Kayser–Fleischer ring).

Recording of ocular muscle imbalance on a **Hess's chart** is also valuable in the investigation of cases of diplopia, since repeated recordings may give an objective assessment of the patient's progress.

Ophthalmodynamometry, a technique of measuring the pressure in the retinal arteries by applying a simple instrument to the globe of the eye, is occasionally helpful in the diagnosis of occlusion or insufficiency of the internal carotid artery, since the ophthalmic artery is a direct branch of the internal carotid and the retinal artery pressure on the affected side is reduced.

Auditory and Vestibular Function

The simple tuning-fork tests for the assessment of auditory function are described in Chapter 2. For a more accurate assessment of degrees of deafness **audiometry** is necessary. In this method, each ear is tested independently and sounds of different frequencies are used, produced by an electronic instrument which gives pure tones. At each frequency, the intensity of sound (measured in decibels) is steadily increased until the patient can just hear it. By this method it is possible to determine the degree of deafness, if any, which is present in each ear and also whether it is a deafness for all frequencies.

In disease of the cochlear end organ (as in Menière's syndrome), the phenomenon of **recruitment** may occur. This means that an impairment of hearing in the affected ear decreases progressively as the intensity of the stimulus is increased so that eventually it is heard equally loudly in the unaffected and diseased ears. Recruitment does not occur in patients with lesions of the auditory nerve (e.g. acoustic neuroma) so that a test for recruitment is of value in differential diagnosis.

Vestibular function can be tested by **caloric tests.** The head is tilted backwards 60° so that the lateral semicircular canal is vertical and the ear is then irrigated with cold water (at 30° C.) This produces nystagmus with the quick phase to the right if the left ear is irrigated or vice versa. The test is then repeated using warm water (44° C), when the quick phase of the nystagmus occurs in the opposite direction, that is to the side of the ear which is being tested. The two ears are stimulated independently and the total duration of the nystagmus obtained in each of the four tests is recorded. In lesions of the peripheral vestibular system (Menière's disease) or of the vestibular nerve, stimulation of the affected labyrinth by caloric tests will either produce no nystagmus at all or else its duration will be greatly reduced (**canal paresis**). This finding is often of diagnostic value. In certain patients who have lesions of the brain stem or of the temporal or parietal lobes of the contralateral cerebral hemisphere, the duration of the nystagmus occurring to the side away from the cerebral lesion is greatly reduced, whether it is produced by warm water in one ear or cold water in the other. This finding, which is known as **directional preponderance,** is not due to a labyrinthine lesion but to a lesion of the central pathways which are responsible for conducting and recording labyrinthine stimuli.

PSYCHOLOGICAL TESTING

Simple tests of intellectual function have already been described in Chapter 1. A great variety of methods for assessing intelligence and personality are available. Detailed consideration of these psychometric tests is beyond the scope of this volume, but it is worth noting that they can be used to assess objectively the mental changes which occur in organic neurological disease. The Wechsler–Bellevue series are particularly valuable in confirming the presence of early dementia and in assessing degrees of deterioration. A comparison of verbal and performance tests will sometimes reveal specific defects in the utilisation of language or in the execution of skilled motor activity which may not be clearly apparent on routine clinical examination. In neurological medicine these tests are of most value in confirming objectively subjective impressions of early intellectual deterioration. Other tests designed for the assessment of personality rather than intellect, such as the Rorschach ink-blot test, have more application to psychiatry than to neurology.

REFERENCES

BULL, J. W. D., 'Diagnostic neuroradiology', in *Modern Trends in Neurology*, Ed. Feiling, A., Chapter 20, 1st series (London, Butterworth, 1951).

GILLIATT, R., 'Clinical electromyography', in *Modern Trends in Neurology*, Ed. Williams, D., Chapter 5, 2nd series (London, Butterworth, 1957).

HILL, J. D. N. and PARR, G., *Electroencephalography*, 2nd ed. (London, Macdonald, 1963).

KILOH, L. G. and OSSELTON, J. W., *Clinical Electroencephalography* (London, Butterworth, 1961).

LICHT, S., *Electrodiagnosis and Electromyography*, 2nd ed. (Baltimore, Waverley Press, 1961).

MERRITT, H. H. and FREMONT-SMITH, F., *The Cerebrospinal Fluid* (Philadelphia, Saunders, 1938).

ROBERTSON, E. G., *Pneumoencephalography* (Springfield, Ill., Thomas, 1957).

SWEET, W. H., 'Formation, absorption and flow of cerebrospinal fluid', in *Modern Trends in Neurology*, Ed. Williams, D., Chapter 3, 2nd series (London, Butterworth, 1957).

WALTON, J. N. (Ed.), *Disorders of Voluntary Muscle*, Chapters 21-25 (London, Churchill, 1964).

WOLSTENHOLME, F. E. W. and O'CONNOR, C. M., *The Cerebrospinal Fluid* (London, Churchill, 1958).

CHAPTER 4

PAIN

PAIN is one of the most common and disturbing of human experiences. While it may result from a great many causes, the appreciation of painful sensations depends upon the stimulation of pain-sensitive nerve endings in the skin, muscles, skeleton, blood vessels, viscera and membranes, and upon the conduction of nerve impulses into the central nervous system where the sensation finally enters consciousness. The central pathways along which impulses conveying painful sensations travel and the effect of disease of the central nervous system upon its appreciation will be considered in Chapter 10, while methods used for the relief of pain are discussed in Chapter 20. In this chapter a number of common neurological syndromes of which pain is a prominent symptom will be mentioned, with particular reference to the mechanism of its production.

It should first be remembered that patients vary widely in their response to painful experiences, some remaining relatively impassive when experiencing sensations which would produce in others an intense reaction. This individuality in emotional responses to painful stimuli means that although the threshold intensity of stimulus required to give the appreciation of pain (the pain threshold) is relatively constant, the reaction to painful stimuli which exceed the threshold intensity may be specific to the individual and can even vary in the same patient, depending upon circumstances.

There are no specific sensory receptors in the skin which are concerned with the perception of pain; it is now apparent that painful cutaneous stimuli are recorded by multiple fine cutaneous nerve endings and that it is the pattern and frequency of stimulation of a series of anatomically-related nerve endings which determines the character and severity of the pain. In general nerve-fibre networks of this type are most luxuriant in those areas of skin which are most sensitive. Analysis of the pain which follows cutaneous stimulation has shown that it has two components, the first immediate and the second delayed; probably these two forms of the sensation are conveyed by nerve fibres which conduct at different rates. A sensation of deep pain is also experienced after stimulation of deeper structures such as tendons, blood vessels and the periosteum. Painful lesions of the muscles or viscera sometimes give pain in the overlying skin, or else this symptom can be experienced in a cutaneous area which is comparatively remote (referred pain). The mechanism of reference of painful sensations is still not fully understood, though some believe that a spread of activity between sensory neurones within the spinal cord is responsible.

A great many different types of pathological change can give rise to pain, through stimulation of pain-sensitive nerve endings in the organ or organs which are diseased. Thus, trauma and inflammation are two of the most important causes of cutaneous pain, while pain of skeletal origin is often similarly produced; malignant disease, including metastases in bone, can also be very painful. Visceral pain, particularly that arising in the abdominal organs, most often results from excessive contraction of plain muscle, giving rise to the passage of pain-carrying impulses along afferent fibres accompanying sympathetic nerves, though distension of hollow organs or inflammation of their enveloping membranes (such as the peritoneum) may also be painful; in the latter case the impulses are often carried by somatic afferents. Pain arising in skeletal muscle is commonly due to prolonged over-activity, cramp or fatigue, though repeated activity of a muscle which has an inadequate blood supply (ischaemic work) can also be responsible; this principle probably applies also to cardiac muscle (angina of effort).

Since the sensory nerve fibres and central structures concerned in the reception and appreciation of painful stimuli are themselves sensitive to inflammation or irritation, and since there are a number of other pain-sensitive structures within the cranium and spinal canal, it is apparent that pain can be a relatively common symptom of disease of the nervous system. We must therefore consider in turn headache, facial pain and the characteristics of pain in the back, trunk or limbs which may result from nervous disease. It should be noted at this stage that a reduction in the ability to perceive painful stimuli is known as **hypalgesia;** an excessively painful response is called **hyperalgesia,** while a painful sensation which has peculiarly unpleasant or abnormal characteristics is referred to as **hyperpathia.**

HEADACHE

Headache is produced by the stimulation of pain-sensitive structures within the cranium or in the extracranial tissues of the head and neck. Sensitive structures lying extracranially include the occipital, temporal and frontal muscle groups, the skin of the scalp, the arteries which traverse the subcutaneous tissue, and the periosteum. The cranial bones themselves are insensitive. Within the skull the sensitive areas are the meninges, particularly the basal dura mater and that which forms the walls of the venous sinuses, as well as the large arteries which lie at the base of the brain, forming the circle of Willis and its branches. The greater part of the cerebral substance itself is relatively insensitive to stimuli which are normally painful if applied to appropriate receptors.

One of the commonest causes of **headache of extracranial origin** is emotional tension. So-called **tension headaches** are characteristically occipital, but sometimes frontal, in situation, and result from continuous partial contraction of the muscles which are attached to the scalp. Typically headaches of this nature come on towards evening when the patient is tired; the posterior neck muscles are often tender and this symptom may be relieved by rest if the patient can be taught to relax properly. The headaches of so-called **eye-strain** are probably similar in aetiology; if an uncorrected visual refractive error is present, then the continuous effort required to compensate for this defect will also result in muscular tension, giving rise to headaches which can be relieved by the provision of appropriate spectacles. Headache of purely **psychogenic origin,** of the type which occurs in neurotic, hypochondriacal or hysterical individuals, is often vertical in situation and is typically described in over-elaborate terms, perhaps in order to impress; a common example is to say that the top of the head feels as if it were being lifted off. Not uncommonly patients of this type also experience true tension headaches towards the end of the day. Headaches described as being like 'a sense of pressure' or like 'a tight constricting band' are usually of this type and it should be noted that depressed patients may complain of headaches occurring in the mornings when depression is often at its worst.

Disorders of the **extracranial arteries** can also give rise to headache and indeed the symptoms of migraine, one of the commonest of headache syndromes, which will be discussed in detail below, may be attributed in part to alterations in calibre occurring in the branches of the external carotid artery. Other 'vascular' headaches, such as that of a 'hangover', or of hypertension, can probably be attributed at least in part to dilatation of extracranial rather than intracranial arteries. The pain of temporal arteritis is also clearly extracranial in origin, being the result of inflammatory changes in the temporal arteries. Other causes of headache which must also be considered to be in a sense extracranial are **paranasal sinusitis** and **middle-ear disease** in which the pain results either from the increasing tension of pus in a confined space or from spread of inflammation to the bone and its coverings.

Headache of intracranial origin is due to inflammation, compression, and distortion of or traction upon the pain-sensitive meninges and blood vessels within the skull. Such headaches are usually referred to the frontal or occipital regions or both, though a unilateral lesion will sometimes produce a unilateral headache, say, in. one or other temple. When this is the case it can be assumed with reasonable confidence that the lesion concerned lies upon the side of the head where the headache is experienced.

The headache of **diffuse meningeal inflammation,** as occurs in meningitis, subarachnoid haemorrhage and following air encephalography, is generally severe, continuous and unvarying and associated with neck stiffness. Like the headache of **increased intracranial pressure,** whether the latter results from a single space-occupying lesion or from diffuse brain swelling or hydrocephalus, it is characteristically made worse by sudden movements of the head, by stooping, or by coughing and straining. Each of these mechanisms is likely to increase even further the distortion of pain-sensitive structures which is already present, either through movement, or through a sudden brief increase in the intracranial pressure produced by delaying the outflow of venous blood from the cranium. Typically this type of headache is throbbing in nature, perhaps owing to the transmission of arterial pulsation to tissues which are already under increased tension. It is present as a rule on waking but tends to improve as the day wears on. If a cerebral abscess or tumour is the cause, then vomiting and papilloedema may also be present.

A headache which is very similar in character to that described above is due to a comparable mechanism in cases of **reduced intracranial pressure,** in which there is again traction upon pain-sensitive arteries and meninges. This is the basis of the **post-lumbar puncture headache** which is presumed to be due to continued leakage of C.S.F. through the hole in the spinal dura left by the lumbar puncture needle. The headache of dehydration has a similar cause and some believe that a clinical syndrome of **intracranial hypotension,** characterised by this type of headache, can occur spontaneously, but this is by no means certain, as the pressure in the spinal theca on lumbar puncture may be remarkably low in healthy patients who make no complaint of headache. A benign syndrome of 'cough headache' does, however, occur in which severe headache, typically of 'intracranial' type, accompanies coughing. While some such patients have emphysema and may be presumed to have an unusually large increase in intracranial pressure during coughing owing to delayed venous return to the heart, others have no evidence of severe chest disease and in these cases the aetiology of the syndrome remains obscure. While the possibility of intracranial tumour should always be borne in mind in such patients, many cases of this type carry an excellent prognosis, though little can be done to relieve this symptom except to advise avoidance of the circumstances which give rise to coughing.

Migraine

Migraine is one of the commonest of neurological disorders and may at the same time be one of the most disabling. It occurs in both sexes, but is more common in women, and generally begins in adolescence or early adult life, often in patients who have suffered from bilious attacks in childhood. Rarely migrainous headaches begin for the first time at about the time of the menopause, usually in hypertensive women, and attacks are particularly liable to occur during or just before the menstrual periods. Often there is a strong family history of the condition, while it is seen most frequently in the more intelligent, industrious and energetic, though intense and obsessional, members of the community. Attacks of migraine have a tendency to be more frequent during or after episodes of overwork or emotional stress.

Migraine has been defined as a paroxysmal unilateral headache, preceded by visual and sensory phenomena and accompanied or followed by nausea and vomiting. While this may be a description of a 'typical' case, there are many patients with undoubted migraine in whom no visual or sensory aura is ever experienced and in whom the headache is never one-sided. The paroxysmal occurrence of this symptom is its most important feature.

The mechanism of production of the migrainous headache is now well understood. The initial disturbance is one of vasospasm in the extra- and intra-cranial arteries and their branches, often on one side of the head, and this is followed some ten to thirty minutes later by a dilatation of the same vessels. The arterial constriction is responsible for the symptoms of the aura, the dilatation for the headache. The aetiology of these alterations in vascular tone, however, remains obscure. There is evidence of excessive fluid retention in the body before each attack, followed by a subsequent diuresis, a finding which raises the possibility of a metabolic or endocrine cause. Certainly there is no definite evidence that allergy or a disorder of the autonomic nervous system is responsible. Paroxysmal headaches of migrainous type may be a prominent symptom in patients harbouring intracranial arteriovenous angiomas or even aneurysms, but in these individuals the headache is usually strictly unilateral, occurring on the same side of the head as the vascular anomaly; the reason for this association is not known.

Usually the migrainous attack begins soon after waking in the morning. A visual aura is the most common, resulting from spasm of the retinal arteries or of branches of the posterior cerebral artery supplying one or both occipital lobes. The patient will then experience either a hemianopic field defect, a less well-defined scotoma or rarely transient blindness, jagged lines ('fortification spectra'), or bright, dancing or shimmering lights (teichopsia) in one half-field. Alternatively a sensory aura, with paraesthesiae (tingling, numbness and pins and needles) in the corner of the mouth and in the arm, or less commonly in the leg on the same side, may occur, presumably due to spasm of those branches of the middle cerebral artery which supply the sensory cortex. In occasional patients the aura (vertigo, diplopia, bilateral paraesthesiae) suggests that the hind-brain rather than the fore-brain circulation is involved (basilar artery migraine) and sometimes fainting occurs either during the aura or at the height of the headache. Very rarely there is actual transient weakness of one arm and leg (hemiplegic migraine) or a paresis of one oculomotor nerve (ophthalmoplegic migraine); however, most patients with the latter condition have an aneurysm of the internal carotid artery compressing the nerve trunk within the cranium.

As the aura passes off the headache begins and mounts in intensity. It can be unilateral and frontal (above one or other eye), bifrontal, bioccipital, or generalised. Sometimes it is comparatively mild, though accompanied by lassitude and depression, but more often it is prostrating, and there is photophobia, so that the patient must lie down in a darkened room. Typically the headache will last all day, passing off after a night's sleep, but sometimes it wanes in an hour or two. Alternatively, it may persist, though with diminishing intensity, for a few days or even for as long as a week. Characteristically the headache is accompanied by nausea, sometimes by vomiting and occasionally by retching. There are some individuals in whom an aura never occurs, and others who occasionally have the aura without the headache; indeed numerous variants occur, the above being the typical clinical picture. 'Bilious attacks' in childhood are almost certainly a migrainous variant, while some believe that the same is true of recurrent attacks of abdominal pain or cyclical vomiting in children and adolescents.

Attacks of migraine can be mild and infrequent, occurring once every few months and constituting little more than a nuisance, but in other cases they are severe and prostrating, occurring every few days, and are then the cause of serious disability. There is a tendency for the condition to improve as the patient approaches middle age and to disappear at the menopause, but the form which first develops in post-menopausal women may be particularly intractable. A temporary exacerbation with frequent attacks often accompanies a paramenopausal depressive illness. Treatment is considered in Chapter 20.

Migrainous Neuralgia

There exist a group of patients who experience episodes of severe and continuous pain, often burning in character, in, around or behind one eye or in the cheek, forehead and temple. These attacks tend to occur in bouts lasting a few weeks or months and during a bout the patient suffers one or several attacks, lasting from fifteen minutes to several hours, each day. Not uncommonly the attacks recur at the same time of day or night and they may waken the patient from sleep. There is often suffusion of the conjunctiva and blocking of the nostril on the affected side during the attacks. The aetiology of this condition, which has been variously referred to as **histamine headache, ciliary neuralgia,** or **cluster headache,** is unknown, but it has certain affinities with migraine and is probably best referred to as periodic migrainous neuralgia.

FACIAL PAIN

Pain in the face is a common symptom which may present formidable difficulties in understanding and interpretation. Whereas it sometimes results from obvious local causes such as maxillary sinusitis, neoplasia of the maxilla, mandible or soft tissues, caries, dental abscess or parotitis, it can also be due to a variety of pathological lesions involving the trigeminal nerve, its branches and central connexions. Thus a plaque of demyelination or a syrinx (cavity) in the brain stem may give a continuous unilateral facial ache through irritation of the central connexions of the trigeminus, as may a tumour (acoustic neuroma, meningioma, nasopharyngeal carcinoma) or aneurysm which is compressing the Gasserian ganglion or the intracranial portion of the fifth cranial nerve. Similarly, herpes zoster of the Gasserian ganglion, which tends to affect particularly the ophthalmic division of the nerve, gives severe and continuous pain in the eye and forehead. Even more frequent, however, are the syndromes of intermittent facial pain, including trigeminal neuralgia and atypical facial neuralgia.

Trigeminal Neuralgia (Tic Douloureux)

Trigeminal neuralgia is an intermittent, brief, lancinating pain in the face, confined to the area of cutaneous distribution of one trigeminal nerve, and often evoked by movement of the face or by touching the skin. It is equally common in the two sexes and is most commonly seen after middle-age, particularly in the elderly, though it rarely occurs in early adult life.

The aetiology of the 'idiopathic' form of the syndrome is unknown, though the pain may sometimes occur in classical form as a symptom of disseminated sclerosis, resulting from a plaque of demyelination at the point of entry of the trigeminal root into the brain stem; very rarely it can be the first symptom of a posterior fossa tumour, such as an acoustic neuroma lying in one cerebellopontine angle. The increasing incidence of the condition in the elderly has given rise to the suggestion that ischaemia of the trigeminal nerve or ganglion, resulting from atherosclerosis, is the principal aetiological factor, but comparatively few cases have been studied pathologically and no consistent histological changes have been demonstrated.

The pain of tic douloureux is characteristically sudden, excruciating and brief, 'like the stab of a red-hot needle'; a continuous pain in the face, or one lasting for several minutes, is not tic douloureux, though some patients experience a background of dull aching pain between the paroxysms. The pain does not extend outside the territory supplied by the trigeminal nerve, nor does it cross the midline. It can occur in the distribution of any one or all of the divisions of the trigeminus; if the ophthalmic division alone is involved, this syndrome is often referred to as **supraorbital neuralgia.** The intensity of the pain can be judged from the apparently involuntary spasm of the facial muscles on the affected side and the agonized expression which accompany each attack. The patient often holds one hand in front of the face to protect it and will not allow it to be touched as he knows that movement, as in speaking, or chewing, or touching the face, and as in shaving or washing, may provoke an attack. Neurological examination is rarely informative, though a few patients have slight objective diminution of sensory perception on the affected side of the face.

Characteristically, tic douloureux is a periodic disorder. It tends to occur in bouts lasting several weeks or months, during which the pain occurs with variable frequency and severity. Long remissions of weeks, months or even years may separate the bouts but these remissions tend to become progressively shorter. The condition, though intensely distressing, is essentially benign, and does not shorten life, though some few patients are occasionally driven to suicide to find relief from their agony. Fortunately, most patients now respond to drug treatment (*see* Chapter 20), but in unresponsive cases effective treatment, in the form of alcohol injection of the Gasserian ganglion, or neurosurgical division of the trigeminal sensory root, is available, at the expense of permanent facial anaesthesia.

Atypical Facial Neuralgia

Apart from the local causes of facial pain to which reference has already been made, other painful syndromes of intermittent character can affect the face. One of these is migrainous neuralgia which has already been considered.

Costen's syndrome is a condition in which a severe shooting type of pain radiates down the lower jaw or up into the temple whenever the patient chews. It differs from trigeminal neuralgia in that chewing is the only 'trigger' which produces the pain, and touching the face, for instance, has no effect. This condition is believed to be due to dental malocclusion, resulting probably in compression of branches of the auriculotemporal nerve in the neighbourhood of the temporo-mandibular joint. The pain can be relieved by building up the 'bite'.

One of the commonest forms of **atypical facial pain** is an inter-mittent but long-lasting pain of aching character which affects the cheek and upper jaw and occurs almost without exception in young and middle-aged women. In such a case it is wise to exclude dental sepsis, sinusitis and other organic lesions as a possible cause of the pain, but investigations are almost always negative. This type of pain, which responds poorly to treatment, is generally believed to be a manifestation of psychiatric illness, particularly depression or anxiety. Unquestionably the pain is sometimes improved by psycho-therapy, by tranquillisers and even by electroconvulsion therapy, but in some patients it is quite intractable. Whereas in most cases there is positive evidence of psychiatric disturbance, the pathogenesis of this condition is poorly understood. Attempts which have been made to relieve the pain by cervical immobilisation or by sectioning the greater auricular nerve have no rational basis, and this trouble-some condition remains very unsatisfactory from the point of view of management.

GLOSSOPHARYNGEAL NEURALGIA

This rare condition is in many respects similar to trigeminal neu-ralgia as the pain occurs in periodic bouts and is brief and lancinat-ing in character. It occurs in the tonsillar fossa, back of throat and larynx and may radiate to the ear on the affected side. Swallowing is the stimulus most likely to produce the pain. The aetiology of this syndrome is unknown. Like trigeminal neuralgia it may respond to drug treatment, but if intractable it can be cured by division of the affected glossopharyngeal nerve in the posterior fossa.

PAIN IN THE SPINAL COLUMN AND LIMBS

While there are a great many skeletal and ligamentous lesions which can produce pain in the spinal column, some lesions involving nervous tissues also give rise to pain in this situation. Diffuse inflammatory conditions such as ankylosing spondylitis, or metabolic disorders producing osteoporosis, may give a dull aching pain involving the greater part of the spinal column, while osteomyelitis of a vertebral body or a metastasis in one or more vertebrae give severe and continuous pain which is localised to the affected area of the spine. As a secondary effect of these conditions, distortion and deformity of the bony architecture can occur, resulting in compression of the spinal cord (this is in general painless) or of spinal roots (giving pain in the distribution of the root concerned). Similarly, lesions of the spinal cord and its roots, whether they be intramedullary (e.g. disseminated sclerosis, syringomyelia), intrathecal (meningioma, arachnoiditis) or extradural (prolapsed intravertebral disk) may irritate or compress sensory tracts or fibres or nerve roots, producing a similar type of pain. Furthermore, a neoplasm such as a neurofibroma which may begin by producing pain due simply to compression of its parent spinal root, will later grow sufficiently large to erode the bone of the vertebral body, giving a dull continuous 'skeletal' type of pain in the affected area of the spine. It should also be remembered that root irritation often produces a 'protective' spasm of the overlying spinal muscles and this spasm may itself be painful, while the muscles concerned become tender. Voluntary contraction of these muscles will then increase the pain as will nervous tension.

NERVE AND NERVE-ROOT COMPRESSION

When nerve fibres or trunks concerned with the transmission of pain-carrying impulses are compressed or irritated, whether in the spinal cord, spinal roots or peripheral nerves, a characteristically intolerable, continuous, burning pain is produced. If fibres concerned with touch and proprioception run in the same nerve, then associated paraesthesiae (tingling, numbness, pins and needles) also occur. Some of these features may be due to direct nerve irritation, others to ischaemia. Paradoxically, vasodilatation due to warmth can so increase the volume of the nerve which is being compressed that its effective blood supply is further reduced and the pain is made worse, while excessive cold, resulting in vasoconstriction, will also increase ischaemia and hence the symptoms. Pain due to peripheral nerve compression is referred to the cutaneous area from which the nerve concerned receives sensory fibres. Similarly, root pain radiates throughout the dermatome of the root concerned, but it is less well recognised that deep muscular pain due to the same cause may be more widespread, corresponding broadly to the muscles supplied by the homologous motor root. Root pain has other special characteristics; thus it is affected by sudden movements of the spinal column which would be likely to cause movement of the root or of the pathological lesion which is compressing it. Similarly a sudden increase in the cerebrospinal fluid pressure, as in coughing or straining, will cause a sharp, shooting paroxysm of pain in the appropriate distribution. When symptoms of this type are of long standing, the trunks of peripheral nerves which contribute to the sensory root or roots involved often become tender on pressure.

CAUSALGIA

Causalgia is the name given to a particularly unpleasant burning type of continuous pain which may follow peripheral nerve injuries, or root lesions, particularly those in which severance of a nerve has been incomplete and some regeneration has occurred. This type of pain is most common in the hand and arm but does occur occasionally in the leg; it is most frequent of all after lesions of the median nerve. The skin area in which this spontaneous pain occurs is usually shiny and the seat of excessive perspiration; there is often intense hyperaesthesia and the patient will not allow the skin to be touched as this greatly accentuates the pain. Although the exact mechanism of this syndrome is not fully understood it is clear that autonomic pathways play an important role, as blocking or section of somatic sensory nerves from the skin area concerned do not relieve the pain, but sympathectomy is usually effective.

PHANTOM-LIMB PAIN

It is well recognised that after amputation of a limb (or removal of an ear, the penis or some other member), sensations may be experienced for several months or years suggesting that the part concerned is still *in situ*. Not infrequently, pain of a curiously unpleasant and intolerable nature, resembling causalgia in many respects, develops in this phantom member. Usually such patients are found to have plexiform neuromas in the amputation stump, resulting from regeneration of fibres from the severed ends of peripheral nerves, and digital compression of such a neuroma will reproduce the patient's spontaneous pain. Repeated percussion or sometimes excision of the neuroma may relieve the pain.

POST-HERPETIC NEURALGIA

Pain in the distribution of the affected root, whether it be the ophthalmic division of the trigeminus, or a cervical, dorsal or lumbar posterior root, is a striking feature of herpes zoster. In younger patients the pain generally resolves within a few weeks at the most, but in the elderly a severe continuous burning pain may persist for years afterwards. It seems that this pain must depend upon the reception of sensory stimuli from the skin area concerned, since in the early stages it can sometimes be relieved by subcutaneous infiltration with a local anaesthetic. However, relief from these measures is only temporary and it appears that a progressive facilitation occurs in those synapses within the central nervous system which are concerned with the transmission of these sensory impulses, for eventually the pain continues to occur apparently spontaneously, despite division of the peripheral pathways. The pain may be so intolerable that some patients are driven to suicide. Eventually in most cases spontaneous improvement occurs, but nevertheless the condition presents serious problems in management (*see* Chapter 20).

THALAMIC PAIN

We have discussed above the mechanisms by which irritation or compression of peripheral nerves or sensory roots may give rise to pain, and it was mentioned that lesions within the spinal cord which affect the spinothalamic tracts can also give rise to pain in the limbs. Similarly, a lesion of the thalamus itself (usually an infarct) may be the cause of severe pain in the contralateral face, arm and leg. So-called thalamic pain is intense, burning and continuous in character and has other peculiarly unpleasant qualities, often described by the patient with such adjectives as 'tearing' or 'grinding'. Pain of this type is fortunately rare as it is comparatively unaffected by any but the most powerful analgesics. Neurosurgical measures occasionally utilised in cases of this type are mentioned in Chapter 20.

CONCLUSIONS

It can be concluded that headache and pain in the face, spine and limbs are among the most common symptoms of nervous disease. A rational approach to differential diagnosis and treatment of these manifestations must depend upon a working knowledge of the anatomy of the sensory pathways and of the applied physiology of pain. It is also essential to assess the patient as an individual so that the importance of emotional factors in the genesis of his symptoms, as well as the significance of his emotional reaction to the pain he is experiencing, may be taken into account.

REFERENCES

KEELE, C. A. and SMITH, R. (Eds.), *The Assessment of Pain in Man and Animals* (Edinburgh, Livingstone, 1962).

KUNKLE, E. C. and WOLFF, H. G., 'Headache', in *Modern Trends in Neurology*, Ed. Feiling, A., Chapter 3, 1st series (London, Butterworth, 1951).

MARSHALL, J., 'The applied physiology of pain', in *Physiology of the Nervous System*, Ed. Walsh, E. G., Chapter 3 (London, Longmans, 1957).

WHITE, J. C. and SWEET, W. H., *Pain, its Mechanisms and Neurosurgical Control* (Springfield, Ill., Thomas, 1955).

WOLFF, H. G. and TITZELL, A. P., *Headache and other Head Pain*, 2nd ed. (New York, Oxford University Press, 1963).

CHAPTER 5

DISORDERS OF SPEECH, APRAXIA AND AGNOSIA

To achieve an understanding of the means by which the function of speech is developed and controlled and of the ways in which it may be disordered, is an endeavour in which many students are compelled to admit defeat. Even less comprehensible to some are the functions of praxis and gnosis, the first of which is concerned with the performance of complex willed movements, the second with recognition of people, objects and symbols. Admittedly the anatomical and physiological organisation of these functions is complex and far from being wholly understood. The multiplicity of views expressed concerning localisation of speech function within the cerebral hemispheres, along with the profusion of minutely varying disorders of speech which have been described, each with its own title, have added to the confusion. And yet, at the risk of over-simplification, it can be said that an appreciation of a number of simple basic principles may bring a degree of clarity to what has long been a singularly difficult field. First it is necessary to understand something of the way in which speech and other higher cerebral functions are acquired and developed and it will then be possible to mention some of the ways in which they are disordered by disease.

THE ORGANISATION OF SPEECH

Control of Speech in the Cerebral Cortex

The young infant takes his first steps towards the acquisition of speech function when he begins to associate particular sounds with particular objects in his environment. These sounds are subsequently organised into words which are symbols used to identify the objects concerned. Nouns, therefore, are first acquired, and subsequently conceptual or abstract powers of thought are developed in the utilisation of adjectives, verbs and adverbs to qualify these nouns or to describe activities instead of things. As the psychological concept of a word symbol is developed, so too the proprioceptive sensory impulses derived from the muscles of articulation come to be unconsciously associated with the expression of the word concerned, so that the child appreciates that a group of movements of the larynx, lips and tongue will result in the production of this word. Gradually, as additional words are acquired, these symbols lose some of their importance as individual entities but acquire new significance or meaning from their association with other words. In this way meaningful phrases and sentences are built up. When the child begins to read, visual symbols take their place alongside the appropriate sounds and in the process of writing (visual speech), these same symbols acquire new associations in proprioceptive sensations derived from the fingers of the writing hand. Similarly, in learning a new language, the words utilised in a foreign tongue develop associations with words of the same meaning in the individual's native language. Words have now acquired new and abstract meanings and are utilised not only for the communication of thoughts to others, but also for so-called 'internal speech' or the conscious logical process of abstract thought. Not all thought is verbal; some depends upon the conjuring up of visual or auditory images within the mind, but the more complex problems are generally dealt with by the thinker in verbal form. The scientist or the musician may, by contrast, think in terms of mathematical or chemical formulae or of musical sounds, but these too are symbols, either auditory or visual, which are comparable to the written or spoken word.

It is therefore apparent that many sensory and motor activities are concerned in the understanding and production of words, whether spoken or written, and of other auditory or visual symbols. Thus in order to speak a sentence, it is necessary first for the person concerned to formulate the thought he wishes to express, then to choose the appropriate words (a choice which depends upon his acquired knowledge of the significance of these symbols), and then to control the motor activity of the muscles of phonation and articulation, a process which involves the reception and correlation of proprioceptive sensory impulses from the muscles concerned. If the message is to be written rather than spoken, the motor and sensory impulses from the hand are also involved. Similarly, in the understanding of speech, whether spoken or written, the accurate recording of auditory or visual stimuli is essential before the significance of the symbols utilised can be appreciated.

If we then consider the parts of the brain which control speech function it can be seen that those areas of the cerebral cortex which are particularly concerned with the production or understanding of spoken or written verbal symbols must have connexions with those areas which control the motor activity of the muscles of articulation and writing and with the areas dealing with the reception of auditory and visual stimuli. These connexions are in fact achieved by means of a profusion of subcortical association fibres which not only pass between various areas of cortex in one cerebral hemisphere but also communicate, via the corpus callosum, with comparable cortical areas in the other hemisphere. The process of learning of speech, as of other functions, presumably depends upon the repeated passage of impulses along stereotyped pathways in these association tracts, a process which involves a progressive facilitation of the synapses which are traversed, so that the ease of passage of impulses is greatly increased. The function of memory and the ability to recall words or other symbols, as well as the emotional responses or visual images conjured up by particular words or phases, presumably depend upon the reactivation, either involuntarily or at will, of particular association pathways in which the necessary information has been 'stored'.

It is thus apparent that the function of speech cannot be said to be 'localised' in any particular part of the brain, as so many different cortical areas and association pathways are concerned in its integration. It is, however, true that in nearly all persons (90 per cent of the population) who are right-handed, the overall control of speech function is subserved by the left cerebral hemisphere. In some of the remaining 10 per cent who are left-handed or ambidextrous, the left hemisphere remains dominant and controls this faculty, but in others it is controlled from the right side. Furthermore, it is also apparent that the area of the dominant hemisphere which lies at the posterior end of the inferior frontal convolution (Broca's area), just in front of that part of the motor cortex controlling movements of articulation, is particularly concerned with production of the spoken word. Similarly the posterior third of the superior temporal convolution on this side (Wernicke's area) exercises important influences upon the understanding and interpretation of word symbols (Fig. 4c). Nevertheless, lesions other than in these two areas, and particularly in the posterior half of the dominant hemisphere, can have a profound influence upon speech function, possibly through the involvement of association fibres.

The Peripheral Neuromuscular Control of Speech

There are two essential processes, namely phonation and articulation, by which the voluntary musculature is able to convert the thought conceived in the cerebral cortex into the spoken word. Phonation, or the production of sound, results from the controlled passage of a column of air across the vocal cords, and the sound so produced is increased by resonance in the sounding-box of the larynx and pharynx. The sound is then modified by movements of the lips and tongue which subserve the function of articulation. These processes can be disturbed by lesions of the motor pathways controlling the voluntary muscles concerned and the clinical features so produced will be discussed below.

APHASIA

Although the term 'aphasia', if strictly interpreted, means absence of speech, it is usually utilised instead of the more correct 'dysphasia' to identify any disorder, however mild, of the use of words as symbols. Aphasia occurs in various forms and degrees, depending upon the situation, extent and severity of the cerebral lesion which is responsible.

In general, aphasic disturbances fall into two principal groups. The first, **motor or expressive aphasia,** generally results from a lesion in the neighbourhood of Broca's area. In its severest form the patient loses the power to speak completely or may say little more than 'yes' or 'no'. He nevertheless understands fully the spoken word, and will readily obey commands. His inability to express his thoughts in words may be the cause of severe distress and it is often apparent that he is well aware of what he wishes to say, but is unable to find the appropriate words. The writing of words, a form of motor speech, is usually similarly affected **(agraphia).** When expressive aphasia is less severe, the patient uses far fewer words than his normal vocabulary would allow and these are utilised hesitantly and sometimes repetitively (perseveration) with slurring and long pauses, but nevertheless the words which are used are appropriate to the thoughts being expressed. **Palilalia** is a name given to an increasingly rapid repetition of stereotyped words or phrases; it probably bears some relationship to expressive aphasia, though it is most common in disorders of the brain stem such as postencephalitic Parkinsonism, a fact which is difficult to understand.

So-called **nominal or amnestic aphasia** is regarded by some as the least severe form of expressive aphasia; in this condition the patient is unable to identify people or objects by their proper names though he is well aware of their nature and significance. In other words it is the association between a particular object and a particular word which is lost; the patient, when shown a pencil for instance, is unable to recall the word 'pencil', though he will say and demonstrate that the object is used for writing and will recognise that the word 'pencil' is correct when it is offered to him. Although it is true that nominal aphasia will sometimes be produced by a lesion in the neighbourhood of Broca's area, it is probably more correct to regard this condition as a form of sensory or receptive aphasia as it is the recognition of the significance of names and the ability to recall them which is impaired rather than their spontaneous utterance. Indeed, this sign most often results from a lesion in the dominant superior temporal convolution, where it may be presumed to have affected association fibres joining the so-called 'motor' and 'sensory' speech areas. A disorder in some ways similar may rarely occur in polyglots or in immigrants, who lose the ability to utilise the language of their adopted country but retain fluent control of their native tongue, an indication that the more recently acquired patterns of speech organisation are more easily disturbed than those which have been long established. Usually, however, in aphasia all languages which the patient knows are equally impaired. Also, in some patients with motor or expressive aphasia, whereas speech can no longer be utilised at will for the formulation of the patient's thoughts, its emotional control remains unimpaired, so that the patient is able to swear or to produce expletives in response to an appropriate stimulus.

Sensory or receptive aphasia is essentially an inability to appreciate the significance of words, whether spoken or written, as symbols. The patient with this condition, which is generally produced by a lesion in the neighbourhood of Wernicke's area of the dominant cerebral hemisphere, shows a complete failure to comprehend the meaning of words which he hears or sees. The appreciation of musical sounds may also be lost (**amusia**). The patient still has words at his command and his speech is often fluent and voluble but he uses them inappropriately so that what he says or writes may thus be agrammatic and unintelligible; this form of speech disorder has sometimes been called **jargon aphasia. Echolalia** is a name which has been given to a related disorder in which the patient repeats a meaningless phrase. **Word-deafness** is a fractional form of receptive aphasia in which the patient is totally unable to understand the meaning of words spoken to him, but yet his own speech, reading and writing are normal and he himself is able to use words appropriately. Similarly, in **word-blindness,** he cannot recognise written words or letters. In 'pure' word-blindness it is only the ability to recognise verbal symbols which is impaired, but sometimes the patient is also unable to appreciate the significance of numbers and even of colours. These rare varieties of aphasia can result from lesions of association pathways in the dominant temporal, parietal or even occipital areas.

Other lesions of association pathways can give rise to the fractional disorders of speech which have been called agraphia, alexia and acalculia. **Agraphia,** the inability to write, is simply a form of expressive aphasia and occurs in lesions near Broca's area, but it can rarely occur in patients whose spoken speech is unimpaired. Similarly **alexia,** an inability to understand the written word, is a form of receptive aphasia but can occur as an isolated phenomenon in isolated discrete lesions of the dominant parietal lobe. **Acalculia,** or the inability to calculate, is a closely related phenomenon resulting from lesions in the same neighbourhood; the patient is unable to appreciate the symbolic significance of figures rather than of letters and words; a similar disorder may derange the understanding of musical or scientific symbols.

It is thus apparent that the organisation of speech function in the dominant hemisphere is a complex mechanism, depending not so much upon 'localisation' in specific cortical areas but upon a large series of neuronal pathways and cell stations in which patterns of speech and related functions are stored and can be recalled at will. Pathological lesions may impair these functions by destroying cell-stations or their intercommunicating pathways, and a great many different forms of speech disorder are thus produced. Hence, speech can be regarded as being a function of almost the entire dominant cerebral hemisphere, but nevertheless an understanding of the principles involved is of great assistance in the clinical localisation of cerebral lesions, for certain specific disturbances in the use or understanding of words are consistently produced by lesions in different areas of the brain.

DYSARTHRIA

Complete loss of speech function due to a disorder of the neuro-muscular mechanisms responsible for articulation is known as **anarthria**; it is quite different from aphasia in that the patient's understanding of speech, his reading and writing are intact, but he is unable to speak owing to the fact that the muscles of the lips and tongue cannot so control the movements of the expired air that words are formed. Anarthria is rare, but dysarthria, or impaired articula-tion, is relatively common. The speech of a patient with dysarthria is slurred and indistinct, but his use of words is appropriate and his understanding unimpaired. The muscles responsible for articulation are those of the face (supplied by the seventh or facial nerve), the larynx and pharynx (supplied by the tenth or vagus nerve), the jaw (supplied by the motor root of the fifth or trigeminal nerve) and the tongue (supplied by the hypoglossal nerve). Lesions giving rise to dysarthria can be classified as, first, upper motor neurone lesions, secondly, disorders of co-ordination and of the extrapyramidal system, thirdly, lower motor neurone lesions, fourthly, lesions of the myoneural junction, and lastly myopathic lesions. A unilateral lesion involving one pyramidal or corticospinal tract, say, in the motor cortex of one cerebral hemisphere, will occasionally give some degree of dysarthria, though this is not usually severe. Bilateral pyramidal tract lesions are usually necessary to produce dysarthria of upper motor neurone type, as in patients with lesions of the upper brain stem; total anarthria and often dysphagia may occur in a patient who has a hemiplegia due to a unilateral cerebral infarct and then develops a second one on the opposite side. There is often a pathological emotional reaction, with inappropriate laughing and crying in such a case (**pseudobulbar palsy**). Dysarthria can also result from lesions of nervous pathways which influence, without directly promoting, muscular activity. Thus disorders of the cerebellar system may give inco-ordination of the articulatory muscles, causing a jerky or explosive speech with undue separation of syllables (e.g. 'scanning' speech, which is sometimes seen in disseminated sclerosis). Extrapyramidal disorders such as Parkinson's disease give rise to rigidity of the muscles subserving speech, as of the limbs, and the speech therefore becomes slow, quiet and monotonous.

Lower motor neurone lesions, as in patients with motor neurone disease affecting the bulbar musculature (progressive bulbar palsy), or in patients with polyneuritis (say, after diphtheria), bulbar polio-myelitis, or syringobulbia, can also give dysarthria. Depending upon the severity and extent of the muscular atrophy and weakness, the speech is slurred and indistinct and eventually becomes un-intelligible. Usually dysphagia, or other evidence of weakness of the bulbar musculature, is also present.

A similar type of dysarthria, again due to weakness of the articulatory muscles, is seen in myasthenia gravis, and here the slurring increases markedly with fatigue. In patients with myotonia, stiffness of the tongue may give a certain 'spastic' quality to the speech, while in facioscapulohumeral muscular dystrophy, inability to close the lips makes it impossible for the patient to pronounce labials, so that a characteristic dysarthric speech is produced.

MUTISM

Mutism is a total inability to speak, sometimes seen in a person without any demonstrable organic disease of the central nervous system. It can occur in psychotic patients (e.g. schizophrenia) and is an occasional manifestation of hysteria. Mutism combined with the loss of volitional movement of the trunk and limbs (akinetic mutism) is a rare result of an upper brain stem lesion.

APHONIA

Patients with aphonia have lost the ability to phonate but are still able to articulate, so that they speak in a whisper. While aphonia may be the result of disease of the larynx and vocal cords (laryngitis, tumour or paralysis of the vocal cords) it is most often a hysterical manifestation, the unconscious motivation being usually an attempt to escape from a stressful situation. Often it is necessary to inspect the vocal cords in order to establish the diagnosis of hysterical aphonia and to exclude organic disease, but apart from a history of previous hysterical manifestations or of recent stress, the most useful diagnostic pointer is that the patient is still able to phonate when coughing.

SPEECH DISORDERS IN CHILDHOOD

Developmental disorders of speech form a small but important group of disorders in which accurate diagnosis is of paramount importance, since many children with this type of condition may be wrongly regarded as mentally defective and many will respond to appropriate treatment.

Deafness

The totally deaf child will remain completely mute unless properly trained, as the normal channel for acquiring speech (i.e. through hearing) is not available to him. Usually the diagnosis becomes apparent when it is observed that the child, who has caused concern to his parents through his failure to speak, also fails to respond to external noise of whatever character. High-tone deafness is more difficult to diagnose, as the child with this condition does acquire speech, though this is unintelligible to any but his parents as he fails to utilise those vowel sounds and consonants (e.g. *e* and *t*) which depend upon high tones for their recognition. Audiometry is usually necessary for confirmation of the diagnosis.

Developmental Dysarthria

Dysarthria in childhood can be a manifestation of local developmental abnormalities such as cleft palate, or of cerebral palsy, in which case there are usually other neurological signs which indicate its nature. There are, however, a small group of children in whom dysarthria, associated with inco-ordinate or clumsy movements of the tongue and palate, is the only neurological abnormality. The condition may be due to a congenital apraxia of the muscles of articulation. Cases of this type respond well to long-continued speech therapy.

Developmental Aphasia

Congenital **word-deafness** or auditory imperception is a rare form of speech defect in which the patient fails to acquire normal speech

D*

function, is not deaf, as he responds to sounds, yet shows no interest or attention when spoken to. After a number of years many patients acquire a vocabulary of their own which, though meaningful to them, is incomprehensible to all except their nearest relatives. This type of defective speech is sometimes identified by the obsolete terms 'idioglossia' or 'lalling'; it may be difficult to distinguish from the defective speech of high-tone deafness except by audiometry.

Developmental alexia, or reading defect, occurs also in various degrees of severity, being commonest in left-handed children, or in those, naturally left-handed, who have been persuaded to write with the right hand. In broad terms it appears to be due to a defect in the establishment of speech function in one or other cerebral hemisphere, and is often associated with 'mirror-writing'. It may be an inherited disorder and commonly occurs in children who are in other respects intelligent.

Dyslalia

Dyslalia is a benign and not uncommon form of speech disorder occurring in childhood. The child develops speech at the normal age and speaks fluently though unintelligibly, as he tends to substitute one consonant for another in many words. Usually cases of this type acquire normal speech within three to twelve months of beginning speech therapy, but without treatment the abnormal speech pattern may persist for many years.

Stammering

Stammering is a disorder of articulation characterised by the repetition of sounds or syllables and by prolonged pauses which punctuate speech. It is much more common in boys than in girls. Dentals (t, d), labials (p, b) and gutturals (k) are the sounds which seem most difficult to pronounce, and severe facial grimacing may accompany the attempt to utter words containing these letters. While many have suggested that this condition is of psychogenic origin, the fact that it is very common in left-handed children and particularly in shifted sinistrals (who are naturally left-handed but have been persuaded to write with the right) suggests that it has an organic basis and, like reading defects, it may be related to an incomplete localisation of speech function in one or other cerebral hemisphere. It can be present from the age of two or three years, but quite often begins at the age of six to eight years when a child who has previously spoken fluently is beginning to read and write. While many stammerers seem shy and introspective, this mental attitude is most probably the result rather than the cause of their disability. Certainly there is no evidence that stammering is a result of organic brain disease, though it may develop for the first time in some adult patients who become aphasic following a cerebral lesion. It is more properly regarded as a functional disorder of the organisation and establishment of speech function. It can often be controlled to a remarkable degree by the use of syllabic speech.

APRAXIA

Apraxia is the inability to carry out a willed voluntary movement despite the fact that the motor and sensory pathways concerned in the control of the movement are intact. In other words no actual paralysis, ataxia or sensory loss may be present. Thus a patient who is asked to put out his tongue may be completely unable to do so on request, though a moment later he will spontaneously lick his lips. Hence the condition can be regarded as a loss of acquired motor skills, or an inability to reactivate those nervous pathways in which the memory and technique of specific movements (**praxis**) have been recorded. It can be considered to be a defect of the 'association' areas or fibres concerned with volitional motor activity. The supra-marginal gyrus of the dominant parietal lobe appears to contain an important cell-station in this organisation of movement, and lesions of this area commonly produce bilateral apraxia. A lesion between this cortical area and the motor cortex of the left cerebral hemisphere will lead to an apraxia of the right limbs, while a lesion of the corpus callosum dividing those fibres which are passing to the right motor cortex will give rise to a left-sided apraxia.

Apraxia of the lips and tongue is relatively common, while in the extremities apraxic disturbances may be revealed as an inability to dress or undress (**dressing apraxia**) or to construct models from blocks or letters with matches (**constructional apraxia**).

AGNOSIA

Presumably visual, auditory and tactile stimuli are perceived in the occipital, temporal and postcentral areas of the cortex, respectively, as crude physical phenomena which only acquire significance when related to past sensory experiences which have been collated and 'stored' as sensory memories in the appropriate association areas of the cortex. This process of recognition of the significance of sensory stimuli is known as **gnosis**. Lesions of the appropriate association areas of the cerebral cortex impair this faculty of recognition, even though the primary sensory pathway is intact; the syndrome so produced is called **agnosia**. Visual agnosia is an inability to recognise objects seen, in a patient who is not blind; auditory agnosia is a failure to appreciate the significance of sounds in a patient who is not deaf (a condition which shows some resemblance to receptive aphasia). A patient with tactile agnosia (often called **astereognosis**) cannot identify objects which he feels. Usually an agnostic defect involves only vision or hearing or touch in isolation, so that a patient who cannot recognise a pen, and may not even see that it is an object with which to write (unlike the patient with nominal aphasia) will name it at once if it is placed in his hand.

THE BODY IMAGE

A constant stream of sensory impulses from the special senses, skin, muscles, bones and joints informs us of the condition and situation of the parts of our body in relation to each other and in relation to our external environment. From these stimuli we build up almost unconsciously an image of our body which is continually varying. Certain parts of the body such as the hands and mouth play such important roles in our everyday activity, and are so well endowed with highly-developed sensory receptors, that their share of the body image is proportionally much greater than, say, the small of the back. A skilled craftsman or the driver of a motor vehicle may become so attuned to the use of his tools or vehicle that in a sense these become a part of his body image and he then unconsciously relates himself plus the tool or vehicle and not himself alone to his environment. This concept of the body image is 'stored' in the association areas of the parietal lobes, and when the performance of motor skills is included it becomes clearly related to the function of praxis mentioned above. Certain lesions of the parietal lobe tend to distort the body image so that the patient is unable to distinguish right from left (**right–left disorientation**). He may neglect the opposite side of his body and the whole of extrapersonal space on that side (**autotopagnosia**) while he may even deny that the contralateral limbs are paralysed (**anosognosia**) and sometimes attempts to throw them out of bed. The term 'anosognosia' is sometimes used to describe denial of other gross neurological manifestations. Often the patient with a parietal lobe lesion will perceive normally sensory stimuli applied independently to the two sides of the body, but if bilateral stimuli are simultaneously applied, one may be ignored (**tactile inattention**). It has been said that disorders of the body image occur only with lesions of the non-dominant parietal lobe, but it now seems that this suggestion has resulted from the fact that in lesions of the dominant hemisphere they are obscured by aphasic, apraxic or other defects. Commonly, because of the contiguity of important association areas in the dominant parietal lobe, multiple defects occur;

thus **Gerstmann's syndrome** is a combination of right—left disorientation, finger agnosia (an inability to identify individual fingers) and constructional apraxia.

DEVELOPMENTAL APRAXIA AND AGNOSIA

Specific learning defects other than developmental dyslexia, to which reference has already been made, have been recognised increasingly in recent years and appear to be the result of either minimal brain damage due to birth injury or defective physiological organisation of cerebral dominance. In contradistinction to the dyslexics, these 'clumsy children', who are often wrongly regarded as being mentally defective, show a higher verbal than performance level on the Wechsler intelligence scale for children. Defects of sensory perception as well as of skilled motor activity may be recognised in these children who often improve to some extent as they grow older; but many require patient individual tuition in the particular skills (e.g. writing) in which they are defective.

CONCLUSIONS

It can be concluded that an understanding of the many complex disorders of speech, of movement and of recognition which occur in patients with cerebral lesions must depend upon a working knowledge of the means by which these functions are organised and controlled in the brain. If it is recognised that these functions depend not upon the activity of isolated specific cortical areas but upon a complex network of association fibres joining a series of cortical cell-stations, it will then be apparent that lesions in varying situations will affect these individual functions in various ways, often giving fractional disorders of function to which certain specific names have been applied. It is, however, necessary to understand the whole before identifying the particular, and from this understanding, information of considerable value in the localisation of cerebral lesions may be derived. In considering disorders of the peripheral neuromuscular mechanisms subserving speech, it is also apparent that a systematic approach to the problem will aid in identifying the situation and nature of the lesion responsible.

REFERENCES

BRAIN, W. R., *Speech Disorders* (London, Butterworth, 1961).
BRAIN, W. R., *Diseases of the Nervous System*, 6th ed., (London, Oxford University Press, 1962).

CRITCHLEY, M., *The Parietal Lobes* (London, Arnold, 1953).

MORLEY, M., *The Development and Disorders of Speech in Childhood* (Edinburgh, Livingstone, 1957).

NEILSEN, J. M., 'Agnosias, apraxias, speech and aphasia', in *Clinical Neurology*, Ed. Baker, A. B., 2nd ed. (New York, Hoeber-Harper, 1962).

PENFIELD, W. and ROBERTS, L., *Speech and Brain Mechanisms* (Princeton, N. J., Princeton University Press; London, Oxford University Press, 1959).

CHAPTER 6

DISORDERS OF CONSCIOUSNESS

CONSCIOUSNESS is a state or faculty which almost defies definition. It implies a state of awareness of one's self and of one's surroundings, and its content includes a variety of recurring sensory experiences combined with emotions, ideas and memories which are the product of thought processes. Whereas it is clear that the cerebral cortex plays an important role in maintaining and determining the content of the conscious state it is now apparent that cortical mechanisms of motor or sensory activity are by no means autonomous and that they can be activated or suppressed through the activity of the reticular substance of the upper mid-brain and by hypothalamic mechanisms. This reticular–hypothalamic complex thus exercises important influences upon the state of awareness and it is becoming increasingly apparent that disturbances of consciousness which are observed in clinical neurological practice are largely dependent upon lesions, either functional or structural, of these areas of the brain or of the pathways which connect them to the cerebral cortex. In this chapter we shall consider some of the commoner physiological and pathological alterations in the conscious state, their pathogenesis and their importance in neurological diagnosis.

SLEEP

Sleep is a periodic physiological depression of consciousness which results from changes in the activity of the reticular substance and hypothalamus. That this is the case can be demonstrated by the fact that extensive destruction of the cerebral cortex and even massive lesions of both frontal lobes may not interfere with sleep regulation so long as the function of basal midline structures is unimpaired. During sleep the cardiac output, pulse rate, blood pressure and respiration fall, the tendon reflexes may be lost and the plantar responses may even become extensor.

A number of disorders of the sleep rhythm are known, some of which are semi-physiological and of no serious pathological significance, while others are produced by organic lesions in the neighbourhood of the mid-brain and hypothalamus. Many of the less ominous disorders can be regarded as resulting from 'uneven' activity of the various parts of the reticular–hypothalamic complex so that in a sense the activity of one part of the brain may be suppressed or reactivated before another.

Thus **sleep paralysis** is a condition in which the patient, when falling asleep, or more commonly on waking, finds himself completely unable to move a muscle, though motor activity will return immediately if he is touched. This experience can be very alarming, but movement generally returns within a minute or less and the condition is of no serious significance. The so-called **night-nurse's paralysis,** which some have believed to be a psychogenic or fear reaction, is probably closely related. Another related disturbance may take the form of so-called **hypnagogic hallucinations,** a series of visual or other hallucinations which are of brief duration, though sometimes terrifying in character, and which occur as the patient is falling asleep. Presumably this condition is due to persisting activation of association areas of the cerebral cortex; **night terrors** in children are probably similar. **Nocturnal myoclonus,** a sudden jerk of the voluntary musculature which occurs as the patient is drifting into sleep, is another condition which is essentially physiological and presumably results from a sudden transient reactivation of the motor system. Myoclonic jerks occurring repeatedly in sleep, however, must often be regarded as pathological, as many such patients develop epileptic seizures; however, in some such cases it is difficult to know where to draw the line between the physiological and the pathological.

Insomnia is a common disorder of sleep which occurs so frequently in the elderly that it is again difficult to know when it should be considered pathological. In younger patients it is usually the result of anxiety, an emotional disturbance which must clearly influence the reticular–hypothalamic system. **Somnambulism** or sleep-walking is also related to emotional stress and can in a sense be regarded as a reactivation of complex co-ordinated muscular movements occurring while consciousness remains impaired.

Narcolepsy is another relatively common disorder which appears to result from a functional disturbance occurring in the reticular–hypothalamic system. Patients suffering from this condition experience attacks of almost irresistible sleep which develop during the day, most often in the afternoons. The desire to sleep can be resisted if the patient gets up and moves around, but if sitting down the somnolence is overwhelming and he falls asleep, usually only for a few minutes, but sometimes for several hours. He can, however, be aroused with ease, as from normal sleep. Males are affected more often than females and the condition usually begins in adolescence or early adult life; it is generally benign, and can be regarded as an exaggeration of the physiological drowsiness which develops under appropriate circumstances. Many patients who experience attacks of this nature also suffer from **cataplexy,** a name which has been given to episodes of sudden loss of power in the voluntary muscles, which cause the patient to go 'weak at the knees' and even to slump suddenly to the ground; he may be unable to move a muscle for several seconds or even for as long as a minute. These attacks are commonly precipitated by sudden emotion such as laughing, crying, fear or excitement. The condition can be regarded as a transient inactivation of that part of the reticular substance controlling motor activity and is again an exaggeration of the physiological, as normal people sometimes become 'weak with laughter'.

It is true that organic lesions, whether neoplastic or inflammatory, in the region of the third ventricle and hypothalamus or upper brain stem, occasionally give rise to symptomatic narcolepsy, but more often they produce **hypersomnia,** a condition in which the patient sleeps for long periods, is difficult to rouse and may then be confused for a variable period of time. **Akinetic mutism** is a name given to a syndrome which can follow injury to the upper brain stem, and in which the patient is apparently asleep, with a relaxed musculature; although his eyes may open and follow objects moved in his field of vision, or he may respond to sounds, he cannot speak or be aroused by powerful sensory stimuli. Certain other lesions of the mid-brain and contiguous areas, and particularly those of encephalitis lethargica, produce **reversal of the sleep rhythm,** so that the patient sleeps by day but is awake and restless at night. Disorders of this type cease to be physiological variants and are closely related to the pathological states of stupor and coma which can result from structural or metabolic disorders affecting similar areas of the brain.

STUPOR

Stupor is a disorder of consciousness in which the patient gives every appearance of being asleep but from which he cannot be fully aroused; he may open his eyes and on vigorous stimulation will show some responses which indicate a degree of awareness of his surroundings. The condition of akinetic mutism referred to above can probably be regarded as a form of stupor. While this state sometimes results from injury, compression or disease of the upper brain stem and hypothalamus, it can also occur as an effect of drug intoxication, metabolic disorders, anoxia or severe infections such as typhoid fever, although in these conditions delirium, to be described below, is more common. Subdural haematoma, giving rise probably to brain stem compression, is a common cause of a stuporous state.

COMA

Coma has been defined as complete unconsciousness with no response to sensory stimuli, even at the reflex level. In other words the comatose patient does not show even reflex withdrawal following a painful stimulus. A patient who is semicomatose, however, while seeming to be completely unconscious, with no awareness of his surroundings, will respond to painful stimuli by groaning or simply by withdrawal of the affected part.

While coma can result from a variety of conditions, some of which are primarily cerebral disorders, while others are generalised metabolic disturbances, it is becoming apparent that the disturbance of consciousness, whether it is due to a structural or a biochemical lesion, is again produced by a disorder of function in the reticular–hypothalamic complex. Thus a lesion of one cerebral hemisphere can give rise to coma through pressure upon or ischaemia of the upper brain stem and hypothalamus, while metabolic causes of coma also have a profound effect upon the functioning of these structures.

The **differential diagnosis** of the causes of coma is a problem with which the clinician is frequently faced and deserves brief consideration here. Where an adequate history is available from friends or relatives who have observed the progress of the illness leading to coma, the diagnostic problem is often eased considerably, but when a patient is found comatose and no accurate history of the onset is available, diagnosis may bristle with difficulties. Thus **head injury,** an important cause, is generally identified by the history, but even if this is lacking there is usually some external evidence of laceration or contusion. In cases of **subdural haematoma,** however, the causal injury may have been trivial and the patient may gradually have become drowsy and eventually comatose over a period of several weeks or months. Some patients with this condition are stuporose rather than comatose. In **subarachnoid haemorrhage** a history of sudden onset with severe headache and neck stiffness, and the presence of blood-stained cerebrospinal fluid is revealing; however, the clinical picture of **primary cerebral haemorrhage** is not dissimilar, though in such cases a profound hemiplegia is usually present from the onset. When **cerebral thrombosis** is the cause, the onset is generally more gradual with less severe clouding of consciousness, though if the infarct is extensive, the patient can be comatose and hemiplegic, a clinical picture which is little different from that of cerebral haemorrhage. The onset of **cerebral embolism** is of course abrupt, and there is often clinical evidence of a source of emboli, generally in the heart (mitral stenosis, bacterial endocarditis, cardiac infarction). **Encepha-**

litis and **meningitis,** being inflammatory disorders, are usually accompanied by fever, and the patient's comatose state is usually the end-result of an illness which has lasted for a day or two or longer, with headache, neck stiffness (in meningitis particularly), drowsiness and confusion. In such individuals, cerebrospinal fluid examination is of the greatest importance. Similarly, sudden coma is uncommon in patients suffering from **cerebral tumour,** most of whom have experienced previous headache, focal fits or the gradual development of paralysis, and papilloedema will often be present. In patients with **cerebral abscess,** too, the onset is generally gradual and there will often be an evident focus of infection in the middle ear, nasal sinuses, skin or lung. The relatively uncommon **hypertensive encephalopathy** is generally recognised through the retinal and urinary changes of malignant hypertension combined with the blood pressure reading. The recognition of the coma which follows an attack of **epilepsy** rests upon the absence of physical signs and a history of previous fits.

Turning to toxic and metabolic causes of coma, **anoxia** will generally be identified by a history of carbon-monoxide poisoning, whether from coal gas, a coke brazier or exhaust fumes, or by a history of partial drowning or difficult general anaesthesia. **Acute alcoholism** will be suspected from the smell of alcohol on the breath and confirmed by urine or blood-alcohol estimation, but it should be remembered that partially intoxicated patients are particularly liable to head injury, while cerebral vascular catastrophes not uncommonly occur during an alcoholic debauch. Deep, hissing, 'acidotic' respiration with acetone in the breath, glycosuria and ketonuria, will usually establish a diagnosis of **diabetic coma,** while a pale, sweating and flaccid patient with bilateral extensor responses may be shown by blood-sugar estimation to be suffering from **hypoglycaemia** due either to insulin administration or to a tumour of the pancreatic islet cells. Patients with **uraemia** tend to have deep acidotic breathing like those with diabetic coma, but the breath has a uriniferous smell, and hypertension, retinal changes and albuminuria are usually present. **Liver disease** is easily overlooked as a cause of coma, but the patient, while becoming comatose, will usually have shown the characteristic 'flapping' tremor of the outstretched hands, and there may be jaundice, dark urine and stigmata of hepatic cirrhosis such as 'liver palms' and cutaneous spider naevi. Other rare causes of a comatose state include **malaria, Addison's disease, myxoedema** and **hypopituitarism.** Finally, **drug intoxication** must also be remembered as an increasingly common cause of a type of coma which may show no specific clinical features, especially if **barbiturates** have been taken, say, in an attempt to commit suicide.

Salicylates, by contrast, tend to produce a characteristic deep cyanosis with acidotic breathing, while **opiates** give characteristic pin-point pupils. However, in any patient with coma of unknown cause, when no history is available, poisoning should be borne in mind and the patient's belongings should be searched for a bottle or carton which may have held the offending tablets, while it will sometimes be necessary to wash out the stomach or to examine the urine for the presence of barbiturates or other drugs.

DELIRIUM AND CONFUSION

There are a great many physical illnesses which are accompanied by mental symptoms of varying degree, most of which take the form of **clouding of consciousness,** with or without other more specific manifestations. This group of disorders may be referred to as the **symptomatic psychoses.** They occur not only as a symptom of cerebral lesions but also in a variety of infective and metabolic disorders. These are not primarily diseases of the nervous system but they affect its functioning to a greater or lesser extent, even though they may not produce histological changes in the brain which can be identified by present techniques. The clouding of consciousness or lack of awareness which results is sometimes no more than the minimal disinterest and 'fuzziness' in the head which accompanies mild influenza, but it can take the form of a severe psychotic reaction with grossly disturbed consciousness and bizarre disorders of thought. There is some evidence that the type of reaction an individual shows may depend partly upon his previous personality and constitution.

Delirium is a term which has been used to identify a state of severely clouded consciousness in which the patient is disorientated in time and place, and his attention-span is brief. His thought processes are disordered so that he is unable to appreciate his present circumstances and to relate them to past experiences; he may be living in a fantasy world peopled by the products of his imagining. Hence delusions or false imaginary ideas are frequent, as are hallucinations, usually visual, which can be vividly real and frightening and may result in an intense fear reaction with restless or even violent behaviour. Fluctuation in the mental and physical state is common, so that periods of shouting and restlessness alternate with others of apparent somnolence, punctuated by low muttering. Commonly the speech is slurred. There is a tendency for drowsiness to be most frequent during the day, while the patient becomes excited, hallucinated and uncontrollable at night. The stage of true delirium is often preceded by a stage of restlessness and irritability, insomnia, lack of concentration and pathological brightness or euphoria, a stage which may last for several hours or days, depending upon the cause. Frequently there are accompanying motor manifestations; the patient is tremulous, and spontaneous twitching or jerking of the voluntary musculature occurs, even in sleep. Often a return to restful sleep is the first sign of resolution of the delirium, but even after apparent recovery, some delusions may persist and these often have a paranoid character, encompassing ideas of persecution or ill-treatment.

Delirium occurs in classical form in patients with chronic alcoholism after a debauch or after the withdrawal of alcohol and is then known as **delirium tremens.** The condition which follows withdrawal of barbiturates or amphetamine in patients who have been taking excessive quantities of these drugs over a long period is essentially similar, and is also characterised by the occurrence of drug-withdrawal convulsions. Less severe and specific delirious states, differing only in detail but not in overall pattern, are observed in patients with encephalitis or meningitis, in severe infections such as septicaemia or typhoid fever, in metabolic disorders such as liver disease and pernicious anaemia, in some cases of bronchogenic carcinoma without cerebral metastases, in treatment with ACTH or cortisone and in a great many other disorders. Delirium of mild degree is a common manifestation of febrile illnesses in childhood and is then observed particularly at night.

When the mental disturbances are less striking in character but yet the patient shows fluctuations in awareness, with incoherence of thought and variable disorientation ('where am I'), but usually without frank delusions or hallucinations, the condition is often referred to as **confusion** or a **confusional state,** of mild, moderate or severe degree. The condition differs from delirium only in detail and in fact these disorders merge with one another so that the frankly delirious patient generally passes through a phase of confusion during recovery. In recovery from a head injury giving rise to coma, for instance, the patient may be delirious and later confused as consciousness slowly returns. Hence some authorities have suggested that the term confusion should be dropped and that the condition to which it refers is better referred to as **subacute delirium.** Other terms which have been utilised to identify this group of conditions include toxic-infective psychosis, metabolic or exhaustion psychosis, or organic reaction state, as these disorders are essentially mental reactions resulting from organic disease which is disordering brain function. From the standpoint of convenient clinical usage it is probably justifiable to retain the term 'delirium' to identify the severe disturbance and 'confusion' the less severe, provided it is appreciated that there is no essential difference between the two.

Derangement of memory is a feature of many of the grades of disordered consciousness referred to above and is responsible for some of the spatial and temporal disorientation which is so frequent. Presumably, the structural or metabolic abnormalities concerned produce their effects by impairing the efficiency of the cerebral association pathways upon which, as we saw in Chapter 5, our memory of objects, of events and of language depends. Hallucinations may result from fractional reactivation of some parts of these pathways. A syndrome which is frequently identified as an independent entity, though it has some affinities with confusion and even delirium, is **Korsakoff's syndrome,** or the so-called 'amnestic syndrome'. The salient feature of this condition is that the patient loses the ability to record and retain new impressions. He will at one minute appear alert and his conversation is lucid, but within a moment or two he will have forgotten the interview completely. The memory of his remote past may be intact. As a result he becomes disorientated, certainly in time and often in place, and in order to conceal this memory defect he confabulates; for instance, he will describe in detail fantastic activities which he claims to have carried out some few hours or days earlier, though he may never have left his bed. Usually his descriptions have some basis in fact in the remote past but he is utilising these previous experiences to fill in the recent period for which his memory is defective. Though Korsakoff's syndrome occurs most frequently in patients with alcoholism and polyneuropathy, it sometimes complicates other metabolic and infective illnesses; it may develop during recovery from head injury or subarachnoid haemorrhage or indeed in patients who are recovering from delirium resulting from a variety of causes. It is of some interest that lesions of the hypothalamic region and particularly of the corpora mamillaria may give rise to this clinical picture and it is therefore presumed that these structures are important cell stations in the cerebral pathways concerned with the establishment of memory patterns.

That psychological as well as physical causes can seriously impair memory is apparent from the occurrence of **hysterical amnesia,** a syndrome in which the patient, who is apparently alert, may have no recollection whatever of his identity, of his address or of any other details concerning himself. The condition, which is usually of acute onset, so that the patient is found wandering aimlessly, is presumably due to some process of psychological inhibition resulting in an inability to reopen voluntarily the pathways where memories are retained. Usually the condition develops as a method of escape from undue stress. Sometimes a similar impairment of memory is the sole effect of a discrete **temporal lobe lesion.**

CEREBRAL IRRITATION

In addition to the manifestations of delirium or confusion which occur in patients with diffuse brain disease such as meningitis, encephalitis and subarachnoid haemorrhage, these individuals often show a typical behaviour pattern which is characteristic of so-called 'cerebral irritation'. They lie curled up on one side in bed, often with their eyes away from the light, and resent being disturbed, so that they may pull back the bedclothes when the doctor attempts to remove them. If the meninges are inflamed, neck stiffness will generally be apparent as well.

TRANSIENT DISORDERS OF CONSCIOUSNESS

One of the commonest problems which a doctor is called upon to solve is the significance of brief disorders of consciousness, commonly referred to as 'blackouts'. Are these fits or faints, that is, are they epileptic or syncopal? No distinction can be more important for social and occupational reasons and, at times, none can be more difficult to make with confidence.

EPILEPSY

Epilepsy is difficult to define in view of the many guises which it may assume. Many definitions have been offered, varying from the frankly mechanistic (a recurrent cerebral dysrhythmia) to the unrealistically psychoanalytical (a manifestation of an unconscious desire for unconsciousness). Though no definition can possibly be sufficiently broad and at the same time exclusive of disturbances of consciousness which are essentially different, it is possible to regard epilepsy as a recurrent disorder of consciousness which is characteristically transient, ceases spontaneously, and is often preceded or accompanied by motor or sensory phenomena. Though a definition of this type would embrace most cases of epilepsy it could unfortunately also be utilised to describe certain cases of syncope and other conditions which are certainly not epilepsy and must be distinguished from it. Furthermore, loss of consciousness is not invariable in some attacks which are unquestionably epileptic.

In considering **aetiology** it is possible to divide cases of epilepsy into two broad groups, namely so-called *idiopathic* epilepsy and *symptomatic* epilepsy. In cases of idiopathic epilepsy there is no evidence of any organic brain lesion which is responsible for the attacks, nor do these usually have a focal onset in any part of the body. Because idiopathic attacks are believed to result from a functional disturbance in the basal areas of the brain which exercise some control over cortical activity (such as the reticular substance), they are often referred to as 'central', 'centrencephalic', or 'crypto-genic' epilepsy. In symptomatic epilepsy, the attacks are a symptom of organic disease of the brain, whether it be the effects of fever (febrile convulsions), diffuse degenerative brain disease, an infarct, encephalitis or abscess, a cerebral tumour or a scar following head injury (post-traumatic epilepsy), anoxia, hypoglycaemia, hypocalcaemia or even drug withdrawal. Some would suggest that seizures occurring as a result of overt brain disease should not be regarded as epilepsy, and that this term should be reserved for the 'idiopathic' condition. This view would seem to be untenable as the nature of the seizures may be essentially similar in the two types of case and more and more cases previously considered to be suffering from idiopathic epilepsy are being discovered to be cases of the symptomatic variety, in which unsuspected cerebral lesions are responsible for the attacks. Many apparently normal individuals would have fits if their brains were subjected to a pathological or biochemical insult of sufficient degree, but this tendency is a variable one which is probably specific to the individual. The so-called 'convulsive threshold' shows considerable variation from one person to another. Those with a very high threshold would never suffer a convulsion, no matter how severe the stimulus, while those with a low one presumably make up the majority of 'idiopathic' epileptics who have attacks without apparent cause. But it is very difficult to draw a clear line of demarcation between the epileptic and non-epileptic in persons whose 'convulsive threshold' falls between these two extremes. Thus a maximum of 50 per cent of patients with pene-trating brain injuries develop post-traumatic epilepsy. Hence it seems reasonable to regard all seizures of epileptic type as epilepsy, but always to consider the possibility of an organic cause and only to regard the patient as a case of idiopathic epilepsy if the search for such a cause is negative. How assiduous this search should be de-pends upon the age of the patient and the severity and frequency of the attacks; this problem will be considered in Chapter 20. With present techniques of investigation it is probable that many patients with symptomatic epilepsy are wrongly diagnosed as suffering from the idiopathic variety.

The convulsive threshold is clearly dependent to a considerable extent upon the patient's constitution, and a hereditary factor is probably important as many epileptics have epileptic or otherwise unstable relatives. Even so, no clear pattern of inheritance emerges and the chances that an epileptic may have a child who is similarly affected are not very great statistically if the other partner of the marriage is normal. Although certain analeptic drugs (picrotoxin, leptazole, bemegride) may have the effect of producing epileptic seizures, as may fluid retention in the body, no consistent biochemical or other abnormality has been found in patients with idiopathic seizures. Although attacks are common in some women just before or during the menstrual period, endocrine factors are unlikely to be important.

A second factor to be taken into account, in addition to the so-called 'convulsive threshold', is the resistance of the brain to the spread of the epileptic discharge, a property which may be independent of the former. If this resistance is low and the spread is rapid, a focal lesion will give rise to a generalised convulsion with immediate loss of consciousness and no localising features, while if the resistance is high, the epileptic manifestations will remain localised to the appropriate area of the body (*focal* or *Jacksonian epilepsy*) and consciousness may be comparatively unimpaired throughout the attack. In cases where the resistance is intermediate between these two extremes the onset of the fit may be focal but it will then develop into a generalised seizure.

Hence one satisfactory method of classifying cases of epilepsy is on an aetiological basis, but this can only be done with confidence in a comparatively small proportion of cases. More often it is necessary for practical purposes to adopt a *clinical classification* depending upon the character of the seizures. From this point of view, attacks may be divided into the following categories—

1. Minimal seizures (petit mal).
2. Minor seizures (including Jacksonian epilepsy, akinetic attacks and many 'psychomotor' or 'temporal lobe' attacks).
3. Major seizures (grand mal).
4. Myoclonic epilepsy.

MINIMAL SEIZURES

Attacks of true **petit mal** begin only in childhood, occur in either sex and sometimes continue into adult life, though they usually cease in adolescence. Often patients with this type of epilepsy also have occasional major seizures and in others when minimal attacks cease they are replaced by major ones. True petit mal must be regarded as the classical example of idiopathic epilepsy; it is practically never symptomatic, although attacks which are clinically identical are sometimes observed in children with diffuse brain disease or cerebral birth injury; in such cases there are also major attacks as a rule.

Petit mal can often be identified by the characteristic generalised spike-and-wave discharge in the EEG.

An attack of petit mal is generally momentary, lasting only a few seconds; the child's expression suddenly becomes blank, his eyes roll upwards and there may be a brief spasmodic jerk of the limbs (**myoclonus**); within a moment he is normal again. The loss of consciousness is so transient that the child does not fall, and his attention span is so briefly disrupted that he may, for instance, continue to read aloud after an almost imperceptible pause. In very occasional cases the attack is sufficiently prolonged for the child to fall to the ground, only to pick himself up again immediately (**akinetic epilepsy** —a purely descriptive term implying loss of consciousness without spasmodic movements). However, attacks of this nature should generally be included in the group of minor seizures as they are variable in aetiology and are most often unusually brief episodes of major epilepsy. Attacks of petit mal can occur as often as twenty to thirty times daily and are sometimes made more frequent by emotional stress. This form of epilepsy has usually a good prognosis as many sufferers lose their attacks in adolescence and remain well, but others go on to develop major seizures.

MINOR SEIZURES

This group embraces a great variety of epileptic manifestations, including most of the forms of **focal** or **Jacksonian epilepsy** in which the spread of epileptic discharge is not sufficiently rapid to give a major convulsion. The pattern of the seizures depends entirely upon the area of the brain which is being irritated by the organic lesion whether it be a tumour, a scar of previous injury, or some other pathological lesion, and upon the direction of spread of the epileptic discharge. Focal epilepsy must always imply the presence of a localised lesion of the brain, even though in some cases techniques of investigation at present available are inadequate to demonstrate its nature. In cases of focal epilepsy, the EEG may show focal spike or sharp-wave discharges, or localised slow activity.

If the lesion lies in or near the motor cortex, then the attack usually consists of intermittent rhythmical (clonic) jerking of a hand and arm and this may spread to the face or leg, depending upon which part of the cortex is involved. If the discharge continues for hours or even days, these manifestations can be prolonged (*epilepsia partialis continua*), but more often the attack subsides in seconds or minutes. It may be followed by transient weakness of the affected member (Todd's paralysis). Though consciousness is often temporarily clouded during the attack it sometimes remains unimpaired throughout. *Sensory epilepsy* will result from lesions near the sensory cortex,

when paraesthesiae rather than jerking are the primary manifestation, though the latter may develop if spread to the motor cortex
follows. When epileptic discharges begin in the occipital lobe, crude
visual phenomena result (bright lines or flashes of light), while if
visual association areas are involved the patient can experience
formed visual hallucinations of people or of past events. Similarly a
lesion near the speech areas may give transient aphasia and one near
the auditory cortex auditory hallucinations, either crude or highly
organised, depending upon whether the actual auditory cortex or its
association areas are primarily affected. Should the spread of the
epileptic discharge be rapid, any of these manifestations can constitute the brief aura of a major seizure and will give useful information concerning the situation of onset of the epileptic discharge.

The commonest and most important form of focal epilepsy is
temporal lobe epilepsy, which has often been referred to previously as
psychomotor epilepsy or 'epileptic equivalents'. Many patients with
minor seizures and many with major ones have foci of epileptic
discharge in one or other temporal lobe, a fact which may be
indicated either by the content of the seizure or by the aura or
sequelae of a major attack. It has become increasingly apparent in
recent years that the very high incidence of this form of epilepsy is
due to the frequency with which pathological changes occur in the
anterior and medial parts of the temporal lobes (uncus, hippocampus,
amygdaloid nucleus, Ammon's horn). These changes can result from
birth injury, with 'moulding' of the head and herniation of the
medial part of the temporal lobe through the tentorial hiatus, or from
cerebral anoxia of whatever cause.

Although the lesions responsible are often present from birth, and
some attacks of temporal lobe epilepsy begin in childhood, these
seizures sometimes do not develop until late adolescence or even
adult life, though acquired lesions may be responsible in some older
patients. The number of manifestations which may develop in cases
of this type is legion and is clearly dependent upon the many important physiological functions which are subserved by the temporal
lobes. Thus the attack may include intense *emotional experiences*
(fear, depression, anxiety), feelings of unreality (*depersonalisation*)
and a sensation of intense familiarity as if the patient were living
through a vivid past experience (*déjà vu*). There may also be unpleasant hallucinations of smell or taste (*uncinate seizures*), *vaso-
motor manifestations* (sweating, salivation, palpitation and 'butter-
flies in the stomach'), or *vertigo*, while *irrational speech or behaviour*
(automatism, such as undressing in public) or even episodes of
violence or *temper* can occur. It is in cases of this nature that *permanent mental changes* of psychotic type may develop. Sometimes,

with spread of discharge to the lower end of the motor cortex, there are smacking of the lips or twitching of the corner of the mouth, while if it spreads more posteriorly there may be distortion of visual images so that objects look smaller (*micropsia*) or larger (*macropsia*) or appear to be fading into the distance. Any of these manifestations occurring in an episodic manner, without warning, either in isolation or in succession, should suggest a diagnosis of temporal lobe epilepsy, particularly if there is some accompanying clouding of consciousness and certainly if they are followed by a major convulsion. Nevertheless, it may sometimes be difficult to distinguish between temporal lobe seizures on the one hand and episodes of phobic anxiety (with panic and depersonalisation) on the other, as fainting may result from the hyperventilation which often occurs in panic attacks. It should be noted that any irritative focal lesion in the temporal lobe can produce the features described above and whereas this may be a scar of long standing, it is sometimes an expanding lesion such as a tumour.

It is of some interest that powerful sensory stimuli can sometimes provoke focal epileptic discharges in patients who have foci in the appropriate area of the brain. Thus activation of epileptic seizures by music (*musicogenic epilepsy*) or intermittent light flashes (photic stimulation) has been observed and some children with '*self-induced*' *epilepsy* find that they can produce attacks by passing their fingers rapidly between their eyes and a bright light. Conversely, it is sometimes possible to abort an epileptic seizure by means of sensory stimuli which presumably compete for the occupancy of the fibre pathways along which the epileptic discharge is spreading. Some patients find that they can shorten minor attacks by means of powerful concentration, while others, for instance, who experience seizures with an aura of uncinate type (see above) can stop the attack by sniffing a substance with a powerful odour.

While it is impossible to describe all the possible manifestations of focal or minor epilepsy, the principles outlined will indicate that almost any symptom of disordered cerebral function can occur as a manifestation of this condition.

MAJOR SEIZURES

A major convulsion or grand mal attack will result from a focal cerebral lesion, in the temporal lobe or elsewhere, if the spread of the epileptic discharge occurs rapidly throughout the two cerebral hemispheres. It can also be a symptom of diffuse brain disease, but there are a considerable proportion of cases in which no cause can be found and the attacks are presumed to be idiopathic or 'centrencephalic' in origin. The younger the patient, the more likely this is to be the case. Most cases of idiopathic major epilepsy first develop attacks in childhood or early adult life, whereas in middle age the proportion of patients who are found to have cerebral tumours or vascular disease as a cause of the fits is considerably greater; however, even in late life no aetiological factors are demonstrable in a considerable proportion of cases.

The typical major attack may begin with an aura or warning which indicates the situation of onset of the discharge but quite often this sensation is indefinable and little more than a 'sinking feeling' or an 'odd sensation in the head'. It is rare for an aura to last for more than a second or two and very often there is no warning at all. Consciousness is lost, the patient falls to the ground and may injure himself in the process, particularly, say, if he were to fall on to a fire. Cuts and bruises and falls downstairs are relatively common. The muscles then go rigid (the tonic phase), the teeth are clenched, the tongue is often bitten, the patient becomes cyanosed, and froths at the mouth. Within a few seconds, the musculature relaxes and rhythmical repetitive jerking of the limbs and trunk occurs (the clonic phase). The patient is often incontinent of urine and occasionally of faeces. Sometimes the clonic phase is absent and indeed the attack is so brief that the patient falls and then jumps up almost immediately (akinetic seizures). More frequently the jerking continues for a minute or two and is followed by relaxation. Often the patient will fall into a deep sleep, but if roused he is temporarily confused, or confusion may even last for several minutes or hours. In other cases he is lucid and co-operative almost immediately. Often there is a headache and muscular aching which persist for some hours afterwards and vomiting occasionally occurs.

Death in a major convulsion is a very rare complication indeed if the airway is kept clear, but if repeated convulsions occur without recovery of consciousness between them (*status epilepticus*) there is some danger to life and treatment is an urgent matter.

It has long been considered that mental disease may be a sequel of long-continued epileptic seizures, and that there is a specific 'epileptic personality' in which paranoid traits are prominent. While it is true that some patients with temporal lobe epilepsy become psychotic, it is questionable whether it is the epilepsy itself or the primary pathological changes in the temporal lobe which are responsible. Similarly there is no evidence that idiopathic epilepsy influences the mentality, but many diffuse cerebral disorders which give rise to dementia or psychosis can produce epileptic seizures as a symptom. Diffuse brain damage resulting from anoxia occurring in repeated attacks of severe major epilepsy can, however, also produce dementia.

MYOCLONIC EPILEPSY

Myoclonus, a momentary jerking movement of the voluntary muscles, can accompany attacks of petit mal, but similar manifestations occur sporadically and repetitively in certain cases without apparent impairment of consciousness. Occasional myoclonic jerks occurring when falling asleep can be considered to be physiological, but frequent nocturnal myoclonic jerks are often an epileptic manifestation and many such patients also have major seizures. Repeated myoclonic jerking may also be a symptom of diffuse and progressive brain disease, in such conditions as cerebral lipidosis (when it occurs particularly on startle), subacute encephalitis (when there is also progressive dementia) and the rare condition of progressive myoclonic epilepsy of Unverricht (in which the myoclonus becomes progressively more frequent and severe, dementia also occurs and the patient eventually dies from exhaustion and inanition). Paramyoclonus multiplex is probably just another name for progressive myoclonic epilepsy; in such cases degenerative changes and intranuclear inclusions may be found in the dentate nucleus of the cerebellum and abnormal mucopolysaccharides may be found in the serum.

CONCLUSIONS

It can be concluded that epilepsy may be classified from the aetiological standpoint into idiopathic and symptomatic varieties and that the idiopathic group is one which is diminishing steadily, as newer techniques reveal more organic disorders of the brain which produce epilepsy as a symptom. From the clinical point of view true petit mal (minimal seizures) is to be distinguished as a separate entity, at present of unknown aetiology; in many patients with major seizures, too, the condition must still be regarded as 'idiopathic'. A considerable proportion of patients with grand mal, however, and most of those with minor seizures, are suffering from focal organic brain disease, frequently affecting the temporal lobe. As we shall see in Chapter 20, accurate diagnosis is of the greatest importance from the point of view of treatment.

SYNCOPE AND OTHER BRIEF DISORDERS OF CONSCIOUSNESS

It is sometimes very difficult to differentiate clinically between simple faints or syncopal attacks and epileptic seizures. Syncope is most common in young patients, particularly in adolescent girls, and is often produced by long periods of standing in one position, by an emotional shock ('the sight of blood'), or by 'stuffy' atmospheres. It is particularly liable to occur in early pregnancy, while it can develop at any age in patients with uraemia or blood loss, or with heart block **(the Stokes–Adams syndrome)**. In the latter condition, syncope with pallor occurs during a period of cardiac asystole, and when the circulation is restored, the patient's face flushes and there may even be convulsive movements. Indeed, syncope of whatever cause can rarely result in transient epileptic manifestations, including transient twitching of the limbs and urinary incontinence, if cerebral anoxia is sufficiently prolonged. **Micturition syncope** is not uncommon, particularly in the elderly male patient who gets up during the night with a full bladder and loses his senses in the toilet.

In general terms, syncope is due to cerebral ischaemia, resulting usually from pooling of blood in the skin and viscera. Generally the patient feels a 'swimming in the head' and a sensation of heat; he then begins to perspire and is usually able to reach a place of safety before consciousness is lost (unless he is standing on parade). The loss of consciousness is generally brief, the patient's skin is deathly pale, cold and clammy, and his pulse is often thin and rapid, but occasionally it is slow. The aura of a syncopal attack is usually considerably longer than that of an epileptic seizure, there are generally emotional or physical precipitating factors, and injury is uncommon, while convulsive movements and incontinence are rare. The attacks usually occur when standing and not when sitting or lying. Often they are brought on by standing up abruptly. These are the principal points upon which differential diagnosis is based.

So-called **vaso-vagal attacks** have been described in which the patient becomes flushed and his pulse is slowed, while gastric or cardiac discomfort may occur. There is considerable doubt as to whether attacks of this nature ever occur in a stereotyped manner, and it now seems improbable that they should be afforded separate identification as they are merely one form of syncopal attack.

Drop attacks are episodes in which the patient's legs give way and he falls but does not lose consciousness. They tend to occur late in life and are probably due to transient brain stem ischaemia.

Hysterical convulsions are generally bizarre and florid with more violent and varied and less stereotyped movements than occur in epilepsy, while tongue-biting, injury and incontinence do not occur and the patient shows other manifestations of hysteria. However, in young women, hysterical attacks may take the form of sudden falling with, apparently, transient loss of consciousness and without convulsive movements. Similar attacks are not uncommon in some male patients who develop a so-called accident neurosis after minor injury. When, as occasionally happens, these attacks occur in young females who have also had genuine attacks of epilepsy, differential diagnosis can be very difficult. Hysterical hyperventilation (rapid panting respiration) which is often accompanied by panic and which leads to paraesthesiae in the lips and tongue and even to tetany, may also give rise to syncope and is often misdiagnosed. **Spontaneous hypoglycaemia** can give rise to attacks of light-headedness, fatigue, sweating, giddiness and even confused and irrational behaviour. Rarely, major epileptic convulsions result, particularly in those patients who have a tumour of the islets of Langerhans, with excessive insulin production. When reactive or functional hyperinsulinism is the cause, due to an excessive fall in blood sugar following the peak produced by a high carbohydrate meal, or after rapid gastric emptying, the symptoms are as a rule less severe. Nevertheless this condition, too, must be considered in determining the cause of transient disturbances of consciousness.

REFERENCES

ADAMS, R. D., 'Faintness, syncope and episodic weakness'; 'Coma and related disturbances of consciousness'; 'Sleep and its abnormalities'; and 'Recurrent convulsions'; in *Principles of Internal Medicine*, Ed. Harrison, T. R., 4th ed., Chapters 33-36 (New York, McGraw-Hill, 1962).

BRAIN, W. R., *Diseases of the Nervous System*, 6th ed., (London, Oxford University Press, 1962).

FORSTER, F. M., 'The epilepsies and convulsive disorders', in *Clinical Neurology*, Ed. Baker, A. B., Chapter 18 (London, Cassell, 1955).

GASTAUT, H., *The Epilepsies* (Springfield, Ill., Thomas, 1954).

JACKSON, J. H., *Selected Writings of John Hughlings Jackson*, Ed. Taylor, J., Vol. 1 (London, Staples, 1958).

MATTHEWS, W. B., *Practical Neurology*, Chapters 3-4 (Oxford, Blackwell, 1963).

MAYER-GROSS, W., SLATER, E. and ROTH, M., *Clinical Psychiatry*, 2nd ed. 291-318 (London, Cassell, 1960).

PENFIELD, W. and JASPER, H., *Epilepsy and the Functional Anatomy of the Human Brain* (London, Churchill, 1954).

WILLIAMS, D., 'The temporal lobe and epilepsy', in *Modern Trends in Neurology*, Ed. Williams, D., 2nd series (London, Butterworth, 1957).

CHAPTER 7

DISORDERS OF THE MIND

A COMPLETE appreciation of the brain–mind relationship has defied the understand of philosophers and physicians for centuries and is likely to do so for many years to come. Though much has been learned concerning the disorders of thought processes which result from disease of the brain, and the Freudian discipline of psychopathology has cast light upon some of the factors which may be responsible in part for mental disease, we still know little of the means by which cerebral activity subserves and controls human thought. It is this lack of fundamental knowledge concerning the physiology of thought which has led to the wide divergence of opinion between groups of psychiatrists, some of whom believe that virtually all mental disorder can be accounted for by physical changes, some as yet unidentified, which affect the functioning of the brain, while others, and particularly the psychoanalysts, consider that psychological influences are all-important. In fact, it seems probable that it is a combination of factors, psychological, physical and constitutional, which generally account for the development of symptoms of mental disorder in any individual case. So many varieties of mental disease (in the broadest sense) can result from the interplay of these aetiological factors that the concept of specific mental diseases is gradually disappearing, to be replaced by a more flexible terminology which takes account of psychiatric syndromes, their variability and their interrelationship. Thus it was once agreed that a **neurosis,** characterised usually by anxiety and related symptoms, and resulting from psychological causes, was totally different aetiologically and prognostically from a **psychosis,** a term generally implying insanity, and typified by serious derangement of the processes of thought. It is now apparent that the distinction between these two disorders is not absolute and that neurotic or psychotic reactions may occur in response to organic disease.

A detailed survey of the minutiae of psychiatric classification and differential diagnosis would be out of place in a work on neurology, and for this information the reader must turn to a textbook of psychiatry. However, so many mental symptoms can accompany or simulate brain disease that a brief survey of some of the commoner psychiatric syndromes is essential in order to assist in the identification of neurological disorders which may be complicated or imitated in this way.

E　　　　　　　　　　109

As disorders of consciousness and of memory, including the symptomatic psychoses, have been considered in the preceding chapter, it will be convenient to consider first developmental or constitutional disorders such as mental deficiency (**amentia** or **oligophrenia**), which can be considered to be a disorder of physical development, then **abnormalities of personality and character,** disorders which are primarily abnormalities of psychological development. Secondly we must discuss **dementia,** which can be regarded as a diffuse disintegration of mental function, involving intellect, memory, thought, emotions and behaviour, and depending usually upon organic brain disease. Next we shall consider a number of **fundamental psychiatric reactions** which occur in response to a variety of physical or mental stimuli, some of which are known, others unknown. Commonest of these are the **disorders of mood or affect,** sometimes called the affective disorders, of which the most prominent symptoms are anxiety and/or depression. **Hysteria** is another common psychiatric reaction, in which there are symptoms of mental or physical type, unaccounted for by organic disease, but activated by the desire to gain profit from the symptom or to escape from stress. Another type of neurotic reaction is the **obsessive–compulsive** variety, in which insistent thoughts so occupy the patient's mind that they may compel him to carry out actions which he knows are foolish or unnecessary but which he cannot resist. The **schizophrenic** reaction is characterised particularly by introversion, severe distortion of thought processes and by paranoid features which imply ideas of persecution; this disorder is essentially constitutional and is not usually the result of exogenous factors. Finally, brief mention must be made of some so-called **psychosomatic disorders,** a group of physical conditions in which psychological factors clearly play an important aetiological role.

MENTAL DEFICIENCY

Amentia or mental defect implies an intellectual deficit which is present from birth and can be confirmed by psychometric testing, by means of which the intelligence quotient (I.Q.) and 'mental age' of the patient are assessed. Low-grade mental defectives may be divided into the idiots (mental age of up to three in an adult) and imbeciles (mental age of up to seven). Idiots are incapable of guarding themselves against common dangers and must usually be confined in institutions. Imbeciles are also incapable of managing themselves or their affairs, but are occasionally able to live satisfactorily in a protected domestic environment and may even be able to do work of a low-grade nature. High-grade mental defectives or morons, some of whom have I.Q.s approaching the lower normal limit of ninety, are very common and mostly live outside institutions. Some few can be educated in ordinary schools but others must attend schools for the educationally subnormal. The diagnosis of high-grade mental defect can readily be overlooked and the patient is often regarded as being 'rather stupid', 'incapable of giving a reasonable history', 'hypochondriacal'. Character defects seem to be particularly common in morons and many habitual petty criminals, prostitutes, sexual offenders and murderers fall into this group.

In many idiots and imbeciles, as well as in a proportion of morons, there are associated congenital abnormalities involving other organs, while epilepsy or signs of 'cerebral palsy' may coexist. In **mongolism,** there is a characteristic facial appearance and disorders of skeletal development are also seen. This condition is now known to result from a disorder of chromosomal constitution in that an extra chromosome may be attached to one of the pairs ('trisomy'). Sometimes mental defect is a result of an inborn error of metabolism affecting the nervous system as in **amaurotic family idiocy** (Tay-Sachs form of cerebral lipidosis) or **phenylpyruvic oligophrenia** (a disorder of phenylalanine metabolism), but more often the amentia appears to be due to a combination of genetic influences and not to a single factor or to any definable physical or metabolic disease.

ABNORMALITIES OF PERSONALITY AND CHARACTER

We can recognise in the shy, introverted and absent-minded idealist, or in the fanatical adherent of outlandish cults or causes, differences in personality which distinguish him from his fellow men though he may not necessarily be regarded as abnormal. Such an individual is often referred to as **schizoid,** as this type of personality is common in relatives of schizophrenic individuals. We shall consider the **hysterical** and **obsessional** characters and the **cyclothymic** personality below. Here, however, it is important to mention **psychopathy.** Psychopaths are persons who, though not insane or mentally defective, behave in a socially abnormal manner. This appears to be a constitutional defect of personality, in which genetic influences play a considerable part. That structural abnormalities of the brain cannot be entirely excluded as a possible cause of psychopathy is indicated by the fact that similar defects of moral sense can occur as a sequel of encephalitis lethargica, but no consistent pathological changes have been found in the majority of psychopaths. A common variety of psychopathy is seen in the so-called unstable or constitutionally inadequate indivi-dual, lacking in determination and diffuse in his efforts, who is incapable of holding down any job for more than a short period. Many such patients are socially irresponsible, and become embezzlers, alcoholics or petty criminals. Flagrant antisocial behaviour is common in certain other psychopathic individuals and some are inherently aggressive, being liable to sudden outbursts of temper in which they may commit crimes of violence. Education, discipline and punishment have little effect upon these patients, who are essentially lacking in conscience and moral sense, but as they are not insane or mentally defective their management presents a formidable problem to society.

DEMENTIA

Dementia, or progressive disintegration of the intellect, of memory and of the powers of abstract thought, is a disorder of the mind which results from organic disease and generally from physical or metabolic disturbances affecting the brain. The first sign of a dementing process may be an error of judgement incompatible with the patient's previous ability, or a failure to grasp all the facets of a difficult situation. It may simply be said that Mr. X is 'losing his grip'. Subsequently, memory, particularly for recent events, becomes impaired, so that the patient is forgetful, unable to concentrate and his attention wanders freely. Increasing emotional lability with inappropriate laughing or crying or with irritability and irrational impulsive acts may follow, and striking changes in mood, taking the form of elation in some cases and apathy in others, often occur. By the time the patient becomes neglectful of his personal appearance and dirty in his habits, the diagnosis is usually obvious, but in the earlier stages it is much more difficult to make. Increasing unpunctuality, neglect of detail, and longer periods spent alone in the bathroom may be useful pointers. It is nevertheless remarkable how often patients with severe degrees of dementia continue to hold responsible jobs, despite increasing so-called 'eccentricity', until some major error of judgement or *faux pas* brings matters to a head. In the late stages, delusions occasionally occur, taking the form of grandiose imaginings ('I am the King of Spain') or ideas of hostility or persecution towards relatives or business associates.

A great many forms of organic brain disease give rise to progressive dementia. Many of these disorders are progressive and incurable, but others are eminently treatable and some show no very specific clinical features so that these possible causes should always be borne in mind. The first of these is **neurosyphilis** (particularly general paralysis of the insane), in which a fatuous euphoric dementia is common and there may also be Argyll–Robertson pupils and rarely spastic paresis of the limbs. Diagnosis can be made by cerebrospinal fluid examination. Another possible cause is ˙**intracranial tumour,** either primary or secondary, and involving particularly the frontal lobes. In such a case it is common for memory and intellect to be severely affected when other aspects of behaviour and personality are reasonably well preserved, while there may be features (headache, vomiting and papilloedema) to indicate that the intracranial pressure is raised. A number of **toxic and metabolic disorders** can also result in a progressive dementia; **drug intoxication** and **alcoholism** are usually self-evident causes if the history is adequate, but **pernicious anaemia** and **myxoedema** are other treatable conditions which are easily overlooked and in which the dementia is entirely reversible with appropriate treatment. When intellectual deterioration follows upon severe diffuse **head injury, inflammatory disease,** such as encephalitis or meningitis, long-standing **temporal lobe epilepsy** or a **chronic psychosis,** the cause is generally apparent and little can usually be done. This also applies to cases of cerebral lipidosis, diffuse cerebral sclerosis and other **degenerative disorders** which cause dementia in childhood. The same is unfortunately true of cases of **cerebral atherosclerosis** in which, however, the dementia, though progressive, is usually step-like, rather than insidious in its advance, being accompanied by transient episodes of confusion, aphasia and/or motor or sensory disturbance, indicating minor 'strokes' due to focal cerebral ischaemia.

Another group of conditions in which progressive deterioration of personality and intellect occurs in an insidious manner and which are unfortunately uninfluenced by treatment, are the group of degenerative cerebral disorders of unknown aetiology known as the **presenile and senile dementias. In Alzheimer's disease** and in **Pick's disease,** as in **senile dementia,** there is degeneration of cortical neurones and deposition of argyrophilic material in the form of plaques ('senile plaques') in the cerebral cortex. In senile dementia, the patient is usually in the seventh or eighth decade, the intellect and personality deteriorate hand in hand and very often there is characteristic nocturnal restlessness, so that the patient wanders about in the middle of the night. Alzheimer's disease is, in a sense, a premature senility of the brain, and in such cases progressive dementia develops in the forty to sixty age group. In the late stages, aphasia and spasticity of the limbs may develop. In Pick's disease, again a condition of late middle life, there is often affection of more than one member of a family and the pathological changes are more circumscribed, often beginning in one or other frontal lobe. As the changes are initially focal, epilepsy or neurological signs suggesting a localised brain lesion are occasionally seen, while aphasia and defective memory are common at a time when the personality remains reasonably well-preserved; eventually, however, a global dementia supervenes.

Huntington's chorea must also be mentioned as a cause of presenile dementia of relatively non-specific type. In such cases there is generally a clear-cut family history of the condition and the characteristic involuntary movements of the limbs and face are seen, though rarely dementia alone is the first manifestation. In the rare degenerative condition sometimes known as **Jakob–Creutzfeld disease,** a presenile dementia is associated with signs of bilateral pyramidal tract dysfunction, with clinical features suggesting Parkinson's disease, and often with weakness and wasting of peripheral limb muscles.

Hence a multitude of possible causes must be considered in any case of dementia; accurate diagnosis is of considerable importance, for in some conditions the prognosis is grave, while in others (neurosyphilis, intoxication, pernicious anaemia, myxoedema and benign intracranial neoplasms) the condition may be reversible with appropriate treatment.

DISORDERS OF MOOD (AFFECTIVE DISORDERS)

An individual's mood at any one moment of time can broadly be considered to be synonymous with the state of his emotions. As the hypothalamus, and probably certain areas of the cerebral cortex, exercise considerable control over the emotions it is apparent that disorders of mood will result from certain organic lesions of the brain. It is equally true, however, that the prevailing mood or mood changes may also be substantially influenced, not by physical disease, but by the patient's emotional constitution and by a variety of psychological factors.

The principal mood disturbances which result from organic cerebral disease are emotional lability, apathy, euphoria, excitement, depression and anxiety; those of psychogenic origin are similar but include mania, hypomania and depression (manic-depressive psychosis) and anxiety (anxiety neurosis). **Emotional lability,** characterised by laughing or crying in response to minor or inappropriate emotional stimuli, and by rapid alternation of these emotional responses, is seen usually in patients with extensive bilateral cerebral lesions, particularly when both frontal lobes are involved. It rarely occurs as a result of unilateral frontal lesions but is most often observed in patients with diffuse cerebral atherosclerosis and the syndrome of 'pseudobulbar palsy'. **Apathy,** or progressive loss of interest in one's personal surroundings, leading sometimes to stupor, is an emotional state which generally results from lesions in the hypothalamic region. It occurs in patients with severe post-encephalitic Parkinsonism and in diffuse degenerative cerebral disorders, including the presenile dementias, while a similar mental state is also seen in certain psychoses such as schizophrenia. **Euphoria** is a feeling of cheerful well-being, verging sometimes on elation. It occurs in some patients with general paresis and in some with disseminated sclerosis, who remain excessively cheerful, sometimes fatuously so, despite their disability; transient euphoria may also result from drugs such as amphetamine and alcohol. **Excitement,** or mental over-activity, which can take the form of elation, rage or excessive volubility, is related to the emotional state of euphoria on the one hand and mania on the other and is often accompanied by agitation and physical restlessness. It is often a feature of the delirious state, and may rarely result from lesions in the hypothalamic region. **Depression** is probably more often psychogenic than due to organic disease, but can be seen in patients with head injury, general paresis, temporal lobe lesions, bronchogenic carcinoma and rarely in disseminated sclerosis. Although this mood disorder is sometimes a psychogenic reaction to the presence of incurable illness, there can be little doubt that severe depression may occasionally be physically determined, as in that which typically follows a severe attack of influenza. **Anxiety,** too, is a natural reaction to many physical illnesses but there is some evidence that it is occasionally a direct result of organic pathological change, as in the fear and apprehension which may colour delirious states or that which occurs during recovery from a severe head injury. The sensation of *angor animi*, or fear of impending doom, typically accompanies an episode of cardiac infarction and it is of interest that a similar sensation or alternatively depression or apprehension can occur as a part of the aura of temporal lobe epilepsy.

Turning to the primarily psychogenic disorders of mood, the **manic-depressive psychoses** are essentially endogenous, that is, they develop primarily as a result of constitutional or other influences arising within the subject. Anxiety, on the other hand, is usually a result of exogenous stress, though constitution has a profound influence upon the development of this symptom. Depression, too, may be the result of exogenous factors, in which case it is known as **reactive depression.**

The true manic-depressive varies between a state of mania on the one hand and intense depression on the other. This disorder is essentially constitutional; when similar but less florid mood swings occur the condition is referred to as **cyclothymia.** The **manic patient** is initially gay, talkative, cheerful and elated, restless and excitable.

As the state of mania develops he may become increasingly distressed, aggressive and even violent, and his mind flies from one idea to another without obvious connexion between the two ('flight of ideas'). A less severe degree of mania, or hypomania, is evident in the vigorous, active and voluble extravert who is 'the life and soul of the party' and some degrees of hypomania are compatible with successful social adaptation and material gain. In true mania, however, if the patient is not sedated, exhaustion supervenes.

The depressive, by contrast, is slow, retarded and lacking in interest. In **severe melancholia** the patient will retire to bed in a state of utter apathy and may lie staring fixedly at the ceiling, taking no account of all that goes on around him. There is severe constipation, all motor activity is slowly and lethargically performed and the pulse rate is slow. Less severe degrees of endogenous depression are much more common, particularly in middle age, as in post-menopausal women, and in patients who have never previously shown severe disorders of mood; this condition is often referred to as **involutional depression.** The patient passes his days in a state of gloom and dejection; everything is viewed with a pessimistic air and he looks at the world 'through grey-coloured spectacles'. Interest in home, family and hobbies is lost and he may spend long hours of silence, sitting gazing into the fire. There is often a desire for solitude, friends are shunned, work neglected, and ideas of guilt, unworthiness and inadequacy are common. Suicidal ruminations are frequent, as all joy in living is lost, and indeed suicide is a serious potential hazard in this disease. Physical symptoms (headache, giddiness, indigestion) are common and there is a characteristic form of insomnia in that patients tend to wake in the early morning after falling asleep quickly on retiring. Mild forms of this syndrome are difficult to recognise and are easily confused with an anxiety state by the uninitiated. The distinction is important, for treatment of the two conditions is quite different. Prolonged lethargy, undue fatigue and feelings of vague ill-health and lack of energy in those past middle-age are commonly due to masked depression. Paradoxically, some patients with severe depressive states become remarkably agitated and tears flow readily.

Anxiety is a common emotional disturbance which can be a perfectly normal reaction under conditions of appropriate stress. It is when the feeling of anxiety or apprehension is not clearly related to any particular object or circumstance that it becomes pathological and may then be considered to constitute an anxiety neurosis. Physical concomitants of anxiety are frequent and include sweating, feelings of suffocation or choking, sighing, restlessness, fatigue, 'dizzy bouts', and tension headaches. The anxious patient is often totally unable to rest or to relax. Whereas anxiety is a common feature of many psychiatric syndromes and may accompany depression or even psychotic illnesses, it is those individuals who are constitutionally predisposed to the development of severe anxiety symptoms as a result of minor stress who become neurotic. In such individuals episodes of anxiety may occur acutely in the form of 'panic attacks', or may present with episodes of tension and with physical symptoms of the type outlined above, but with intervening periods when life is lived on a relatively even keel. In the chronic anxiety state, the patient exists in a state of continual worry and is irritable and unhappy. Not uncommonly symptoms are focused upon one particular organ; for instance the patient with a cardiac neurosis or 'effort syndrome' complains of breathlessness, palpitation and precordial pain. Reactive depression frequently coexists with anxiety but self-reproach and suicidal ideas are much less common than in the endogenous variety and patients with this type of depression have difficulty in getting to sleep but do not wake as early in the morning as the true depressive.

Depersonalisation, or a feeling of unreality of the self, can coexist with either depression or anxiety. Such patients can feel so intensely unreal that they believe themselves to be 'floating in air' and may even have delusional ideas that they are soon to die or that their bodies are shrinking. When depersonalisation is severe and combined with panic attacks and with phobias (unreasoning fear of heights, of people, of enclosed places, or of crossing the road) this syndrome has been characterised as a so-called 'phobic anxiety state'. A feeling of chronic instability, with associated light-headedness and a feeling of faintness, often confused with true vertigo unless the history is carefully taken, is commonly due to depersonalisation and is typically more troublesome out-of-doors than in the home.

OBSESSIONAL NEUROSIS

Obsessions are thoughts which compulsively crowd into consciousness, even though, on reflection, the sufferer is aware that they are unreasonable or irrational. Many normal individuals have particular obsessions in that they are ritualistic in their habits. The child who walks on the lines of the pavement, the housewife who repeatedly straightens minutely crooked pictures on the wall is somewhat obsessional, as are most of the excessively tidy and rigidly conscientious members of the community. Obsessional features are very common in childhood but tend to disappear with increasing maturity. The obsessional personality cannot always be regarded as abnormal; it is when compulsive thoughts impose a senseless ritual that the

E*

borderline of normality is crossed. Thus it is normal to wash one's hands several times in the day but the person who does so every few minutes may be obsessed with fear of dirt, of germs, or of disease. Similarly obsessed is the patient who checks up on the fact that the doors and windows are locked at night, not once, but five or six times. Though minor obsessional traits are compatible with reasonable adjustment to life in the community, the severe case of obsessional neurosis is so occupied with his compulsive thoughts that any other occupation than thought is out of the question and he retires into a life of seclusion.

An obsessional neurosis is essentially different in aetiology, nature and prognosis from a simple anxiety state, though many obsessionals are neurotic and many anxiety neurotics have obsessional ideas. A disorder which has affinities with both these forms of neurosis is **hypochondriasis,** a state of mind in which the patient becomes intensely introspective and excessively occupied with his own bodily symptoms, so that he may have no other topic of conversation than his own illnesses, whether imaginary or real. In severe or so-called malignant hypochondriasis the patient's ideas may assume a frankly delusional quality. An example is the patient who is so firmly convinced, say, that he has an abscess in the skull or in the back of the throat that he goes from doctor to doctor in search of one who will operate to remove the offending but imaginary focus of infection.

HYSTERIA

The differential diagnosis between hysteria and organic disease is one of the most difficult in medicine. In neurology the problem is a particularly common one and has been the graveyard of many a professional reputation; for although hysterical symptoms can simulate almost any physical disease it is disorders of the nervous system which are most often imitated. The single most important point in the diagnosis of hysteria is that this condition must not be diagnosed by exclusion, as a label casually applied when clinical examination and ancillary tests have failed to reveal organic disease. On the contrary, there must be positive evidence of hysteria, for hysterical symptoms are always purposive, they arise in order to obtain for the patient some real or imagined gain, either to fulfil an ambition, to realise a phantasy, or to escape from a stressful situation. To lose a job or to fail an examination through illness is much more respectable than to do so through inefficiency; whereas such motivations may not be wholly conscious, the end desired by the patient can usually be uncovered on careful enquiry.

Patients who develop hysterical symptoms tend to have certain characteristic personality traits. They commonly deceive themselves that they are much more able or important than they really are, they are emotionally shallow, easily influenced and unreliable and often utilise hysterical symptoms in order to draw attention or sympathy upon themselves or to dominate their relatives and friends. Hysteria may occur in both sexes but is more common in females; as the basic abnormality is constitutional, symptoms usually develop first in adolescence or early adult life, though much depends upon the severity of the stress to which the individual is subjected.

Anxiety symptoms are often prominent in hysterical reactions, but relatively few neurotic patients exhibit frankly hysterical manifestations. A characteristic group of mental symptoms resulting from hysteria arises from an ability to dissociate one part of the personality from another. Thus, hysterical 'twilight states', trances, or simulation of insanity (Ganser states) may occur, but most common is the **hysterical amnesia** or **fugue,** in which the patient wanders away from home for several hours or days, having lost all sense of his identity.

As a general rule, hysterical symptoms are a result either of suggestion or of an idea or phantasy in the patient's mind. Suggestion is of the greatest importance; thus a hysteric may become paralysed because her mother had a stroke, or a symptom will develop in response to a leading question asked by a doctor, which the patient then endeavours to justify. It is from discrepancies between the patient's idea of a physical illness and the signs of the organic disorder itself that most diagnostic assistance is obtained. Motivation is also important; thus a patient with 'stage-fright' loses his voice, while another who is dreading forthcoming examinations develops hysterical blindness so that he is unable to study. In hysterical **aphonia** the patient is able to cough on demand, while the individual with **hysterical blindness** will blink on threat or avoid obstacles in his path. **Hysterical convulsions** are staged for their histrionic effect and invariably occur with an audience; the patient is careful not to injure himself and tongue-biting and incontinence do not occur unless the patient who has been asked about these features many times decides to oblige by providing them. The convulsion is often preceded by **hyperventilation** and actual tetany may develop through respiratory alkalosis. In **hysterical paralysis,** a single limb is usually involved, though hemiplegia or paraplegia are seen. There are generally discrepancies between the clinical findings and those resulting from organic disease of the nervous system; in particular, the reflexes are generally normal or else they show slight but symmetrical exaggeration, and the plantar responses are flexor. Typically, when the patient tries to move the affected limb, there is a massive apparent expenditure of effort with little result, and careful palpation of the muscles involved generally reveals that agonists and antagonists are contracting simultaneously. Hysterical disorders of **gait** are seen in patients who claim to have paralysis of the lower limbs, but in others there is no abnormality to be detected on examining the patient when lying in bed, although the gait is bizarre, and unlike that associated with any organic nervous disease. Falling may be frequent, but significantly without injury. Caution must be exercised in excluding the broad-based gait of truncal ataxia due to a mid-line cerebellar lesion, in which, too, signs of cerebellar dysfunction may be conspicuously absent in the recumbent patient. Hysterical **sensory loss** is also common; it frequently occurs in 'glove and stocking' distribution, with a clear-cut upper margin (unlike polyneuritis where the transition is gradual) or there may be a total hemianaesthesia affecting all forms of sensation. Loss of vibration sense over one half of the skull is invariably hysterical. Co-ordinated movements are then perfectly good despite apparent complete loss of position and joint sense. In a limb showing hysterical weakness or paralysis the sensory impairment may end sharply at the elbow, knee, groin or shoulder, giving a pattern of sensory impairment which could not be produced by an organic lesion. These patients are often very suggestible and 'islands' of normal sensation can be demonstrated in anaesthetic areas. In any event, the sensory impairment never corresponds with the cutaneous distribution of any peripheral nerve, sensory root or tract. Other less common hysterical manifestations include **dermatitis artefacta,** produced by self-inflicted cutaneous trauma, and hysterical **pyrexia,** which is most common in nurses and is usually an artefact produced by cups of tea, cigarettes or hot water bottles or by substituting thermometers. Some patients go to the extent of producing subcutaneous or intra-articular abscesses by injecting themselves with bath water, in which case the infecting organism is generally *B. coli.* Related to hysteria, but psychiatrically more complex, is the condition often called **'von Munchausen's syndrome';** patients in this category become skilled at feigning organic disease and may seek admission to one hospital after another. Some few are drug addicts but others simply demonstrate 'a desire to be ill'. Along with all these features described above there is, in hysteria, a characteristic **belle indifférence** or seeming unconcern about what, if physically determined, would be a serious disability.

From the description given above it may be asked why the differential diagnosis from organic disease should sometimes be so difficult. Unfortunately the clinical picture is not always so clear-cut. For example, the early manifestations of extrapyramidal disorders such as torsion spasm (dystonia musculorum) can produce abnormalities of gait which initially look hysterical. Furthermore, hysterical manifestations arise in patients with organic disease and it may be difficult to determine how much is overlay and how much genuine. In disseminated sclerosis, for instance, early manifestations of hysterical type are common even before distinctive physical signs have appeared. Hysterical manifestations developing for the first time late in life can be the first symptoms of an organic dementia. The most important principles to follow in establishing the diagnosis are first to seek assiduously for any motivation, unconscious or otherwise, which may be responsible for the symptoms and secondly to look for sources of suggestion which could be determining the pattern of the illness.

SCHIZOPHRENIA

Schizophrenia is a psychosis or psychotic reaction which is so common and yet so variable in its many manifestations that the reader must turn to a textbook of psychiatry for an adequate description of its clinical features. And yet it is a disorder which can occasionally mimic organic nervous disease; for this reason its most common features will be briefly mentioned here.

The disease typically occurs in young adults, often those of shy, dreamy and introverted personality. Emotional disturbances may be early manifestations, taking the form of apathy and disinterest, with shallowness or incongruity of affect; nothing is felt deeply and inappropriate giggling is common. Indecision and lack of initiative are frequent. Gradually the patient becomes more and more withdrawn, with self-neglect and eventual stupor. In the **catatonic** schizophrenic, stupor is accompanied by a curious waxy flexibility of the limbs, which may be placed in bizarre positions and remain there. Lack of ideas is accompanied by a sudden stoppage or block in conscious thought and the patient may yet have sufficient insight to realise that he is unable to think logically. Thought disorders of this type with deterioration in personality and work performance are the salient features of the simple or **hebephrenic** form of schizophrenia. Hallucinations frequently occur and are most often auditory in character, so that the patient hears imaginary voices which are sometimes so vivid that he answers their remarks. Delusions are also frequent; the patient may believe that he is being influenced by electricity or by radio waves. In the **paranoid** schizophrenic these delusions have a flavour of intense suspicion and the patient believes that he is being persecuted, perhaps by a religious group or sect. A paranoid psychosis of this nature developing comparatively late in life is often referred to as **paraphrenia,** and in this condition the personality is relatively well-preserved.

Physical abnormalities, of which cyanosis of the extremities is the most constant, are relatively frequent in patients with schizophrenia, and there is some substance in the idea that this may be essentially an organic disease, although no consistent biochemical or pathological changes have been discovered in such cases. Nevertheless, it is apparent that inherited traits are largely responsible. Whereas the fully-developed case is not difficult to recognise, in the early stages the condition is difficult to distinguish from depression, anxiety with depersonalisation, chronic hypochondriasis, delirium and organic dementia, although the age incidence and natural history of these disorders are generally quite different.

PUERPERAL PSYCHOSIS

A variety of forms of psychotic reaction can occur during the puerperium. Some of these illnesses show features of endogenous depression, many have close affinities with schizophrenia. Whereas the illness is often short and recovery complete, particularly with appropriate treatment, the psychosis persists in a significant proportion of cases.

PSYCHOSOMATIC DISORDERS

That somatic symptoms can be the most prominent or indeed the only manifestations of a psychiatric disturbance is now clearly apparent. Many patients with endogenous depression, for instance, seek medical advice on account of headaches or other symptoms which appear to be physically determined. It is equally clear that many organic diseases are powerfully influenced by psychological factors. Thus thyrotoxicosis may develop after an emotional shock, the symptoms of peptic ulcer, migraine and ulcerative colitis may be greatly increased by anxiety, and there is some correlation between chronic tension and raised blood pressure. The exact means by which psychological factors produce their effects in these disorders is far from clear; it is evident that many of them are consistently more frequent in individuals with certain types of emotional and physical constitution. By dividing humanity into different constitutional types or somatotypes, on the basis of physical characteristics, it is sometimes possible to predict the mental or physical disorders to which they are likely to be subject. Although our understanding of the mechanism by which psychological factors influence organic disease is incomplete, it is apparent that any physician who attempts to treat disease without taking into account all relevant emotional influences and without attempting to alleviate those which appear to be significant, is failing in his duty to his patient.

REFERENCES

ALLISON, R. D., *The Senile Brain* (London, Arnold, 1962).
CURRAN, D. and PARTRIDGE, M., *Psychological Medicine*, 5th ed. (Edinburgh, Livingstone, 1963).
HENDERSON, D. K. and GILLESPIE, R. D., *Textbook of Psychiatry*, 9th ed. (London, Oxford University Press, 1962).
MAYER-GROSS, W., SLATER, E. and ROTH, M., *Clinical Psychiatry*, 2nd ed. (London, Cassell, 1960).
NOYES, A., HAYDON, E. M. and VAN SICKEL, M., *A Text-book of Psychiatric Nursing*, 6th ed. (New York, Macmillan, 1964).

CHAPTER 8

THE SPECIAL SENSES

THE special senses include the faculties of smell, vision, hearing and taste. Closely related to hearing, at least in an anatomical sense, is the maintenance of equilibrium (vestibular function). These functions are mediated through those cranial nerves which convey the sensory impulses concerned in the appreciation of these sensations to the appropriate areas of the cerebral cortex. Thus the first or olfactory nerve contains the peripheral pathway for the sense of smell, while the second or optic nerve carries visual impulses. The ability to see is closely related to mechanisms subserving binocular vision and ocular movement, so that in considering visual processes it is important also to discuss the functions of the third (oculomotor), fourth (trochlear) and sixth (abducens) cranial nerves which control external ocular movement and which in collaboration with sympathetic fibres derived from the autonomic nervous system also influence those intrinsic ocular muscles controlling the size of the pupils as well as the process of accommodation. Hearing and the control of bodily equilibrium are respectively mediated through the cochlear and labyrinthine divisions of the eighth or auditory nerve, while taste sensations from the anterior two-thirds of the tongue travel in the chorda tympani along with the seventh or facial nerve and those from the posterior one-third are conveyed by the ninth or glossopharyngeal nerve. Disorders of function of the special senses, produced by lesions of the primary sensory receptors, of the cranial nerves concerned, or of their central connexions, are common in patients with neurological disease, and an adequate understanding of the means by which these lesions produce their clinical effects is essential for accurate diagnosis.

SMELL

The olfactory receptors are a series of bipolar nerve cells situated in the upper part of the mucous membrane on either side of the nasal cavity. Inhaled gases given off by all odorous materials become dissolved in the nasal secretions which continually bathe the surface of these sensitive cells. Impulses so produced are conveyed by nerve fibres through the cribriform plate of the ethmoid bone into the cranial cavity to join the olfactory bulb which lies on the under-surface of the homolateral frontal lobe. Thence impulses travel posteriorly in the olfactory tracts to reach that part of the hippocampal gyrus of the temporal lobe which can be regarded as the primary rhinencephalic (olfactory) area of the cerebral cortex, although it has profuse anatomical connexions with other areas of the brain.

From the standpoint of clinical neurology it must be remarked that there is a strong relationship between the faculties of smell and taste, which combined give the sensation of flavour. Thus if either faculty is impaired so too may be the ability to appreciate flavours; in such a patient it is not sufficient to test taste sensation alone, as an inability to perceive olfactory sensations may be the primary abnormality. Furthermore, it should be remembered that disease of the nasal mucosa such as rhinitis, a severe coryza, or sometimes excessive smoking, can so impair the sensitivity of the olfactory nerve cells that the sensation of smell is lost or greatly impaired (**anosmia**). Bilateral loss is thus not always significant, though it may follow a head injury with tearing of the olfactory nerve fibres as they traverse the ethmoid bone. Unilateral impairment of sense of smell is, however, an important physical sign, since in the absence of a primary nasal abnormality it may indicate compression of one olfactory bulb or tract, possibly by a tumour underlying the homolateral frontal lobe. Olfactory hallucinations, as previously mentioned, sometimes occur in patients with lesions in one or other temporal lobe, as in some cases of temporal lobe epilepsy, presumably as a result of irritation of the hippocampal cortex.

VISION

The Visual Pathways

Visual impulses recorded upon the retina are conveyed by the optic (second cranial) nerves through the optic chiasm. In the chiasm, fibres from the nasal half of each retina decussate, whereas temporal fibres do not. Hence each optic tract carries fibres from the temporal half of the homolateral retina and from the nasal half of the contralateral one (Fig. 2). This means that impulses from the right half-field of both eyes are carried in the left optic tract and vice versa. The tract continues to the lateral geniculate body where the axons concerned synapse with nerve cells which give origin to the optic radiation. The optic radiation then travels backwards through the temporal lobe, hooking around the tip of the temporal horn of the lateral ventricle in the process, and onwards to that part of the cerebral cortex which lies in the lips and in the depth of the calcarine

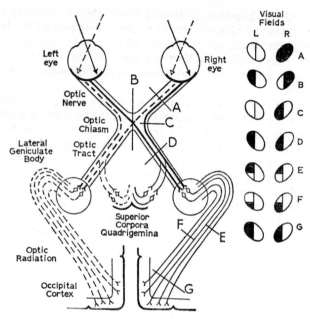

FIG. 2. A diagram of the visual pathways. On the right are examples of visual field defects produced by lesions interrupting these pathways at the points signified by the letters *A* to *G*.

fissure of the occipital lobe. This is the primary visual receptive area and has profuse connexions with the surrounding association areas in which, it appears, visual sensations are recognised and interpreted.

The light-sensitive receptors in the retina itself are the rods which are found diffusely throughout the retina except in the fovea centralis or macular area, and the cones which are concentrated largely in the region of the fovea but are scanty elsewhere. The cones seem to be responsible for finer degrees of visual appreciation at or near the fixation point (visual acuity) and probably for colour vision, while the rods are related to general visual sensitivity and play a particularly important role in subserving visual functions in conditions of poor illumination (as at night). Impulses received by the rods and cones then pass to the ganglion cells which lie in the superficial layers of the retina, whose axons form the fibres of the optic nerve and become gathered together in the optic disk or nerve-head.

In the optic nerve there also travel afferent fibres from the retina and from the muscles of accommodation, which influence pupil size; these synapse in the lateral geniculate body and in the superior corpora quadrigemina of the upper mid-brain, whence fibres arise which travel to the third, fourth and sixth nerve nuclei and to a sympathetic centre in the hypothalamus nearby. It is these pathways which are responsible for constriction of the pupil in response to light or fixation on near objects, and dilatation when the visual field is darkened or when distant objects are being observed. A similar reflex pathway, controlled by visual impulses from the retina, influences the ocular movements necessary for ocular convergence and fixation and for following objects with the eyes.

Visual Acuity

The visual acuity in each eye can be measured independently by means of test-types of the Snellen and Jaeger type (*see* Chapter 3). The acuity is essentially a measurement of the efficiency of macular or central vision as it depends very largely upon normal functioning of this part of the retina and of its nervous connexions, provided the mechanism for focusing light upon the retina is intact. Thus peripheral retinal lesions rarely influence acuity, but a small lesion of the macula or of the fibres of the optic nerve which come from the macular area may seriously affect the ability to read or to distinguish small objects. This is seen particularly in retrobulbar neuritis (*vide infra*) which often produces a central field defect or scotoma. Disorders of refraction (myopia, presbyopia, astigmatism) can seriously impair visual acuity as may other primary abnormalities of the eye (iridocyclitis, cataract, vitreous haemorrhages) which influence the passage of light to the retina, as well as disorders which damage retinal sensitivity (retinal detachment, glaucoma, etc.), but these local causes are usually self-evident and refractive errors can generally be corrected by the use of appropriate lenses.

Colour Blindness

Colour blindness is an inherited defect which occurs in 8 per cent of the male population and in less than 0·5 per cent of females. It is generally inherited as a sex-linked recessive character; though it occurs in many forms, the commonest variety is red–green blindness, either partial or complete, in which the affected individual finds it difficult to distinguish reds from greens. Many such patients are unaware of this defect, as they recognise 'colours' by their brightness, but the diagnosis can be confirmed with the Ishihara charts. The defect is of no serious significance except in those occupations where the recognition of coloured lights or signals, say, is important. It is, however, of some interest that in patients with minimal lesions of the visual pathways, field defects for coloured objects (red is commonly used) can be demonstrated at a time when the field for white objects is complete. The field for red is normally smaller than that for white.

The Visual Fields

Defects of the peripheral visual fields as charted by perimetry, or of the central fields as recorded with the Bjerrum screen, may be of the greatest value in neurological diagnosis (Fig. 2). From a knowledge of the anatomy of the visual pathways it is generally possible to localise with a considerable degree of accuracy the site of the lesion which is responsible. Circumscribed defects of the central fields are referred to as scotomas. In each central field there is a normal 'scotoma', medial to the fixation point; this is the caecum or 'blind spot', corresponding to the optic nerve head or disk in which there are no visual receptors. A scotoma which surrounds the fixation point or macular area is known as a **central scotoma,** and generally results in serious impairment of visual acuity. It is most commonly seen as a sequel of **retrobulbar neuritis,** an inflammatory lesion of the optic nerve which is frequently a feature of disseminated sclerosis. A central scotoma can rarely result from **compression of one optic nerve,** presumably because macular nerve fibres may be the most sensitive to pressure ischaemia, in patients with a tumour (usually a meningioma) behind the orbit. They may also be observed in **pernicious anaemia,** or in **neuromyelitis optica,** an acute demyelinating disorder related to disseminated sclerosis, and in retrobulbar neuritis due to a variety of toxic and metabolic causes, of which **methyl alcohol poisoning** is a good example. **Tobacco amblyopia,** which is a cause of progressive visual failure in smokers of certain brands of pipe tobacco, usually gives a **centro-caecal scotoma,** joining the fixation point to the blind spot.

A severe lesion of one optic nerve will, of course, give complete blindness of the homolateral eye, while the peripheral field of the other eye will be full. This may be seen, for instance, following severe head injury or following occlusion of the central retinal artery due to embolism, atherosclerosis or cranial arteritis. Lesions of the optic chiasm can give a variety of field defects, depending upon the character and situation of the causal lesion. Atherosclerotic ischaemia of the chiasm is occasionally responsible, but the lesions in this area which most commonly give rise to field defects are those which compress the chiasm, namely **parasellar neoplasms** and **aneurysms. Tumours of the pituitary gland,** as they protrude from the sella turcica, will first of all compress the decussating fibres from the lower nasal portions of the retinae, producing defects in the upper temporal field of both eyes, and eventually a **bitemporal hemianopia.** A lesion which compresses the chiasm asymmetrically from above, such as a suprasellar meningioma, a craniopharyngioma or a suprasellar aneurysm of the internal carotid or anterior communicating artery, may produce first a defect in the nasal field of one eye, progressing to complete unilateral blindness and followed by a defect in the temporal field of the other eye. Other possible variations can readily be deduced on anatomical grounds.

A complete lesion of one **optic tract** will give rise to a contralateral **homonymous hemianopia,** that is a complete loss of the nasal field of the ipsilateral eye and of the temporal field of the contralateral eye. Thus in a lesion of the left optic tract, which can be produced by lesions similar to those mentioned as compressing the chiasm, the right half-field of both eyes is lost. However, since optic tract compression is frequently asymmetrical, a progressive increase in size of the defects in these half-fields may be observed over a period of time and the defect may initially be larger in one field than in the other until the hemianopia is complete. When homonymous defects in the two fields are unequal in size and shape they are said to be **incongruous.**

Lesions of the **optic radiation,** whether in the internal capsule, temporal lobe, or occipital lobe, and whether of vascular (infarction, haemorrhage), neoplastic or inflammatory (leucoencephalitis, diffuse sclerosis) aetiology, also give rise to homonymous defects. A large lesion will give a complete homonymous hemianopia, but a smaller lesion, say, one in the temporal lobe affecting the lower fibres of the radiation, may give a contralateral upper quadrantic homonymous defect. As the nerve fibres coming from the retina are closely intermixed in the radiation, so that fibres from homologous portions of the two retinae lie alongside one another, field defects due to radiation lesions are **congruous,** i.e. they are the same in both eyes. It has often been suggested that there is bilateral representation of the macula in the two occipital lobes, so that in a homonymous hemianopia resulting from an occipital lobe lesion the macular area of the blind half-field is spared. This finding is now recognised to be an artefact due to poor fixation during charting of the fields, and in fact in such a case the macular field is actually split. Nevertheless, visual acuity remains unimpaired in a patient with a complete homonymous hemianopia.

Abnormalities of the visual fields may, of course, result from local ocular conditions such as glaucoma and retinal detachment, but these disorders are generally apparent on examination of the eye and rarely give rise to diagnostic difficulty. Some **concentric diminution** of the fields with enlargement of the blind spot is seen in severe papilloedema and less often in optic atrophy due to syphilis or constriction of the optic nerve due to arachnoiditis. Complete loss of the peripheral field with retention of only a small central area (**tubular vision**) is usually an hysterical phenomenon.

The Optic Fundus and its Abnormalities

Ophthalmoscopic examination of the optic nerve-head or disk, of the retinal vessels, and of the retina itself is an essential and often revealing part of a neurological examination. The optic disk is normally slightly pink in colour, but its temporal half is generally somewhat paler than the nasal, while some lack of definition of its nasal margin is common. In the centre of the disk, or slightly more towards its temporal margin, is the physiological cup into which the vessels dip; this cup is frequently much paler than the remainder of the disk and its appearance must not be confused with that of optic atrophy. Excessive cupping of the disk is, of course, seen in glaucoma. Not uncommonly a leash of pale fibres is seen spreading for a short distance across the retina, in fan-like manner, from one part of the edge of the disk; these **medullated nerve fibres** are a common abnormality and have no pathological significance.

The two most frequent abnormalities of the optic disk are swelling (papilloedema) and excessive pallor (optic atrophy).

Papilloedema generally results from some obstruction to the venous return from the retina, so that the first sign may be a distension of the retinal veins, which look unusually tumid. This is followed by obliteration of the physiological cup, and later the centre of the optic disk becomes raised above the level of the surrounding retina, while the disk margins become progressively more blurred and indistinct. When the swelling is severe, haemorrhages and sometimes patches of white exudate develop around the disk margins in a radial manner. A star-shaped patch of white exudate ('macular star') may also develop in the macular area, which is normally a relatively avascular area of the retina, lying about two disk-breadths lateral to the disk. The two principal causes of papilloedema are first, **increased intracranial pressure,** transmitted to the optic nerve sheath and so compressing the veins, as in cases of intracranial tumour, abscess, haemorrhage or meningitis; and secondly, much less commonly, **retrobulbar neuritis.** The latter is an 'inflammatory' neuritis of the optic nerve, due most often to disseminated sclerosis or the related neuromyelitis optica, but rarely resulting from syphilis and from toxic, nutritional and metabolic disorders. These two causes of disk swelling can generally be distinguished by the fact that visual acuity is seriously impaired at an early stage in retrobulbar neuritis. Furthermore, disk swelling is rarely as great in retrobulbar neuritis as in true papilloedema, while haemorrhages and exudates are uncommon in such cases; indeed the optic disk may look surprisingly normal even in the acute stage when the visual acuity is severely impaired. The typical history of this condition is one of progressive failure of vision in one eye, often associated with local pain, and usually leading to partial or total monocular blindness within a few hours or days. There is often complete recovery from this condition after several weeks or months, although a central scotoma may remain. Severe papilloedema due to increased intracranial pressure is often present, by contrast, without loss of visual acuity, though there may be some concentric diminution of the fields with enlargement of the blind spot, and the patient sees flashes of light or 'haloes' around lights, symptoms which may presage impending visual failure. These symptoms indicate that measures to reduce the intracranial pressure should be undertaken urgently, since if visual loss occurs as a result of papilloedema it is often complete and irreversible. Papilloedema can also result from severe arterial disease, as in **chronic nephritis** and **malignant hypertension,** from local lesions giving venous obstruction in the orbit or elsewhere (**central retinal vein thrombosis, cavernous sinus thrombosis, cor pulmonale**), or from **polycythaemia vera.** Occasionally, hyaline bodies lying on or in relation to the optic disk, which are present from birth, can give sufficient blurring of the disk margins (**pseudopapilloedema**) to make diagnosis from true papilloedema a matter of some difficulty.

The optic disk in patients with **optic atrophy** is chalky-white or grey in colour, its pallor being in striking contrast to the surrounding retina. The edges of the disk are clear-cut and often somewhat irregular. The form of optic atrophy which occurs in **disseminated sclerosis** and typically follows an attack of retrobulbar neuritis, although no history of such an episode may be obtained, typically affects the temporal half of the disk much more than the nasal, as the fibres from the macular area of the retina enter this part of the disk. This so-called **temporal pallor,** which is sometimes difficult to distinguish from the normal comparative pallor of the temporal part of the disk, except on the basis of experience, is almost diagnostic of disseminated sclerosis. Optic atrophy may also be an inherited degenerative disorder; it is a feature of **cerebral lipidosis** of the Tay–Sachs type (cerebromacular degeneration), in which case there may also be a cherry-red spot at the macula; it is also a common accompaniment of disease in the **hereditary ataxia** group (*see* Chapter 12). It also occurs in **retinitis pigmentosa,** a genetically-determined disorder which gives rise to progressive bilateral visual failure, usually in adult life, and in which there is also a spidery type of pigmentation of the periphery of the retina and narrowing of the retinal vessels.

Leber's optic atrophy is another inherited condition (usually due to a sex-linked recessive gene) in which bilateral optic atrophy often develops rapidly in young adult males. The history is often reminiscent of that seen in retrobulbar neuritis but vision does not recover. **Syphilis** is also an important cause; as many as 15 per cent of patients with tabes dorsalis, particularly of the congenital type, have very pale disks and the visual fields show peripheral constriction with enlargement of the blind spot. Of more immediate consequence as a cause of optic atrophy in neurological practice is **compression of the optic nerve,** whether by a tumour of the nerve itself or of its sheath, or by a meningioma, pituitary neoplasm or aneurysm which lies in relation to the nerve in its intracranial course. Less commonly a **head injury** will injure one optic nerve with a similar result, while severe papilloedema, glaucoma, choroidoretinitis and occlusion of the central retinal artery may all in time give rise to optic atrophy. When this condition develops as a sequel of long-standing papilloedema, it is often referred to as **secondary** or **consecutive optic atrophy.**

Changes in the **retinal vessels** also have considerable diagnostic value. The venous engorgement which occurs in papilloedema has already been mentioned. In subarachnoid haemorrhage, the rapid inflow of blood into the optic nerve sheath can give such severe venous obstruction that a large brick-red haemorrhage, known as a **subhyaloid haemorrhage,** is to be seen extending from the edge of the optic disk. Early changes of **atherosclerosis** and **hypertension** may take the form of slight 'silver-wiring' of the retinal arteries (Grade I retinopathy) with subsequent narrowing of the veins where the arteries cross them (Grade II); when the changes are more severe, flame-shaped haemorrhages and patches of hard white exudate appear in the retina (Grade III) and eventually papilloedema develops (Grade IV). In **diabetic** patients, small micro-aneurysms are sometimes found on peripheral retinal arteries. **Occlusion of the central artery of the retina** may give sudden unilateral blindness; the arteries are seen to be greatly reduced in calibre and optic atrophy follows. While this syndrome can result from atherosclerosis, in elderly patients it is not uncommonly due to **temporal arteritis,** and some thickening of the temporal arteries and other features of this disease will generally be found. Transient unilateral blindness is often due to embolism of the central retinal artery, and occurs most commonly in patients with carotid stenosis: emboli of platelets or cholesterol may be seen in retinal arteries during attacks.

Among other abnormalities of the retina which are of great diagnostic value are the **retinal angiomas** (tangles of abnormal blood vessels) found in patients with haemangioblastoma of the cerebellum (Lindau–von Hippel disease) and **retinal tubercles** (yellowish nodules, often about half the size of the optic disk) which will help to confirm a clinical diagnosis of tuberculous meningitis or miliary tuberculosis.

The Pupils

The parasympathetic nerve fibres which innervate the constrictor of the pupil travel in the trunk of the third cranial (oculomotor) nerve, while the sympathetic fibres responsible for pupillary dilatation arise in the hypothalamus and travel through the tegmentum of the brain stem and the cervical cord to the lateral horn of grey matter in the eighth cervical and first and second dorsal segments. They leave the spinal cord in the anterior roots and reach the superior cervical ganglion, from which postganglionic fibres arise which enter the skull in the plexus in the wall of the internal carotid artery. Some then pass to the ophthalmic division of the fifth (trigeminal) nerve and enter the orbit with its branches, while others go from the carotid plexus directly to the ciliary ganglion in the orbit, giving rise to the short ciliary nerves.

Both pupils normally constrict when a light is shone upon one retina; the reaction in the illuminated eye is called the direct reaction, that in the opposite eye the consensual one. The afferent pathway for the light reflex travels in the optic nerve to the lateral geniculate body and superior corpora quadrigemina and thence to the third nerve nuclei, whence efferent constrictor fibres arise. Hence a lesion on the afferent side of the pathway (e.g. optic atrophy) impairs both the direct and the consensual reaction to light, while a lesion in the efferent pathway (e.g. third nerve paralysis) to the eye which is being stimulated will affect the direct but not the consensual reaction. Constriction of the pupil also occurs when vision is focused upon a near object, a procedure which involves both accommodation (through contraction of the ciliary muscle) and convergence, and which is subserved by a complicated series of reflexes involving the oculomotor nuclei. Both the light and accommodation reactions of the pupils will be impaired by a lesion of the third nerve. Paralysis of the pupillary reaction to accommodation with preservation of the light reflex is a very rare finding, though it can occur occasionally in lesions of the mid-brain and may seem to be the case when ocular convergence is impaired, as sometimes occurs in post-encephalitic Parkinsonism. Loss of the light reflex with retention of that to accommodation is, however, seen as one feature of the **Argyll-Robertson pupil** of tabes dorsalis, a feature which is also present on occasion in association with general paresis. Additional features in this condition are that the pupils are small, irregular and unequal; there is atrophy of the iris, and loss of the ciliospinal reflex (pupillary dilatation on pinching the skin of the neck). There is some controversy concerning the situation of the lesion responsible for the Argyll–Robertson pupil; some believe it to be in the peri-aqueductal region of the mid-brain, while others have inferred that it is in the ciliary ganglion. In congenital syphilis, the light reflex may be lost, but in such cases the pupils are usually large and are not therefore of the typical Argyll–Robertson type.

A lesion of the **third nerve nucleus** or of the nerve in its intracranial course can give paralysis of the pupillo-constrictor muscles, so that the pupil becomes dilated and fixed. As the parasympathetic fibres lie relatively superficially in the nerve, along with those innervating the levator palpebrae superioris, this pupillary change may be the first sign of a third-nerve lesion, being followed by ptosis and later by external ophthalmoplegia. Pressure upon the nerve trunk by an aneurysm or pituitary neoplasm, and diabetes mellitus, are common causes of a unilateral third nerve palsy. A similar effect can result from herniation of the temporal lobe through the tentorial hiatus so that a unilateral fixed dilated pupil may be an early sign of a space-occupying lesion in or overlying one cerebral hemisphere (such as an extradural or subdural haematoma).

A lesion of the sympathetic pathway gives rise to a constricted pupil (myosis) and is generally accompanied by the other features of **Horner's syndrome** (myosis, ptosis, enophthalmos and loss of sweating on the affected side of the face). The lesion responsible may lie in the descending pathway in the brain stem (as in certain cases of brain stem infarction, e.g. posterior inferior cerebellar artery thrombosis), in the neck, involving one of the cervical sympathetic ganglia, or in the internal carotid artery (e.g. aneurysm). Sympathetic overactivity, due for instance to fright, dilates the pupils.

It should also be remembered that **drugs** have a profound influence upon pupillary size and activity. Myotics, which cause pupillary constriction, include morphine, pilocarpine, neostigmine and eserine, while mydriatics or dilators include the long-acting atropine, homatropine which is used to dilate the pupil for ophthalmoscopy, and cocaine. When the pupils are being examined it should also be remembered that **local ocular conditions** can influence their shape and size. Iridocyclitis, for instance, often gives irregularities of the iris and adhesions to the lens (synechiae), which may restrict the range of pupillary movement. **Hippus** is an interesting phenomenon of intermittent rhythmical pupillary contraction and dilatation; though it is sometimes observed in patients with neurological disease it has no diagnostic value.

Another interesting pupillary abnormality is generally known as the **myotonic pupil.** When, as is often the case, this pupillary abnormality is associated with sluggishness or absence of the tendon reflexes, the condition is referred to as **Adie's syndrome.** Characteristically the syndrome occurs in young women, though it is occasionally seen in males. The patient may notice the sudden onset of slight blurring of vision in one eye or alternatively she observes on looking into the mirror that one pupil is dilated. On examination the pupil is found to be widely dilated and to show a sluggish, delayed reaction to light. The reaction to accommodation is usually better but this too may be impaired and indeed it is occasionally impossible to produce pupillary constriction with either stimulus. The condition is essentially benign but its aetiology is unknown and it is uninfluenced by treatment.

The Eyelids and Orbital Muscles

That part of the levator palpebrae superioris which consists of voluntary muscle is innervated by the third cranial nerve but there is also a smooth muscle component (Muller's muscle) innervated by the sympathetic. Hence a paresis of the third nerve or of the sympathetic can give rise to **ptosis.** Ptosis can also be congenital and is then either unilateral or bilateral; it is also seen in myasthenia gravis when it characteristically worsens as the day wears on, in tabes dorsalis, and in myopathic degeneration of the external ocular muscles (ocular myopathy).

 Lid retraction, or a failure of the upper lid to follow the globe in downward movement of the eye, is typically seen in thyrotoxicosis in which condition **exophthalmos,** or protrusion of the eye is also common. The term **proptosis** is sometimes used to identify a unilateral exophthalmos, particularly when it is asymmetrical. Severe degrees of exophthalmos, sometimes unilateral, but more often bilateral, can result from excessive output of thyrotropic hormone by the anterior pituitary. In this condition there is considerable swelling of the external ocular muscles and orbital tissues and ophthalmoplegia is common (**exophthalmic** or **thyrotropic ophthalmoplegia**). Sometimes in exophthalmic ophthalmoplegia the condition begins with minimal exophthalmos, possibly on one side only and often with weakness limited to one superior rectus muscle. By contrast, severe painful exophthalmos with total paralysis of all ocular movement can develop in acute cases within a few days and papilloedema may ensue, so that urgent surgical decompression may be required. Other conditions which may give rise to exophthalmos include orbital tumour, 'pseudotumour' and other inflammatory lesions in the orbit or paranasal sinuses, retro-orbital intracranial tumours (meningiomas in particular) and thrombosis of, or arteriovenous aneurysm in, the cavernous sinus. A painless, symmetrical exophthalmos, often unilateral, is commonly due to an orbital pseudotumour in which inflammatory swelling of the orbital tissues, sometimes showing histological resemblances to the changes of polyarteritis nodosa, may be found. This condition, too, may require surgical decompression of the orbit, but in some cases there is a good response to treatment with steroid drugs. A mucocele of the ethmoid sinus, by contrast, usually gives a unilateral proptosis with lateral deviation and protrusion of the globe of the eye.

External Ocular Movement and its Abnormalities

Under normal circumstances of visual activity, the eyes do not move independently but a complex mechanism exists for the smooth co-ordination of movement of the two eyes in order that binocular vision may be preserved. Although the cerebral cortex exercises an overall influence upon ocular movement, and stimulation of a part of the frontal cortex produces deviation of the eyes to the opposite side, this mechanism is but poorly understood. It is, however, apparent that centres in the upper mid-brain exercise a controlling influence upon the co-ordinated activity of the nuclei of the third, fourth and sixth cranial nerves. This 'supranuclear' mechanism controls convergence of the eyes and conjugate ocular movements, that is simultaneous movement of the two eyes in an upward, downward or lateral direction. Thus it is that certain lesions of the upper mid-brain can produce a **supranuclear disorder of ocular movement,** so that the patient may be unable to converge or to move the eyes upwards or laterally. Such paralysis of conjugate ocular deviation is seen in tumours of the mid-brain region (glioma, pinealoma) and in mesencephalitis, whether resulting from syphilis or from a virus infection such as encephalitis lethargica. The lesions of Wernicke's encephalopathy resulting from vitamin B_1 deficiency may have a similar effect. A lesion of the pathways which connect the three cranial nerve nuclei concerned with ocular movement, a so-called **internuclear lesion,** may so derange ocular movement that the patient develops diplopia (double vision), possibly with divergence of the ocular axes, but without obvious paralysis of any single external ocular muscle. Internuclear lesions of this type are common in disseminated sclerosis, and often affect the posterior longitudinal bundle, which is the most important of the internuclear pathways. A common syndrome so produced is a failure or impairment of medial movement of either eye when the other looks laterally; often there is gross nystagmus in the abducting eye and this sign, which is virtually pathognomonic of disseminated sclerosis, has been called **ataxic nystagmus** (Harris's sign).

Lesions of the individual **cranial nerve nuclei** themselves (nuclear

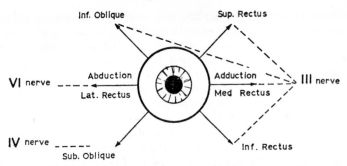

FIG. 3. A diagram of the direction in which the globe of the eye is moved by the muscles which are attached to it; the nerve supply of each of the muscles is also given.

lesions), or of the **nerve trunks** (infranuclear lesions) in their intra-cranial or extracranial course, produce defective ocular movement. This is observed on examination as a squint or strabismus, and the patient has diplopia due to false projection of the visual field by the eye whose movement is impaired. The directions in which the individual external ocular muscles move the globe and their nerve supply are illustrated in Fig. 3. From this it can be seen that observa-tion of the ocular movements when following a finger will generally reveal which muscle or muscles are paralysed and hence which cranial nerve is diseased. A paralytic squint which occurs under these circumstances gives rise to diplopia and must be distinguished from a concomitant squint, which is present at rest, equal in all positions of the eyes, and does not usually give rise to diplopia. Valuable information can also be obtained when diplopia is present, from the relationship of the two images to one another. For instance, if the lateral rectus is paralysed, when the patient looks laterally the object which is projected on to the macula of the normal eye is projected on to the nasal retina and hence to the temporal field of the paralysed eye so that this false image is lateral to the true one. These relationships can be more clearly defined by placing differently-coloured glasses over the two eyes.

Having confirmed which muscle or muscles are affected and hence which nerve is diseased, it is then necessary to decide the nature of the lesion responsible. A great many traumatic, inflammatory, neo-plastic and degenerative disorders arising in the brain stem or in the basal cisterns or orbital foramina can give rise to paralysis of one or more of the oculomotor nerves. In the brain stem itself, **infarcts, gliomas** and **Wernicke's disease** are the most common, while in the basal cisterns, the third, fourth or sixth nerves may be damaged by

trauma, meningitis, meningovascular syphilis, subarachnoid haemor-rhage or **tumour.** A third or sixth nerve palsy of sudden onset in an elderly person may result from compression of the trunk of the nerve by an **atherosclerotic artery** and these palsies generally clear up spontaneously in from three to six months. They are particularly common in patients with **diabetes mellitus.** The third nerve in particular is also vulnerable in patients with basal **arterial aneurysms** or **pituitary tumours,** while it can be paralysed as a result of a cerebral hemisphere lesion giving **tentorial herniation.** When complete third, fourth and sixth nerve palsies develop and are associated with sensory loss in the upper face, then an **aneurysm in the cavernous sinus,** compressing also the first and second divisions of the trigeminal nerve, which accompany these nerves within the sinus, is probable. A somewhat similar syndrome results from lesions in the neighbour-hood of the **superior orbital fissure.**

It should also be remembered that lesions of the myoneural junction and of the ocular muscles themselves can give rise to ptosis, strabismus and diplopia. In **myasthenia gravis,** for instance, drooping of the eyelids towards the end of the day and intermittent or fluctuant strabismus and diplopia are common. An uncommon condition in which there is a slowly progressive bilateral ptosis, with, eventually, impairment of ocular movement in all directions, is **ocular myopathy.** Most cases of this type were previously referred to as **progressive nuclear ophthalmoplegia** on the assumption that the disease was one of the oculomotor nuclei, but it is now recognised to be a progressive dystrophy of the external ocular muscles.

NYSTAGMUS

Nystagmus is a term applied to an oscillatory movement of the eyes which is often rhythmical and repetitive; it is sometimes present with the eyes at rest, but may only appear when they are moved conjugately, or, if present at rest, it may be accentuated by ocular movement. It can be rotary in type (occurring in more than one plane) or may occur only in a lateral or vertical direction. Occasion-ally both phases of the to-and-fro oscillation are of equal duration but more often there is a quick phase in one direction succeeded by a slower recoil; in this case the nystagmus is said to be occurring in the direction of the quick phase. This phenomenon is essentially a dis-order of the posture of the eyes and can be produced by disease of the reflex pathways which influence ocular posture. Stimuli from the retina and labyrinths play an important role in the maintenance of posture of the eyes as of other parts of the body and cerebellar activity is also of importance, so that lesions of any of these structures can give rise to nystagmus.

Congenital nystagmus, which may be familial, is a benign disorder of unknown aetiology in which a continuous pendular movement of the eyes occurs at rest and is often accentuated by movement of the head and eyes in any direction. It is usually asymptomatic. **Optokinetic nystagmus** is a physiological disturbance which occurs when the eyes are fixed upon a moving object such as a rotating drum or the landscape observed from a moving vehicle. The slow phase occurs in the direction in which the object moves and is followed by a quick recoil. Optokinetic nystagmus to one side may be lost as a result of a lesion of the contralateral temporal or parietal cortex and this has been used as a diagnostic test. **Nystagmus of peripheral origin** may be seen in any local ocular condition (such as amblyopia or optic atrophy) which impairs visual fixation; it may then be monocular, occurring only in the affected eye, and is generally pendular in type. Impairment of ocular fixation resulting from ocular muscle weakness, as in polyneuritis or rarely myasthenia gravis, may occasionally give a similar type of nystagmus. **Miner's nystagmus,** which is generally gross and pendular in type, has been attributed to impairment of visual fixation due to a disorder of macular vision which results from long periods of work in conditions of poor illumination, but there are usually many associated symptoms (headaches, giddiness) and there is no doubt that neurosis is an important complicating factor in many cases of this condition.

Nystagmus of labyrinthine origin can be evoked by caloric stimulation of the semicircular canals; if only the horizontal canals are stimulated it is lateral in type, but involvement of the vertical canals gives a rotary type which is therefore more common in disease of the internal ear, and the quick phase of the nystagmus takes place in a direction away from the affected ear. This is seen in acute labyrinthine vertigo (*vide infra*); the amplitude of the nystagmus is increased on looking to the side away from the lesion. Sometimes nystagmus is produced only by sudden movement of the head in a particular direction; this occurs in the benign disorder of the internal ear which is known as benign positional nystagmus, but is occasionally seen in lesions of the brain stem or in patients with neoplasms in the neighbourhood of the fourth ventricle.

The commonest causes of nystagmus in neurological practice are **lesions of the cerebellum or of cerebellar and vestibular connexions in the brain stem.** In a unilateral cerebellar lesion the nystagmus is increased on lateral deviation of the eyes towards the side of the lesion. So profuse are the structures in the brain stem which are concerned with cerebellar, vestibular and oculomotor function (the posterior longitudinal bundle is one of the most important) that virtually any lesion in this situation, whether inflammatory, neoplastic, degenerative or metabolic, gives rise to this physical sign; it is almost impossible to attribute any specific localising or diagnostic value to the sign under these circumstances, except in the case of the ataxic nystagmus previously mentioned. Often the nystagmus resulting from a brain-stem lesion occurs particularly on lateral movement of the eyes, the quick phase occurring towards the direction of gaze, but many other varieties occur. Statistically, disseminated sclerosis is the commonest cause, but encephalitis, vascular lesions, syringobulbia, Wernicke's encephalopathy and tumours can also produce this sign.

THE AUDITORY NERVE

Auditory impulses are received by the cells of the organ of Corti, travel along the peripheral process of the ganglion cells of the cochlea and thence in the auditory nerve to the cochlear nucleus in the pons; they then cross the midline and travel upwards in the lateral field to the inferior corpora quadrigemina and medial geniculate body; from this relay station they pass to the cortical centre for hearing in the middle and superior temporal gyri. The principal symptoms of disease of the auditory system are deafness and tinnitus. **Conduction or 'middle-ear' deafness** due to inflammation or otosclerosis should generally be distinguished by tuning-fork tests (*see* Chapter 3).

Nerve deafness can result from damage to Corti's organ as in Menière's disease (*vide infra*) or occupational deafness. Spread of inflammation from the middle ear will sometimes damage the cochlea, as may syphilis. Nerve deafness can of course be congenital (deaf-mutism), when it is usually due to an atresia of the cochlea and labyrinth. The auditory nerve in its intracranial course is sometimes damaged by inflammatory lesions (meningitis, meningovascular syphilis), by drugs or toxins (streptomycin) or by tumours, of which acoustic neuroma is the commonest. Nerve deafness resulting from a lesion of Corti's organ can sometimes be distinguished from that due to an acoustic nerve tumour by means of the recruitment test (*see* Chapter 3). Deafness resulting from lesions of the cochlear nucleus in the brain stem is extremely rare, and it is not produced by cortical lesions unless they are bilateral and extensive.

Tinnitus, or noise in the ears, is an important symptom of disease of the auditory nerve, though it can result from wax in the ear, or from Eustachian catarrh or middle-ear disease. Characteristically it is a hissing or machinery-like noise which may be unilateral or bilateral, continuous or intermittent. It is not infrequently severe in elderly people and can be so distressing as to interfere continuously with sleep and hearing, so that some individuals become almost suicidal; perhaps in such cases it is due to atherosclerotic ischaemia of the inner ear, though it is sometimes a manifestation of severe depression. Drugs such as quinine, salicylates and streptomycin will also produce this symptom. When unilateral, however, it may be an important symptom of disease of the labyrinth (e.g. Menière's disease) or of the auditory nerve (e.g. acoustic neuroma).

THE VESTIBULAR NERVE

The end-organs which subserve vestibular function are the semi-circular canals, which are concerned with the appreciation of movements of the head in any direction, and the utricle and saccule which convey information concerning the position of the head in relation to gravity. In the ampullae of the semicircular canals and in the utricle and saccule, where they lie in contact with the crystalline otoliths, are hair cells which transmit impulses to the cells of the vestibular ganglion of Scarpa. Thence they are conveyed by the vestibular nerve to the vestibular nuclei of the pons which have profuse connexions with the cerebellum, with the oculomotor nuclei via the posterior longitudinal bundle, and with the spinal cord via the vestibulospinal tract.

The most important symptom produced by disorders of the vestibular system is **vertigo.** Vertigo is the name which has been applied to a disorder of equilibrium characterised by a sensation of rotation of the self or of one's surroundings. Very often it is the objects around the patient which appear to be moving, either continuously in one direction or in a to-and-fro manner, but sometimes it is the patient who feels that it is he himself that is twisting or spinning or falling. Commonly the sensation is accompanied by staggering or even by actual falling, with clumsiness of the limbs, vomiting, depression and pallor. Nystagmus is generally present and in very severe cases the vision is blurred or momentarily lost while rarely transient loss of consciousness may occur. It is important to distinguish true vertigo from the mild 'giddiness' or 'swimming in the head' which is a common psychogenic disorder, or else may be due to a syncopal episode.

In considering the aetiology and diagnostic significance of vertigo it is important to remember the many functions and pathways which are concerned in the normal maintenance of posture, as disorders of a variety of different nervous pathways may give rise to this symptom. Firstly, visual impulses from the retina and from proprioceptive receptors in the external ocular muscles convey information concerning the relationship between the individual and his surroundings.

F

Thus we can experience transient vertigo when looking down from heights or when observing a rapidly-moving object. Secondly, the importance of the labyrinth must be stressed; the commonest forms of vertigo are of aural origin and will be discussed below. Thirdly, and closely related to labyrinthine function, are the proprioceptive impulses derived from neck muscles, while similar stimuli from the muscles of the trunk and limbs give information concerning the position of the body. Whereas lesions of these proprioceptive pathways do not usually produce vertigo it may, however, result from disorders of the central co-ordinating mechanisms in the brain stem and of the cerebellum; the latter is an important part of the efferent rather than afferent mechanisms controlling posture. Lesions of the cerebral cortex rarely cause vertigo, although this symptom has been described as the aura of an epileptic fit and can occasionally result from tumours of the temporal lobe. Even though the cerebellum is of such importance in the control of posture, it is comparatively uncommon for lesions of this structure, however massive, to give rise to vertigo. Brain-stem lesions involving central cerebellar connexions, however, may produce this symptom in severe form. Whereas it may result from **encephalitis, pontine tumours** or **syringobulbia,** the two most common causes of vertigo due to lesions in this situation are **disseminated sclerosis** and **infarction** or transient ischaemia. Occasionally the first symptom of disseminated sclerosis is a sudden severe attack of vertigo, often lasting for hours or days, and associated with severe nystagmus and perhaps with other signs of a brain-stem lesion. The lateral medullary infarct produced by posterior inferior cerebellar artery thrombosis characteristically produces sudden vertigo, vomiting and prostration as an initial manifestation, while less severe attacks can occur as a feature of the recurrent ischaemic episodes of basilar artery insufficiency.

Lesions of the labyrinth itself are, however, the most frequent cause of vertigo. Whereas some patients with compression or irritation of the eighth nerve, say, by an acoustic neuroma, suffer from it intermittently, disease of the internal ear is usually responsible. The sudden onset of vertigo may result from an extension of a middle-ear infection to the labyrinth, but an **'acute vestibular neuronitis',** often erroneously called 'labyrinthitis', can occur without a preceding middle-ear infection. In such a case vertigo develops suddenly and is generally associated with severe vomiting and prostration, some ataxia of the homolateral limbs, and a rotary nystagmus to the opposite side. The patient is often pyrexial and the illness may last several hours, days or weeks. The condition can occur in epidemic form and some believe it to be an acute virus infection of the brain stem, involving vestibular nuclei, rather than a labyrinthitis, as diplopia and a lymphocytic pleocytosis in the cerebrospinal fluid may occasionally be found. Hence the title 'epidemic vertigo' is often preferred, even for sporadic cases. The distinction between this and a first episode of disseminated sclerosis due to a plaque in the brain stem can be very difficult and often depends solely upon the subsequent course, as acute vestibular neuronitis generally recovers completely, whereas in disseminated sclerosis subsequent manifestations of neurological disease are to be expected. Even in the benign labyrinthine disorder, however, one or more relapses may occur within the first few months.

Menière's syndrome (recurrent aural vertigo) is a condition characterised by the occurrence of recurrent attacks of vertigo, often with vomiting and prostration, and accompanied by unilateral tinnitus and progressive nerve deafness. The condition can occur at any age, but is rare in young children; it is commonest in middle life and is somewhat more frequent in males. It appears to be due to a hydrops of the membranous labyrinth, of unknown aetiology, resulting in dilatation of the endolymph system with consequent pressure atrophy of the organ of Corti. Sometimes the deafness and tinnitus have been present for some time before the attacks of vertigo develop but often the latter are the initial manifestations. Attacks may initially be mild and brief, increasing in severity and frequency, but the manifestations are extremely variable. Typically a sudden attack of vertigo occurs with unsteadiness, vomiting and prostration and can be so violent that the patient is literally thrown to the ground. Pallor, perspiration, depression and tachycardia are common accompaniments and rotary nystagmus is present. Occasionally transient loss of consciousness due to syncope occurs in a severe attack. The attack may last only a few minutes or several hours but the patient is sometimes lethargic, unsteady and depressed for several days afterwards. The episodes can occur at intervals of a few days, weeks or even months, but tend to become increasingly less frequent and eventually to disappear completely when deafness is complete in the affected ear. Unfortunately the contralateral ear is occasionally affected, sometimes concurrently but more often subsequently.

A somewhat similar condition which gives rise to episodic attacks of vertigo is the so-called benign positional nystagmus, which results from a degenerative lesion, again of unknown aetiology, in the otolith of the utricle and saccule. In this condition, however, the attacks of vertigo occur only on certain particular movements of the head (e.g. stooping or lying down on one side) and can be reproduced at will by carrying out this movement. Most patients learn to avoid the offending position which evokes the attacks.

Motion-sickness is also a closely related disorder, and is due to the stereotyped repetitive stimulation of the semicircular canals produced by movement of a motor car, ship, train or aeroplane. There is a wide variation in individual susceptibility. Commonly lassitude, vague depression and drowsiness are the earliest manifestations and are followed by vomiting and vertigo, though the latter is not usually severe. A considerable degree of adaptation usually occurs in the habitual traveller.

TASTE

Taste fibres from the anterior two-thirds of the tongue travel through the lingual nerve to the chorda tympani, joining the facial nerve at the geniculate ganglion and proceeding to the pons in the pars intermedia which lies alongside the facial nerve. Taste sensations from the posterior one-third of the tongue are conveyed by the glossopharyngeal nerve. In the pons the fibres of these nerves enter the tractus solitarius, cross the midline and proceed in the gustatory fillet to the optic thalamus whence they are conveyed to the lower end of the postcentral gyrus.

Loss of taste (**ageusia**) on the anterior two-thirds of the tongue can result from lesions of the geniculate ganglion. A facial paralysis due to a lesion at or proximal to this point is usually associated therefore with loss of taste, while one resulting from a more distally-situated lesion is not. A lesion of the glossopharyngeal nerve will result in loss of taste on the posterior third of the tongue on the same side, but taste sensation is so difficult to test with even a reasonable degree of accuracy, that disorders of this sense have little value in clinical neurological diagnosis.

REFERENCES

BRAIN, W. R., *Diseases of the Nervous System*, 6th ed., (London, Oxford University Press, 1962).

COGAN, D. G., *Neurology of the Ocular Muscles*, 3rd ed. (Springfield, Ill., Thomas, 1963).

GARDNER, E., *Fundamentals of Neurology*, 4th ed., Chapter 12 (Philadelphia and London, Saunders, 1963).

MAYO CLINIC, SECTION OF NEUROLOGY, 'The cranial nerves, and neuro-ophthalmology', in *Clinical Examinations in Neurology*, Chapters 4 and 5 (Philadelphia and London, Saunders, 1956).

TRAQUAIR, H. M., *An Introduction to Clinical Perimetry*, 3rd ed. (London, Kimpton, 1938).

VICTOR, M. and ADAMS, R. D., 'Vertigo and Disorders of Equilibrium and Gait' and 'Disturbances of Cranial Nerve Function', in *Principles of Internal Medicine*, Ed. Harrison, T. R., 4th ed., Chapters 30 and 31 (New York, McGraw-Hill, 1962).

CHAPTER 9

THE MOTOR SYSTEM

Disorders of movement of the parts of the body produce some of the commonest symptoms professed by patients with disease or disordered function of the nervous system. Sometimes the ability to move a part in response to the will is impaired (weakness or paresis) and sometimes it is lost completely (paralysis). On other occasions, willed movements are clumsy, ill-directed or uncontrolled (ataxia or inco-ordination), or else the part moves spontaneously or independently of the will (involuntary movements). On physical examination the examiner may be able to confirm the presence of these abnormalities and may also discover abnormalities of tone in which the normal response to passive stretching of a muscle is altered; it can be reduced (hypotonia) or increased in one of two ways (spasticity, rigidity). Abnormalities of this type, and particularly weakness or paralysis, are sometimes emotionally determined (hysteria); alternatively they can be apraxic, resulting from a cortical lesion which has impaired the ability to recall acquired motor skills (*see* Chapter 5). More often, however, they are due to a disturbance in function of the motor pathway which begins in the motor area of the cerebral cortex and ends in the voluntary musculature. There are a number of important physical signs which assist in the localisation of lesions within this motor apparatus, but for a full appreciation of their significance a working knowledge of its anatomy, and of the influences which play upon it, is essential.

ANATOMY AND PHYSIOLOGY

The **upper motor neurones,** which constitute the pyramidal or corticospinal tracts, arise in part from nerve cells in the motor cortex of the cerebrum. This area of cortex lies anterior to the Rolandic fissure, in the precentral convolution. Whereas some of these neurones arise from the giant Betz cells which are common in this area, there are far more fibres in the pyramidal tracts than could be accounted for by the axons of all the Betz cells, so that many of the other upper motor neurones must arise from nerve cells in or near this area which are not structurally distinctive. Stimulation experiments have revealed that activation of cells in the lower end of the precentral gyrus will cause bilateral movement of the pharynx and

145

larynx, while just above are others which, if stimulated, give rise to movement of the contralateral half of the tongue (Figs. 4A, B, C). Facial movement can be elicited at a point slightly higher still and it is of interest that stimulation will give bilateral movement of the upper face but unilateral movement only of the lower face. Movement of the contralateral hand, arm, trunk, leg and foot will then be produced in turn as one ascends the gyrus, and in each case 'representation' is strictly unilateral. The leg and foot 'area' in fact lies partly on the medial surface of the hemisphere and partly on its superior aspect. Nerve fibres arising from the cells in this cortical area then come

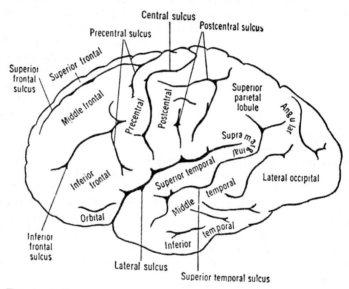

FIG. 4A. A diagram of the lateral aspect of the left cerebral hemisphere.
(From *Fundamentals of Neurology* by E. Gardner, 4th edition, Saunders, Philadelphia and London 1963).

together in the corona radiata and converge upon the internal capsule which lies deep in the hemisphere between the thalamus and caudate nucleus medially and the lenticular nucleus laterally (Fig. 5). The pyramidal tract occupies the posterior one-third of the anterior limb, the genu, and the anterior two-thirds of the posterior limb of the capsule. Behind it lie sensory fibres travelling to the postcentral sensory cortex and then others forming the optic radiation, while anteriorly are fronto-pontine fibres. From the internal capsule the tract passes down in the middle three-fifths of the cerebral peduncle to enter the mid-brain; in the pons it is broken into bundles by transverse pontine fibres, but in the medulla it again becomes a compact tract, the pyramid, which forms an anterior prominence. Throughout the brain stem the tract gives off fibres which travel to the contralateral motor nuclei of the cranial nerves. In the lower part of the medulla, the majority of the fibres in the pyramidal tract decussate to form the crossed pyramidal tract which travels down in the lateral column of the spinal cord on the opposite side, but a small

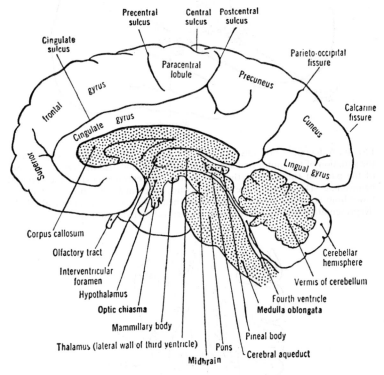

FIG. 4B. A diagram of the medial aspect of the right cerebral hemisphere.
(From *Fundamentals of Neurology*, by E. Gardner, 4th edition, Saunders, Philadelphia and London, 1963).

proportion do not do so and continue downwards in the anterior column of the cord, forming the direct or uncrossed pyramidal tract (Fig. 6). Fibres of the pyramidal tract do not as a rule synapse directly with the anterior horn cells from which the lower motor neurones arise, but rather with internuncial neurones in the grey matter of the spinal cord, which in turn pass on to synapse in the anterior horns.

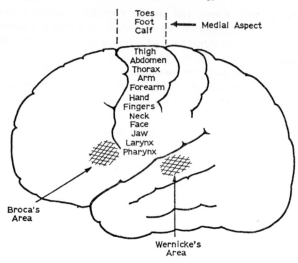

FIG. 4C. A diagram of the lateral aspect of the left cerebral hemisphere indicating the situation of the motor and sensory speech areas and also the 'representation' of the parts of the body in the motor area (precentral gyrus) of the cerebral hemisphere. The areas of the motor cortex concerned with movement of the lower limb lie on the medial aspect of the hemisphere in the paracentral lobule. 'Representation' in the sensory area (postcentral gyrus) is similar.

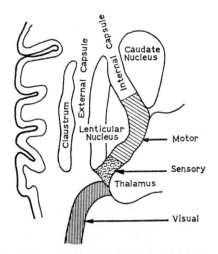

FIG. 5. A diagram of the internal capsule, cut in a horizontal plane, indicating the portions of the capsule occupied by the principal motor and sensory pathways, and the relationship of the capsule to the principal nuclei of the basal ganglia.

(Redrawn from *Introduction to Clinical Neurology*, by G. Holmes, Livingstone, Edinburgh, 1946.)

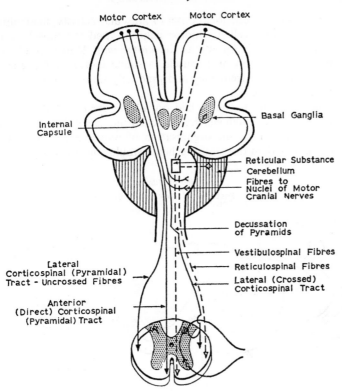

FIG. 6. A diagram of the principal pathways of the motor system. The continuous lines represent pathways of the pyramidal system, the interrupted lines those of the extrapyramidal system. The nuclear masses of the basal ganglia, the brainstem reticular substance, and the dentate nucleus of the cerebellum, which are some of the most important relay stations in the extrapyramidal system, are represented diagrammatically.

(Redrawn from *Fundamentals of Neurology*, by E. Gardner, 4th edition, Saunders Philadelphia and London, 1963.)

The **lower motor neurones,** which transmit impulses from the anterior horn cells of the spinal cord to the voluntary muscles, constitute the final common path of motor activity (Fig. 7). In other words, all nervous mechanisms which influence muscular activity must produce their final effects through impulses which travel along these fibres. The axon of one anterior horn cell never innervates a single muscle fibre, but always a group of fibres which therefore contract simultaneously whenever the anterior horn cell discharges. These muscle fibres may all be gathered together in a single bundle or fasciculus or else they may lie in several fasciculi throughout the

F*

muscle. This basic functional onset of muscular activity, made up of one anterior horn cell, its motor neurone, and the muscle fibres which it supplies, is known as the *motor unit*. During graduated voluntary contraction of a muscle, a single motor unit begins to fire with increasing frequency and gradually more and more of its fellows are recruited.

In the anatomical schema laid out above are outlined the basic functional units through which a muscular movement is initiated and performed. However, the organisation of movement is very much more complex than this simple schema would suggest. For instance,

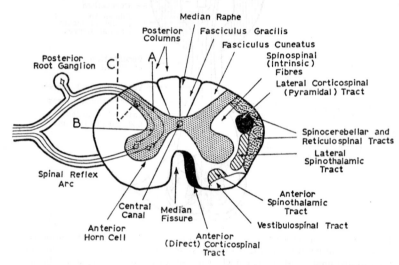

FIG. 7. Diagrammatic representation of the reflex arc and of the principal fibre tracts of the spinal cord. *A*, a simple two-neurone reflex arc. *B*, a three-neurone reflex arc with an internuncial neurone between the sensory and motor neurones. *C*, a corticospinal fibre influencing the activity of the reflex arc.

no single cell in the motor area of the cerebral cortex can be said to innervate any single muscle. Stimulation experiments have revealed that it is not single muscle twitches, but organised movements, which are initiated in the motor cortex. These movements involve several muscles or muscle groups, of which only some act as prime movers or agonists. Others, the antagonists, must be enabled to relax smoothly as the agonists contract, while yet others are required to fix a limb proximally, say, in order to allow a movement which is occurring distally to be efficient. Other muscles, or synergists, may also be brought into play in order to counteract unwanted effects which would be produced by the unmodified action of the agonists. The profusion of internuncial neurones in the spinal cord, which receive impulses from many pyramidal axons and may influence many anterior horn cells, are clearly important in this organisation. However, incoming sensory impulses from stretch receptors (muscle spindles) in the muscles themselves, as well as other proprioceptive sensations which continually inform the individual of the position of the part which is being moved, can also modify this activity through a series of spinal reflexes. Additional modifying influences are exerted through sensory impulses from the eyes and labyrinths which enter the brain stem and initiate activity in the vestibulospinal tracts.

Not only can sensory impulses influence movement in this way, but additional important effects are exerted by the so-called **extra-pyramidal motor system.** Several of the nuclear masses in the basal ganglia and upper brain stem, and particularly the lenticular and caudate nuclei, the subthalamic nuclei, the substantia nigra, the brain stem reticular formation and the olivary nuclei, exercise profound controlling influences upon movement. The details of the complex neural mechanisms subserved by these structures are poorly understood, though the disturbances which appear when they are diseased make their importance manifest. So too with the **cerebellum and its connexions;** this organ has an overall controlling influence upon posture, muscular tone and the co-ordination of movement. These structures all exercise their effects through a series of brain stem and spinal relay neurones which, though they may influence profoundly the activity of the pyramidal tract, are yet quite independent of it and are therefore called extrapyramidal (Fig. 6).

We presume that a particular movement is initiated when the idea of the movement is first invoked in the 'association' areas of the cortex. The appropriate motor cells of the precentral cortex are then activated and impulses travel down the pyramidal tracts, in order to activate the appropriate anterior horn cells and their motor units. Simultaneously the movement is being influenced and controlled by the activity of the cerebellum and of the components of the extra-pyramidal motor system; at the same time as the agonists are being stimulated to contract, the synergists to assist and the fixators to fix, an inhibitory mechanism must be invoked to produce controlled relaxation of the antagonists. Once the movement has begun it will then be subject to continued modification depending upon sensory impulses arriving from the proprioceptors, or from the eyes and labyrinths. Clearly, therefore, in view of its complexity, movement can be disorganised by lesions of many different nervous pathways, and some of the principles which aid in deciding which pathway or pathways are diseased will be considered below.

WEAKNESS AND PARALYSIS

Weakness (paresis) of a group of muscles implies that the power produced on voluntary contraction of the affected muscles is reduced, whereas complete paralysis indicates that the power to move the part concerned is totally lost. Weakness of one limb is referred to as a **monoparesis,** while total paralysis of a limb is called a **monoplegia.** **Hemiplegia** is the term utilised to identify paralysis which afflicts one side of the body, and particularly the arm and leg, while **paraplegia** signifies a paralysis of both lower limbs. When all four limbs are paralysed, the terms **quadriplegia** or **tetraplegia** are used; a symmetrical weakness of all four limbs, affecting the lower more markedly than the upper, and occurring in children with cerebral palsy, is often called a **diplegia.** The term 'palsy' can be used interchangeably with 'paralysis', but is more often utilised in modern neurological practice to identify the paralysis of individual muscles or muscle groups which results from peripheral nerve lesions.

Paralysis may result from a lesion of the upper motor neurone or of the lower motor neurone, and under certain circumstances it can be due to a defect in conduction at the neuromuscular junction or to a biochemical or structural abnormality of the muscle fibre itself. Clinical methods of differentiating between these causes of paralysis will be discussed below.

DISORDERS OF TONE

The tone of a muscle can be regarded as the response it shows to passive stretching. Contrary to the views once held, a completely relaxed and resting muscle is not in a state of continuous partial contraction; it has elasticity, but no tone. Tone can only therefore be assessed when the muscle is moved or when it is concerned with maintaining a posture against an applied force such as that of gravity. **Postural tone** can thus be considered to be that state of partial contraction of certain muscles which is needed to maintain the posture of the parts of the body; clearly the muscles involved and the force of muscular contraction required will depend upon the position of the parts concerned at any one time.

In neurological practice, tone is usually assessed by moving a limb or some other part passively and by observing the reaction which occurs in the muscles which are being stretched. The moment this stretching begins, stretch receptors in the muscle concerned, and particularly the muscle spindles, give out afferent stimuli and reflex partial contraction of the muscle results. Variations in the degree of sensitivity of this reflex, which is also responsible for the tendon reflexes, account for the alterations in tone which occur as a result of nervous disease.

On stretching, the tone of the muscle may be increased (spasticity or rigidity or hypertonia) or it may be reduced (flaccidity or hypotonia) and these alterations are of great value in neurological diagnosis.

Spasticity is one type of increased tone or hypertonia. It occurs in patients with disease or dysfunction of the corticospinal or pyramidal tracts. It appears that the pyramidal tracts normally exercise an inhibitory function over spinal reflexes and when this tract is diseased, stretch reflexes are greatly exaggerated. Thus the affected limb or limbs show an increase in resistance to passive stretching; this resistance is particularly severe initially, but then tends to 'give' suddenly as the movement is continued. Hence this sign, seen particularly well in the legs of a patient with a spastic paraplegia due to bilateral pyramidal tract disease, is known as 'clasp-knife' rigidity. In individuals with spastic weakness, movement is impaired owing to defective conduction of motor impulses by the pyramidal tracts, while there is also 'clasp-knife' rigidity on passive movement. **Rigidity** of extrapyramidal type, in patients with disease of the basal ganglia or substantia nigra, is essentially different. It is seen characteristically in Parkinsonism. In such cases the rigidity is either uniform in degree throughout the entire range of passive movement, in which case it is known as 'plastic' or 'lead-pipe' rigidity, or else it intermittently 'gives' and returns throughout the movement, being then referred to as 'cog-wheel' in type. A particular form of muscular rigidity, known as **decerebrate rigidity,** develops as a result of severe transverse lesions of the upper mid-brain. In such a case all four limbs are rigidly extended, the back is arched and there may be neck retraction, so that the patient, if lying supine, is virtually supported by the back of the head and the heels. This posture is known as **opisthotonus;** the arching of the back can be increased by any sensory stimulus and there is striking resistance to any attempt at flexing the limbs passively.

Flaccidity, or **hypotonia,** is a reduction in tone. In severe degrees of the phenomenon, as in patients with total flaccid paralysis, all resistance to passive stretch is lost and the limbs are limp and flail-like. Lesser degrees of hypotonia in the upper limbs, for instance, can be elicited by asking the patient to hold out his arms horizontally in front of him. The forearms are then tapped briskly; when tone is increased (spasticity) the recoil is sharp, immediate and exaggerated. When one limb is hypotonic the recoil is slower and the arm swings through a wider range. If the patient is asked to contract the biceps brachii against resistance, by bending the arm towards his face, and the examiner's restraining hand is suddenly removed, the patient's hand may strike his face if the limb is hypotonic, whereas if the tone is normal he will be able to stop the movement before it does so. Furthermore, if the subject is asked to raise his arms above his head with the palms facing forwards, the palm of a hypotonic limb will be seen to be externally rotated and facing more laterally than the other. In the lower limbs it is useful to place one's hands beneath the knee and to lift the leg from the bed, then to allow it to fall back quickly; with experience it will soon be possible to judge from the resistance which the limb shows to this movement, whether tone is increased or reduced.

ATAXIA AND INCO-ORDINATION

Ataxia is essentially a clumsiness of motor activity, resulting from an inability to control accurately the range and precision of movement. It can result from a defect in the sensory pathways responsible for the transmission of proprioceptive information from sensory receptors in the periphery. Under such circumstances the appreciation of the position of the parts of the body in space is impaired, and since controlled movement requires continuous and accurate information of this nature for its continued performance, it may be seriously deranged. This phenomenon, which is known as **sensory ataxia,** will be considered in detail in Chapter 10. In such a case, the cause of the unsteadiness will become apparent on sensory examination. Similarly, sensory stimuli from the labyrinths are of great importance in the maintenance of posture and if, as a result of disease of the labyrinths, of the vestibular nerves or of their central connexions, distorted information concerning the position of the head is received, the patient's gait will become grossly unsteady and the movements of his limbs clumsy and poorly controlled. Thus ataxia may also be the result of **labyrinthine dysfunction.**

Perhaps most common of all as a cause of ataxia is **disease of the cerebellum** or of its central connexions in the brain stem. The controlling activity of the cerebellum upon the motor system is concerned particularly with the fine co-ordination of movement and with the judgement of distance; it is these faculties which are selectively impaired as a result of cerebellar disease. Much depends upon which part of the cerebellum or its connecting pathways is diseased, but a detailed consideration of cerebellar anatomy and physiology is beyond the scope of this volume and it will only be necessary to describe a number of general principles which lead one to conclude that the function of the cerebellum or of cerebellar pathways is impaired. In general it can be said that central cerebellar structures, the vermis and flocculonodular lobe, have predominantly vestibular connexions and are concerned particularly with equilibration. Hence lesions in this situation will produce an ataxia which involves central structures of the body and is thus particularly apparent when the patient walks. The patient is unsteady and staggers in a drunken manner; he walks on a wide base and has considerable difficulty in stopping suddenly or in turning. There may also be a rhythmical nodding or 'titubating' tremor of head. In such a case the tests of cerebellar function to be described below, which are concerned with the demonstration of ataxia in lateral structures, such as the limbs, may be singularly uninformative. Because these tests are negative it is a common pitfall to regard such patients as hysterical, particularly if the doctor fails to recognise that a cerebellar lesion which is centrally situated gives this particular type of so-called **truncal or central ataxia.** This type of disturbance is particularly well seen in children with medulloblastomas.

Lesions of the lateral cerebellar hemispheres, affecting the so-called neocerebellum, give rise to a number of physical signs which are more readily identifiable. If the lesion is predominantly unilateral, then these signs are apparent in the limbs on the same side as the lesion. There may also be **ocular signs;** thus in an acute cerebellar lesion *skew deviation* is occasionally seen, in which the eye on the affected side is deviated downwards and inwards, while the contralateral eye is turned upwards and out. *Nystagmus* is also prominent, being of greatest amplitude on looking to the side of the lesion. **Hypotonia** is often present in the ipsilateral limbs, and **ataxia** is evidenced by a striking clumsiness and inco-ordination of movement. The patient is unable to button his clothes and his hand-writing is scrawling and illegible. Judgement of distance is grossly impaired, a phenomenon known as **dysmetria,** and the hand performing a movement may wildly overshoot the mark (**past-pointing**). Tremor of the limbs may be apparent at rest but is greatly accentuated by movement, being worse towards the end of an action (**intention-tremor**). These signs are particularly apparent on carrying out the 'finger–nose' and 'heel–knee' tests and there will also be a gross irregularity of movement if the patient is asked to tap quickly and repetitively upon a smooth surface, or to make dots within a small circle with a pencil. Rapid alternating movements of the limbs, such as pronation and supination of the forearms, are poorly and jerkily performed (**dysdiadochokinesis**). The patient with a unilateral cerebellar lesion also tends to stagger and to deviate towards the affected side when walking. A minimal cerebellar lesion on one side can sometimes be identified most easily by asking the patient to walk a few paces with his eyes closed, when he will deviate to the affected side.

THE REFLEXES

The simplest form of a reflex arc consists of an afferent or sensory neurone and an efferent or motor neurone with whose parent cell the terminal fibres of the afferent neurone synapse (Fig. 7). Stimulation of the sensory neurone will then produce a motor response mediated by the motor neurone. Few reflexes are as simple as this, though the spinal reflex arc by means of which withdrawal of a limb follows upon painful stimulation cannot be much more complex. In many pathways concerned with reflex activity, however, the sensory and motor neurones are separated by connecting or internuncial neurones, most of which lie in the grey matter of the spinal cord; they receive impulses from ascending and descending fibre pathways which exercise important controlling influences upon reflex activity. Unquestionably there are some very long reflex pathways which run a course involving brain stem as well as spinal structures, while some may even traverse the cerebral cortex. There are many reflexes which are concerned with autonomic and visceromotor activity, and even endocrine secretion, but in clinical neurology we are largely concerned with the simpler reflexes which, when activated, result in somatic motor activity.

Clearly reflex activity will be lost or impaired if a lesion is present at any point in the reflex arc. Thus a break in the afferent pathway or in the efferent pathway will mean that a particular form of reflex activity can no longer be obtained. For instance, the **corneal reflex** (the contraction of the orbicularis oculi which follows stimulation of the cornea) may be lost if the cornea is anaesthetic as a result of a lesion of the trigeminal nerve or if the face is paralysed due to a lesion of the seventh nerve. Similarly, the **palatal and pharyngeal reflexes** which result in contraction of the soft palate or pharynx on tactile stimulation may be impaired unilaterally. This occurs if one trigeminal (palate) or glossopharyngeal (pharyngeal) nerve is diseased (the afferent pathway), or if there is a lesion of the vagus nerve (the efferent pathway).

The reflexes which are most informative in the physical examination of patients with nervous disease are the stretch and cutaneous reflexes.

The first of the **stretch reflexes** is the *jaw jerk*, elicited by means of a sharp downward tap on the chin with the mouth held partly open. A positive response consists in contraction of the masseters with elevation of the lower jaw; if this reflex is exaggerated it usually indicates a bilateral pyramidal tract lesion in or above the upper brain stem.

The stretch reflexes normally utilised on examination of the limbs are the so-called **tendon reflexes.** These consist in a reflex contraction of the muscle concerned, produced in practice by a sharp blow upon the tendon of the muscle near its point of insertion. Those commonly elicited have been described in Chapter 2. In the upper limb they are the biceps and radial jerks which obtain their motor innervation from the fifth and sixth cervical roots, the triceps jerk which is mainly innervated by the seventh and the finger jerk which receives its supply from the seventh and eighth roots. In the lower limbs, the knee jerk is innervated by the second, third and fourth lumbar roots, the ankle jerk by the first and second sacral. Any of the tendon reflexes can be diminished or lost if there is a lesion of the sensory pathway which carries afferent impulses from the muscle to the spinal cord, if there is a lesion of the lower motor neurones supplying the muscle concerned at any point along its course, or even if a primary disorder of the muscle itself, a myopathy, has impaired its ability to contract. These reflexes are also lost temporarily during the stage of so-called 'shock' which follows upon an acute destructive lesion of the brain or spinal cord, even if there is no break in the reflex arc. All the tendon reflexes may be symmetrically exaggerated by tension and anxiety or by increased neuromuscular excitability arising from metabolic or other causes, but there is no doubt that the reflexes are most strikingly increased when there is a lesion of the pyramidal tract. A unilateral lesion of this tract is particularly easy to identify, as the reflexes are exaggerated on one side of the body and not on the other. The finger jerk, for instance, is normally present in some patients and not in others; it is only of real significance if it is present unilaterally. The phenomenon of *clonus* is a direct result of exaggeration of the stretch reflexes. It consists of an intermittent muscular contraction and relaxation evoked by sustained stretching of a muscle; it can occur apparently spontaneously in spastic limbs, but is best elicited as a physical sign in the lower limbs by sudden pressure applied in a distal direction to the upper margin of the patella, or by a sharp dorsiflexion of the foot carried out with the leg extended.

Inversion of the upper-limb reflexes may be an important physical sign of spinal cord disease. Thus if there is a lesion of the C5 or C6 segments of the spinal cord, this will break the reflex arc for reflexes innervated by these segments, namely the biceps and radial jerks, which are therefore lost or diminished. If, however, the same lesion is compressing the spinal cord and giving pyramidal tract dysfunction, reflexes innervated by lower segments of the cord (triceps, finger jerks) are exaggerated and can be obtained by stimuli applied over a wide field. Thus tapping the biceps tendon may produce contraction of triceps, while on attempting to elicit the radial jerk, finger flexion, but no radial jerk, is obtained. This so-called inversion of either of these reflexes is diagnostic of a cervical cord lesion.

The **cutaneous or superficial reflexes** which are commonly utilised in neurological diagnosis are the abdominal reflexes, the cremasteric reflex, the anal reflex and the plantar reflex. The *abdominal reflexes* are elicited by stroking the skin of the abdomen (the point of a pin is a suitable instrument) when movement of the umbilicus towards the stimulus should follow. The level of a segmental lesion in the dorsal portion of the spinal cord can sometimes be identified by loss of the lower abdominal reflexes and preservation of the upper. Even more useful is the fact that the abdominal reflexes are unilaterally diminished in amplitude or lost, or may simply fatigue rapidly on repetitive stimulation, when there is a lesion of the pyramidal tract on the same side of the body. There are certain conditions (e.g. disseminated sclerosis) in which the abdominal reflexes may be lost at a comparatively early stage of the disease, whereas in others (e.g. motor neurone disease), in which there also is evidence of pyramidal tract disease, they often survive to a relatively late stage. Total absence of the abdominal reflexes is usually a finding of definite pathological significance, except in the very obese, in multipara with lax abdominal muscles, and in the elderly. The *cremasteric reflex* (contraction of the cremaster on stroking the medial side of the thigh) is also impaired or lost as a result of a pyramidal tract lesion. The *anal reflex* (contraction of the external sphincter on scratching the perianal skin) is particularly likely to be lost when there is a lesion of the cauda equina involving the fourth and fifth sacral roots.

One of the most important reflexes in clinical neurology is the **plantar response.** On stroking the lateral aspect of the sole of the foot from the heel towards the fifth toe, there is normally plantar-flexion of all five toes (the flexor response). The abnormal response which consists of a dorsiflexion of the great toe and a simultaneous downward and 'fanning-out' movement of the remaining toes, is known as an extensor response or the Babinski response. The Babinski response refers only to the abnormal or extensor type of reflex movement and it is semantically inaccurate to say that 'the Babinski was negative or positive'. It is far better to avoid the eponymous term and to refer to the plantar response as being 'flexor' or 'extensor'. An extensor plantar reflex is virtually diagnostic of a lesion of the pyramidal tract at any point in its course from the contralateral motor cortex down through the brain stem and the ipsilateral lateral column of the spinal cord. It is essentially part of a primitive withdrawal response 'uncovered' or 'released' by a pyramidal tract lesion; often, along with the extensor plantar response, there is also contraction of the hamstrings. Indeed, if the spinal cord lesion is severe and complete, stroking the sole will also evoke flexion at the hip and knee and even evacuation of the bladder and bowels (a 'mass' reflex). In such a case the extensor plantar response is readily elicited by a variety of stimuli applied over a wide area (e.g. pressure upon the shin bone, pricking the leg with a pin, etc.).

Among the many other forms of reflex activity which are altered by nervous disease there are few which are of sufficient practical importance to be mentioned here. It is, however, worth noting that in decerebrate patients, as in neonates, the **tonic neck reflexes** may be greatly exaggerated so that on forcibly turning the head to one side the limbs on that side extend while the contralateral limbs flex (Magnus–de Klejn reflex). Persistence of this reflex response after the first three months of life, and of the Moro reflex (flexion of all four limbs on sharply tapping the bed upon which the baby lies) indicates a serious disorder of cerebral development. Similarly, it is apparent that the activity of the frontal lobes in man is sufficient after the first year or two of life to inhibit the reflex grasping and groping which results from stroking the palm of the hand. This **grasp reflex** may, however, return unilaterally as the result of a lesion of the contralateral frontal lobe.

THE CLINICAL FEATURES OF UPPER AND LOWER MOTOR NEURONE LESIONS

Let us take as an example of the effects of an **upper motor neurone lesion** the hemiplegia which is produced by an extensive lesion of the contralateral motor area of the cerebral cortex, or of the internal capsule. If the lesion is an acute one, say, a massive haemorrhage, the paralysed limbs are at first limp and flaccid, immobile and without tone, owing to the phenomenon of so-called 'shock', through which a sudden and extensive lesion produces an abrupt depression of reflexes subserved by relatively remote areas of the nervous system, even though the reflex arc or arcs concerned remain intact. All reflexes are absent at this stage on the affected side. Gradually over the course of a few days or weeks, this flaccidity lessens and the affected limbs become spastic, though there are some few cases in which, particularly if there is also an extensive parietal lobe lesion, the hemiplegia remains permanently flaccid. It should be noted that whereas the affected arm and leg are completely paralysed, those parts of the body which are bilaterally 'represented' in the cerebral cortex can still be moved voluntarily, even on the paralysed side. Thus facial weakness affects mainly the lower part of the face and the upper part slightly or not at all, while no defect in palatal

movement will be apparent. Furthermore, since emotional movement of the face, as in smiling, appears to be controlled not by the
cerebral cortex but by more deeply situated structures, a patient
who is completely unable to move the lower half of one side of the
face at will may yet smile quite symmetrically.

As flaccidity passes off in the paralysed limbs and spasticity makes
its appearance, so the tendon reflexes return, become greatly exaggerated and may be accompanied by clonus. The abdominal and cremasteric reflexes on the affected side remain absent and the plantar
response is clearly extensor. Spasticity is often greatest in the flexor
muscles of the upper limbs and in the extensor muscles of the lower,
so that in a patient with a long-standing hemiplegia, the arm is
flexed at the elbow and at the wrist and fingers, while the leg remains
fully extended.

When the lesion of the pyramidal tract is not sufficiently severe to
cause total paralysis, but only a relatively minor degree of weakness,
it is the finer and more skilful movements, those most recently
acquired by man in the process of evolution, which are most severely
impaired. Thus independent finger and toe movements are very poor,
though the strength of movement at proximal joints such as the
shoulder and hip remains good. So too during the process of recovery
from a pyramidal tract lesion, movement usually returns first at the
proximal joints; it is the cruder movements which are first regained,
while the more delicate activity of the fingers and toes is the last to
return. A patient who is recovering from a hemiplegia resulting
from, say, cerebral thrombosis, may be able to use his hand to grip
or to lift objects, but will often be quite unable to write or to fasten
buttons or shoelaces. He walks with his arm flexed across the front of
his chest and with stiffness, dragging and circumduction of the
affected leg.

Similar physical signs are apparent in patients with bilateral
pyramidal tract lesions giving rise to spastic paraplegia. If the lesion
responsible is an acute transverse lesion of the cord, say, from infection or injury, there is a total flaccid paralysis of the limbs below the
affected segment during the initial stage of spinal shock; subsequently
spasticity, increased tendon reflexes and extensor plantar responses
appear. As the lower motor neurone and the spinal reflex are intact,
severe wasting of muscles does not occur, although when the paralysis
has been present for some time, some degree of disuse atrophy,
affecting all muscles of the limb or limbs, appears. When the spinal
cord lesion is incomplete, the tone of the spastic lower limbs may be
particularly increased in the extensor muscles (paraplegia-in-
extension) but when both pyramidal tracts are severely diseased and
there are also lesions of other spinal pathways, the legs become

progressively more flexed at the knees and hips and stimulation will provoke painful flexor spasms (paraplegia-in-flexion).

Having described the general clinical features of an upper motor neurone lesion it is important to realise that much depends, in an individual case, upon the rate of its evolution. Whereas an acute lesion, e.g. cerebral haemorrhage or cord transection, will give a total flaccid paralysis initially with spasticity slowly evolving over the subsequent days or weeks, a chronic or slowly progressive lesion such as a tumour may give little more initially than a slight impairment of fine movement in one hand, or simply a minimal increase in tendon reflexes in the affected arm; subsequently, however, a spastic monoparesis or hemiparesis slowly develops.

The pathological causes of upper motor neurone lesions are many and varied—too many for their differential diagnosis to be considered in detail in this chapter. Once the lesion has been localised by means of the physical signs, the clinical history should again be analysed carefully to see if any clue can be obtained as to the nature of the pathological process. In this context, the scheme of pathological classification given in Chapter 2 is often useful. Thus if we take the cerebral causes of spastic weakness, these may include traumatic (cerebral contusion, extradural haematoma) inflammatory (cerebral abscess, encephalomyelitis), neoplastic (meningioma, glioma, metastases), and degenerative (cerebral thrombosis or haemorrhage) causes. The natural history of these and of the many other conditions which give pyramidal tract lesions differ considerably, and associated physical signs indicating involvement of other nervous structures or of other systems may be invaluable. Similarly, in spinal cord disease giving rise to spastic paraplegia, many causes are possible. These include trauma (fracture dislocation of spine, haematomyelia), inflammation, either extradural (abscess) or intramedullary (transverse myelitis), neoplasia (meningioma, neurofibroma, glioma, metastases, reticulosis) and a group of common degenerative, demyelinating and metabolic disorders. Of these, disseminated sclerosis is characterised by a remittent course and often by involvement of brain-stem structures; it sometimes gives temporal pallor of the optic disks, nystagmus or diplopia and cerebellar signs as well as signs of a spastic paraplegia with impaired appreciation of 'posterior column' type sensation in the lower limbs. Some few cases, however, run a progressive course with only a spastic paraplegia and no signs of involvement of brain stem structures. In these cases the condition is difficult to distinguish from cervical cord compression due to tumour or cervical spondylosis. In the latter disorder, however, particularly if the long-standing disk protrusions extend laterally, spinal roots are often compressed as well as the cord, and there may be amyotrophy or inversion of upper limb reflexes as well as a spastic paraplegia. Patients with motor neurone disease will usually demonstrate some wasting, weakness and fasciculation of muscles in the limbs, as well as signs of a spastic paraparesis, while in this condition there is no sensory impairment whatever. In syringomyelia, on the other hand, dissociated anaesthesia to pain and temperature sensation with retention of touch is often present in one upper limb, combined with some wasting and weakness of muscles due to a lower motor neurone lesion, while in the lower limbs there are usually signs of a spastic paraplegia. Spastic weakness of the lower limbs is also present in some cases of subacute combined degeneration of the cord, but here sensory symptoms and signs indicating dysfunction of the posterior columns of the cord are usually predominant; there may be tenderness of the calves and absence of certain tendon reflexes owing to a break on the sensory side of the reflex arc, while signs of pyramidal tract disease, though present, are often relatively unobtrusive.

The features of a **lower motor neurone lesion** are quite different. As there is an interruption of the final common path of all forms of motor activity, the muscle or muscle groups involved become totally paralysed and flaccid, and remain so. Any reflex movement for which the paralysed muscles are necessary will be lost. Another invariable feature is that all muscles which are deprived of their motor nerve supply undergo rapid atrophy; they may shrink to half the normal size within about six weeks and will eventually disappear almost completely, being virtually replaced by fibrous connective tissue. Before this stage of total atrophy is reached, and particularly if the lesion responsible lies in the anterior horn cells of the spinal cord (e.g. motor neurone disease), **fasciculation** is commonly seen. The latter is a phenomenon, visible through the intact skin unless the subject is very obese, in which individual muscle fasciculi contract spontaneously, and a continuous flickering of these fibre bundles can be seen to be occurring in a muscle which is apparently completely at rest. Fasciculation, though most often seen in patients with motor neurone disease, is not diagnostic of this condition, as it may occur following old poliomyelitis, and is also observed in polyneuritis and other lesions of the peripheral nerves. Furthermore, it may be benign and of no pathological significance; it is often noticed by doctors in their calf and small hand muscles. A benign condition in which very widespread and coarse fasciculation occurs along with profuse sweating and severe muscular cramps is known as **myokymia.** **Fibrillation,** or spontaneous contraction of individual muscle fibres, also occurs following a lesion of the lower motor neurone, but cannot be seen through the skin, though it can be recorded electromyographically. Hence the clinical features of an acute lower motor neurone lesion are total flaccid paralysis with absence of all reflexes, and rapid atrophy of the affected muscle or group of muscles. In a slowly progressive lesion weakness and atrophy increase gradually, and eventually the reflexes are lost. In such a case it can be difficult to decide whether the lesion involves a single peripheral nerve, several peripheral nerves, a group of spinal anterior roots, or the anterior horn cells of the cord. All-important in making this distinction is a knowledge of the anatomy and innervation of muscles. If more muscles are affected than could be supplied by a single peripheral nerve, it must then be asked whether lesions of one or of a group of spinal roots could be responsible, in which case there may be other evidence of spinal cord disease or dysfunction. If the muscular weakness and wasting is more widespread still, and particularly if it occurs symmetrically in the peripheral muscles of the limbs, the two most likely diagnoses are polyneuropathy (polyneuritis) and motor neurone disease (progressive muscular atrophy). The presence of sensory loss, particularly if present symmetrically in the periphery of the limbs, will confirm the former diagnosis, while if there is widespread fasciculation of muscles, no sensory loss, and some evidence of pyramidal tract disease, motor neurone disease can be diagnosed with reasonable confidence.

Muscular weakness and wasting which can mimic that due to a lower motor neurone lesion may result from a primary disease of the muscles themselves, a myopathy. Here too there is flaccid weakness with atrophy and absence of tendon reflexes. Even in disorders of conduction at the motor end-plate, such as myasthenia gravis, the muscles may be weak and hypotonic, though atrophy is uncommon. In general, however, myopathic as distinct from neuropathic disorders (*see* Chapter 18) tend to affect the proximal rather than the distal muscles of the limbs; fasciculation does not occur. Considerable help in differential diagnosis can be obtained from electromyography, since in polyneuropathy and motor neurone disease the motor unit potentials, though reduced in number, often remain normal or larger than normal in outline, whereas in myopathic conditions, owing to patchy degeneration of individual muscle fibres, they are broken-up and polyphasic.

INVOLUNTARY MOVEMENTS

Movements of parts of the body which do not occur in response to the will and are thus involuntary can be of the greatest importance in neurological diagnosis.

The first type of movement commonly classified in this group, though it is not strictly involuntary, is the so-called **tic** or **habit spasm.** This term covers a variety of twitching or jerking movements which occur irregularly and tend particularly to involve the muscles around the eyes, the remainder of the face and the shoulders. The subject is well aware of the movement, and on close questioning it is generally discovered that it is voluntarily performed as from it the patient obtains relief of tension which would otherwise become almost intolerable. This affliction is clearly related to anxiety. Though initially under the control of the will the movements often become so habitual as to be almost involuntary.

The epileptic fit or convulsion, whether focal or general, clearly involves involuntary movement, but has been previously considered (*see* Chapter 6). A closely related phenomenon, however, is **myoclonus,** a sudden shock-like muscular contraction which can involve a small group of muscles, several muscle groups or even the greater part of the voluntary musculature, either simultaneously or successively. Myoclonic jerks may occur while falling asleep and are not then pathological, though when they occur repeatedly throughout the night the condition is in all probability an epileptic manifestation and many such persons also have occasional major seizures. A brief myoclonic jerk of the limbs is a common accompaniment of an attack of petit mal. Myoclonus in response to startle (say, by noise) is a feature of cerebral lipidosis, while myoclonic jerks also occur in other cerebral degenerative disease such as subacute encephalitis. When myoclonus involves many parts of the body and occurs repetitively or at times almost rhythmically, this clinical syndrome has been called paramyoclonus multiplex, but most such cases go on to develop major epilepsy and dementia as a result of progressive degenerative changes in the cerebrum and cerebellum. This fatal condition is known as **progressive myoclonic epilepsy.** Occasionally in elderly persons a repetitive myoclonus of palate and throat muscles develops. This condition, known as **palatal myoclonus,** also interferes with respiration and speech which then occur in a series of staccato jerks. Though distressing, the condition, which is due to changes in the central tegmental tract of the mid-brain, is not progressive.

Repetitive and sometimes rhythmical twitching of one half of the face should not be confused with either habit spasm or myoclonus, for this condition, **hemifacial spasm** (*see* Chapter 18) is probably due to an irritative lesion of the seventh nerve.

Tremor is a rapid, rhythmically repetitive movement which tends to be consistent in pattern, amplitude and frequency, and usually consists of intermittent contraction of a muscle group and then of its antagonists. It may be *static* (present at rest), *action* (present throughout the range of movement), or *intention* (accentuated towards the end of movement) in type. A *static tremor* of the head and hands, rapid in frequency and small in range, and not generally abolished by movement, constitutes the so-called senile tremor which is seen in a proportion of elderly patients. A more coarse rhythmical nodding of the head is seen in some patients with cerebellar disease. The most typical form of static tremor, however, is the rhythmical 'pill-rolling' movement of the fingers and hands, often affecting also the arms and legs and sometimes the lips and tongue, which is seen in patients with Parkinson's disease. Though accentuated by embarrassment and attention, this tremor is generally abolished by movement, though occasionally in Parkinson's disease an action tremor is present as well. The principal lesion responsible for this tremor appears to be in the substantia nigra of the mid-brain.

Many different forms of disease can give rise to an *action tremor* which is observed particularly well in the actions of writing, of taking hold of an object, or in holding the arms outstretched. The fine tremor of the outstretched hands in patients with thyrotoxicosis is usually easy to recognise, while much coarser movements are seen in individuals with a variety of toxic and metabolic disorders including delirium tremens (alcoholism), mercury poisoning and chronic liver disease; in the latter condition there is a remarkable 'flapping' movement of the outstretched hands, often like the beating of wings. In Wilson's disease (hepatolenticular degeneration), this type of movement of the hands will be seen if the liver disease is sufficiently advanced, but facial grimacing, rigidity and tremor of the limbs are also present as a result of the pathological changes which occur in the lenticular nuclei. In general paresis, tremor not only affects the hands but often also lips and tongue. The condition of so-called *benign familial tremor* is also accentuated by movement. It is remarkable that this form of tremor, though sometimes gross, does not often interfere with fine movements such as threading a needle which would at first sight appear to be impossible. Curiously, this form of tremor, which often develops first in early adult life but occasionally not until middle life, is often relieved considerably by the ingestion of alcohol. The most bizarre and gross form of tremor is often that of hysteria, and is produced for histrionic effect; it is coarse, irregular and variable and tends to diminish when the patient's attention is distracted.

Intention tremor is virtually diagnostic of cerebellar disease. When unilateral it indicates a lesion of the ipsilateral cerebellar hemisphere. Whereas the lesion, if severe, may give rise to some degree of static tremor, this invariably becomes very much worse towards the end of movement, which cannot therefore be accurately controlled, and such activities as writing and feeding are grossly disorganised.

The patient may spill a cup whenever he brings it close to his mouth.

A variety of forms of involuntary movement can result from lesions of the extrapyramidal system, in addition to the Parkinsonian tremor already described. The movement of **chorea,** for instance, though involuntary, may appear at first sight to be semi-purposive and to show a high degree of organisation. Facial grimacing, raising of the eyebrows and rolling of the eyes, curling of the lips and protrusion and withdrawal of the tongue are common. In the limbs the movements are very largely peripheral with intermittent 'wriggling' or 'squirming' of the fingers and toes. Often, too, there is striking hypotonia of the limbs, and the reflexes may be 'pendular' in type in that a single blow on the quadriceps tendon may cause the dependent leg to swing forwards and backwards several times like a pendulum. The limb movements cease during sleep. The exact situation of the lesions responsible for the movements is not known, though the caudate and lenticular nuclei have been implicated. The condition occurs in two principal forms, first rheumatic or Sydenham's chorea, and secondly Huntington's chorea, a degenerative cerebral disease of late adult life, which is inherited as an autosomal dominant characteristic, and in which progressive dementia also occurs. Chorea, particularly the rheumatic form, is often accompanied by excessive emotional reactions and movement is often remarkably uncontrolled and ill-directed with undue expenditure of effort in carrying out some simple action.

Athetosis tends to involve the more proximal limb muscles to give movements which are writhing in character, slower in their execution and of greater amplitude than those of chorea. Often choreiform and athetotic movements are combined in the same patient, when the condition is referred to as choreo-athetosis. Athetosis can be bilateral and of congenital origin due to degenerative changes (*état marbré*) in the corpus striatum. It is sometimes a sequel of birth injury, occurring particularly in those children with cerebral palsy who initially show a flaccid diplegia, and it rarely follows kernicterus due to Rh-factor incompatibility. It may also occur unilaterally in infants with an infantile hemiplegia in whom the lesion responsible has extended to involve the basal ganglia.

Another type of involuntary movement resulting from lesions of the corpus striatum, but in which the trunk muscles are predominantly involved, is the so-called **dystonia musculorum deformans** or **torsion spasm.** In this condition there is a striking increase in tone with frequent irregular spasmodic contraction of the muscles of the neck, back and abdomen, and also of the limbs, giving rise to bizarre alterations in posture. These postural changes are often constant over long periods with superimposed painful spasms and the affected muscles often show a striking degree of hypertrophy. The condition may begin with alteration in the posture of a limb (e.g. inversion of one foot) resulting in a gait which is so remarkable that it may at first be considered hysterical. It is unfortunately progressive, depending upon degenerative changes of unknown aetiology which occur in the corpus striatum. Many believe that **spasmodic torticollis,** a condition of frequent spasm of the sternomastoid and of other neck muscles, which results in a spasmodic turning of the head and neck to one side, is a fractional variety of torsion spasm; there is often a permanent increase in the tone of neck and shoulder muscles, and in some cases the condition progresses to involve other parts of the body, although in others it remains localised. The deficiency of present methods of histopathological study is revealed by the fact that the situation and nature of the lesion or lesions responsible for this condition too, are not yet clearly defined.

One final but characteristic form of involuntary movement which can result from extrapyramidal disease is the so-called **hemiballismus,** a wild, purposeless, 'flinging' movement of one arm and leg which may occur in elderly patients as a result of a lesion, generally an infarct, which involves particularly the subthalamic nucleus of Luys on the opposite side. The movements can be so violent and distressing that if untreated they result in death from exhaustion.

CONCLUSIONS

Although the organisation of voluntary movement is a remarkably complex mechanism which still holds many mysteries, it is apparent that a careful analysis, based upon anatomical and physiological knowledge, of the ways in which it is disorganised in any individual case, whether through weakness or paralysis, ataxia or involuntary movements, can be of the greatest value in localising the situation of the lesion responsible; in this connexion, changes in muscle tone and in the reflexes may give invaluable aid. Once localised, reconsideration of the method of evolution of the lesion will often indicate its nature.

REFERENCES

ADAMS, R. D., 'Disturbances of the motor system. I. Motor paralysis. II. Abnormalities of posture, involuntary movements', in *Principles of Internal Medicine*, Ed. Harrison, T. R., 4th ed., Chapters 26 and 27 (New York, McGraw-Hill, 1962).
BRAIN, W. R., *Diseases of the Nervous System*, 6th ed., Chapters 1 and 12 (London, Oxford University Press, 1962).

DENNY-BROWN, D., *Diseases of the Basal Ganglia and Subthalamic Nuclei* (New York, Oxford University Press, 1946).

FORD, F. R., *Diseases of the Nervous System in Infancy, Childhood and Adolescence*, 4th ed. (Springfield, Ill., Thomas, 1959).

GARDNER, E., *Fundamentals of Neurology*, 4th ed. (Philadelphia and London, Saunders, 1963).

HOLMES, G., *An Introduction to Clinical Neurology*, 2nd ed., Chapters 4-7 (Edinburgh, Livingstone, 1952).

MATTHEWS, W. B., *Practical Neurology* (Oxford, Blackwell, 1963).

PEIPER, A., *Cerebral Function in Infancy and Childhood* (London, Pitman, 1962).

WALSHE, F. M. R., *Critical Studies in Neurology* (Edinburgh, Livingstone, 1948).

WARTENBERG, R., *The Examination of the Reflexes* (Chicago, Year Book Publishers, 1945).

CHAPTER 10

THE SENSORY SYSTEM

THE examination of sensory function and the interpretation of abnormalities in sensory perception present considerable difficulties, since in no part of the neurological examination is the patient's co-operation more important. An objective assessment of the degree and extent of sensory impairment can thus be particularly difficult to obtain and it is often necessary to make considerable allowance for the patient's state of co-operation and intellectual capacity. Areas of cutaneous sensory impairment, particularly to light touch and pinprick, which are subsequently shown to be spurious, are not uncommonly elicited even by the most skilled of observers. Few parts of the clinical examination of patients are as liable to error. In fact, sensory examination is often particularly satisfactory in children and in adults of comparatively low intellect, as it is virtually impossible to achieve uniformity of sensory stimulation in clinical practice. Intelligent patients may perceive and remark upon variations of relatively slight degree which prove in the end to be of no pathological significance, but which nevertheless give rise to some confusion during the course of the examination. Furthermore, it should be remembered that individuals vary considerably in their reaction to sensory stimuli, a sensation which appears acutely painful to one being well tolerated by another. It should also be remembered that whereas it is conventional to examine sensory function and to record the results of this examination independently of those obtained on examining the motor system, motor and sensory functions are intimately connected, the one being largely dependent upon the other. Thus motor activity is grossly impaired if there is a defect in proprioception: a limb from which no afferent stimuli can be received is virtually immobile even though its motor pathways are intact. It is therefore important to realise that a serious disorder of movement can be entirely due to a defect of sensation in the affected part.

THE ANATOMICAL AND PHYSIOLOGICAL ORGANISATION OF SENSATION

The sensory apparatus consists first of a series of sensory receptors in the skin and other organs, secondly of the first sensory neurone, whose cells are located in the posterior root ganglia, and thirdly of additional sensory neurones which are responsible for the conduction of impulses through the spinal cord and brain stem to the thalamus and thence, sometimes, to the cerebral cortex. Visceral sensation, which is conveyed initially alongside fibres of the autonomic nervous system, enters the spinal cord along with somatic sensory impulses and is conveyed centrally in a similar manner.

Sensory receptors can be divided into **exteroceptors** which are largely situated in the skin and are concerned with recording information about the external environment of the body, and **proprioceptors** which are situated in muscles, tendons, joints and viscera and which inform us of the position and condition of these deeper structures. Many of the **exteroceptors** consist of no more than a network of fine nerve endings which terminate in the skin, but there are also more specialised receptors such as the basket-like nerve endings which surround hair follicles, as well as Merkel's disks and Meissner's corpuscles which are believed to record touch sensation, and Krause's bulbs and Ruffini's corpuscles which appear to respond to thermal stimuli. Indeed it was once believed that specific sensory receptors were necessary for the recording of each form of sensation, but recent work on the cornea has shown that touch, pain and thermal sensations can all be appreciated through undifferentiated nerve endings. Each so-called 'sensory spot' on the skin may receive filaments from several branches of a nerve and it is probably the pattern of stimulation and the frequency of discharge in these fibres which determines the nature of the sensation which is perceived, rather than any specificity of the nerve endings themselves. It is, however, true that certain cutaneous 'spots' are particularly sensitive to pain, and others to cold or warmth. This is why there is considerable variation in the sensation evoked by uniform stimuli in contiguous skin areas. Thus a touch on a cold spot will feel cold, or a pin-prick on a pain spot may be more painful than one applied with similar force nearby. Fortunately these fine distinctions are of comparatively little significance in clinical neurology, since sensory abnormalities, to be of practical importance, must generally be relatively crude.

The **proprioceptive receptors** consist of the muscle spindles and the Golgi–Mazzoni tendon organs which respond to tension or stretching of muscles, and the Pacinian corpuscles which are probably responsive to pressure. Comparatively few proprioceptive stimuli reach consciousness; many are concerned with reflex activity mediated through the spinal cord or cerebellum, by means of which posture and movement are controlled.

The Simpler Sensory Modalities

While all forms of sensory experience are interrelated, a number of clearly definable forms of somatic sensation can be recognised whose integrity is customarily assessed during the course of a neurological examination. The first of these is **touch,** which is commonly tested with a light application to the skin of a pledget of cotton wool. Touch may be assessed quantitatively by using von Frey hairs, so graduated that differing pressures are needed to bend them. The threshold for the appreciation of touch varies considerably on different parts of the surface of the body, depending upon such variables as the thickness of the epidermis and the number of hair follicles present. **Pain** sensation is generally assessed by means of a pin-prick, which can also be of graduated severity if an algesiometer is used. Care must be taken that the patient is asked to assess the painful quality of this stimulus and not the sensations of pressure or touch which may be simultaneously evoked. Squeezing of the tendo Achilles or of other deep tendons will determine whether the appreciation of **deep pressure** is intact, but this sensation can also be painful. **Thermal sensation** is generally tested by applying metal test-tubes to the skin, one filled with ice, the other with water at 45° C. Again the patient must be told that it is the feeling of heat or cold he is being asked to note and not the sensation of touch or pressure. The assessment of **position and joint sense** is generally carried out by moving the terminal phalanx of the forefinger or the great toe in a vertical plane and by asking the patient, whose eyes are closed, to describe the direction of movement each time the digit is moved. After making an initial movement of considerable amplitude it must then be decided whether the patient is capable of appreciating movements through a very small range. Another test of position and joint sense is to ask the patient, with his eyes closed, to point towards a part of his body, when the position of the part in space has been altered by the examiner. **Vibration sense,** as tested with a tuning fork of 128-frequency applied to bony prominences, is not a physiological sensation, being compounded of both touch and pressure, but nevertheless the absence of the ability to perceive this form of somatic sensibility, more complex in nature, is commonly tested in the course of the neurological examination. Thus **tactile discrimination** is assessed by recording the threshold distance at which the two blunt points of a compass, simultaneously applied, are independently perceived. The normal threshold for two-point discrimination on the tip of the tongue is 1 mm, on the tips of the fingers 2-3 mm, on the palm of the hand or sole of the foot 1·5-3 cm, and in the centre of the back 6-7 cm. The appreciation of **texture, weight, size** and **shape** of objects can also be assessed somewhat crudely by asking the patient, with his eyes closed, to identify objects placed in the hand, while tactile localisation is tested by asking him to identify on a diagram or model, or on the examiner, the point or points on his body which had been stimulated. He may also be asked to identify figures or letters which are traced with a blunt point on his skin. There is considerable individual variation in the ability to perceive and interpet these more complex sensations, but retention of these functions on one side of the body and their absence on the other is always a finding of pathological significance.

The Sensory Pathways

The cells of the first sensory neurone are situated in the posterior root ganglia and are bipolar in type, having peripheral axons which convey afferent impulses from the sensory receptors, and central axons which enter the spinal cord in the posterior nerve roots. The sensory fibres in the **peripheral nerves** vary in diameter and in their rate of conduction; the large, heavily-medullated, rapidly-conducting *A* fibres are primarily concerned with the conduction of impulses subserving touch, pressure and proprioceptive sensations, while the finer, slowly-conducting *B* and *C* fibres conduct those produced by painful stimuli. Since certain diseases of the peripheral nerves, and particularly various forms of peripheral neuropathy, may have a selective effect upon fibres of one particular size or degree of myelination, there are certain cases in which the appreciation of painful stimulation is more severely affected than that of touch or vice versa. It should also be remembered that whereas cutaneous and pressure sensations travel in pure sensory (cutaneous) and later in mixed sensory and motor nerves, proprioceptive stimuli, particularly from the muscle spindles, travel centrally first of all in motor nerves.

As the central axons of the first sensory neurone enter the spinal cord, some degree of regrouping of these fibres occurs, according to their function. Initially most of them enter the posterior column, lying just medially to the posterior horn of grey matter. The fibres concerned with proprioception, position and joint sense, vibration sense and tactile discrimination, as well as some of those conveying touch, turn immediately upwards in the **posterior columns** and travel to the nuclei of Goll and Burdach in the medulla. Since entering fibres continually displace medially those which have entered the cord at a lower level, it follows that the fibres from the lower limbs lie in the medial part of posterior column (column of Goll), while those from the upper limbs lie more laterally (column of Burdach) (Fig. 8 (*a*)).

A second group of entering fibres, concerned with the appreciation of touch, also enters the most lateral part of the posterior column

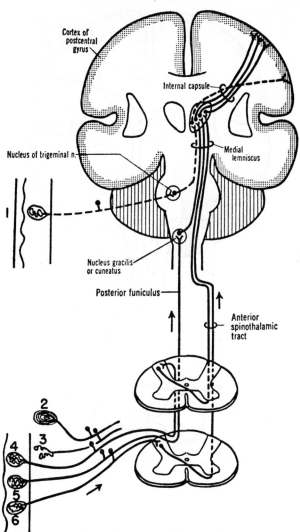

FIG. 8. A diagram of the principal pathways of the sensory system. (*a*) The pathways followed by impulses subserving touch, tactile discrimination, position and joint sense and related sensations.

(From *The Fundamentals of Neurology*, by E. Gardner, 3rd edition, Saunders, Philadelphia and London.)

where they ascend for several segments, then entering the posterior horn of grey matter to synapse with cells in this area. The axons of these cells then cross the midline close to the central canal to end in

G

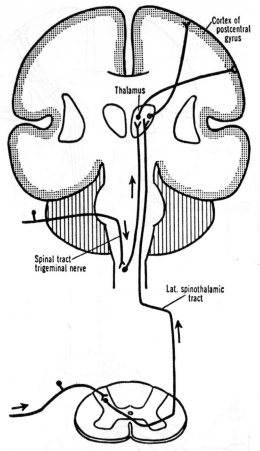

FIG. 8 (*contd.*). A diagram of the principal pathways of the sensory system. (*b*) The pathways followed by impulses subserving pain and temperature sensation.

(From *The Fundamentals of Neurology*, by E. Gardner, 3rd edition, Saunders, Philadelphia and London, 1945.)

the **ventral spinothalamic tract.** Fibres subserving pain and temperature sensation run a very similar course, except that they only ascend in the posterior column for a few segments before crossing the midline to end in the more **lateral portion of the spinothalamic tract** in the opposite lateral column of the cord (Fig. 8 (*b*)). As in the posterior columns, there is some lamination of sensory fibres in the spinothalamic tracts, those from the lower limbs lying nearest the surface of the cord and those from the upper limbs being situated more centrally. This probably explains why a lesion giving rise to spinal cord compression may impair pain sensation first in the lower limbs; the sensory 'level' then ascends steadily but finally becomes arrested on the trunk several segments below the situation of the lesion; presumably the fibres situated nearest to the surface of the cord are the first to be affected by pressure.

When the sensory fibres of the spinal cord reach the medulla oblongata, the spinothalamic fibres enter it laterally and travel directly up through the pons and mid-brain to reach the thalamus. The fibres of the posterior columns, however, terminate in synapses in the nuclei of Goll and Burdach. From the cells of these nuclei new axons arise which immediately cross the midline and then travel upwards as the **medial fillet or lemniscus,** again to enter the thalamus.

The pathway followed by sensory impulses from the face deserves special mention. The fibres of the trigeminal nerve which carry touch and tactile discrimination enter the main trigeminal nucleus and then, in the **quintothalamic tract,** cross the midline to join the medial fillet. Those subserving pain and thermal sensation enter the pons but then travel downwards in the **descending root of the trigeminal nerve** to end in a nuclear mass which extends downwards as far as the second cervical segment of the cord; then they, too, forming another part of the quintothalamic tract, cross the midline and travel upwards in the spinothalamic tract. It is of interest that 'representation' of the parts of the face in the descending root of the trigeminal nerve is inverted; thus a lesion of the lower end of the root in the upper cervical cord will give loss of pain and temperature sensation only, but not of touch, over the area supplied by the ophthalmic division on the same side of the face. It should also be remembered that, as occurs in the peripheral nerves of the limbs, proprioceptive stimuli from the face travel centrally in the motor nerves, such as the facial, so that sense of position in the facial muscles (a difficult faculty to test) is not abolished by a lesion of the trigeminus.

It will thus be seen that all sensory pathways which ascend as far as the brain stem terminate in the thalamus. Throughout their course in the spinal cord and brain stem these fibres have given off collaterals or have synapsed with internuncial neurones. These connexions have completed the sensory side of the arcs concerned with those spinal and brain stem reflexes which are necessary for the maintenance of posture and other functions. There are, for instance, a great many sensory fibres, some of which synapse in Clarke's columns of the posterior horn of grey matter, which ascend the spinal cord in the dorsal and ventral spinocerebellar tracts and which are largely concerned with supplying the information through which the cerebellum exerts control over posture and movement. The thalamus is, however, the first important sensory relay station. It is connected by a series of thalamocortical neurones with the **primary sensory area of the cerebral cortex,** namely the postcentral gyrus; fibres also travel to other parts of the parietal lobe. It is apparent that the cortex is concerned with the appreciation of most of those stimuli which enter consciousness. The integrity of the sensory cortex is particularly important if we are to recognise form, texture, size, weight and consistency of objects, or in order to recognise changes in position of parts of the body. It is also essential for the accurate localisation and recognition of the nature of stimuli applied to the body, for discrimination between two simultaneously applied stimuli, and even more for the ability to relate sensory experiences to others experienced previously, or to sense data perceived through the special senses. Clearly, numerous association pathways are concerned in the appreciation and recognition of these more complex sensory experiences, which may nevertheless be grossly deranged if there is a lesion of the primary sensory cortex, an important cell-station in all sensory association mechanisms. As with the motor cortex, stimulation experiments have revealed that certain specific portions of the postcentral gyrus are concerned with the appreciation of sensations from particular areas of the opposite side of the body. 'Representation' in the sensory cortex corresponds topographically with that in the motor area; thus a lesion of the lower end of the postcentral gyrus will impair sensory perception in the contralateral face and hand, while a lesion on the superior and medial aspect of the hemisphere will result in a failure to appreciate 'cortical' forms of sensation in the opposite leg.

It is, however, important to realise that cortical or subcortical lesions, even if they result in a division of all thalamocortical fibres, do not destroy completely the ability to perceive sensory experiences in the opposite half of the body. In the presence of such a lesion, sensitivity to pain and temperature is affected comparatively little, while crude touch will still be felt, though the finer forms of sensory experience may be greatly impaired. Hence it is apparent that the cruder varieties of sensation can be recorded in consciousness at a thalamic level.

SOME COMMON ABNORMALITIES OF SENSATION

In considering the disorders of sensation commonly noted in clinical neurology, it is first of all essential to understand clearly the meaning of a number of terms which are utilised to describe disorders of sensation. The word **numbness** can have a variety of meanings; when a patient says that a part of the body is numb he may mean that sensation in the part is abnormal, but sometimes this term is used to denote weakness or clumsiness. Hence careful enquiry will be needed in order to determine the significance of this symptom. Many other varieties of sensory abnormality, occurring apparently spontaneously, can be found in patients with neurological disease. Of these, one of the commonest is **pain,** which has been discussed more fully in Chapter 4. Pain may result from inflammation or compression of any pain-sensitive structure; if, for instance, it is due to irritation of a sensory nerve or root, the distribution of the pain will be in the cutaneous area supplied by the nerve or root concerned. Pain can alternatively be felt in the organ or organs which are diseased, while if it is arising in a viscus or in a muscle, it can be referred to an area of skin which sometimes overlies the viscus but may be anatomically remote. The mechanism of referred pain is not fully understood, though it is believed to be due to a spread of impulses to contiguous sensory neurones within the spinal cord. Spontaneous pain in the limbs or trunk can result from lesions of the thalamus, when it has a peculiarly unpleasant burning character, often with additional 'grinding' or 'tearing' qualities. A closely-related sensation of continuous burning, of pricking, of warmth or sometimes of cold, may result from a spinothalamic tract lesion. Disordered sensations of this type, occurring spontaneously, are often referred to as **dysaesthesiae.** In addition to these abnormal sensations, patients who have lesions of the spinothalamic tract often observe that they are unable to feel pain or temperature in the affected part. They have perhaps injured or burned a limb without discomfort or they may admit that they are unable to assess the temperature of water with the affected part.

Another group of abnormal sensations which the patient may feel are called **paraesthesiae.** These include feelings of tingling, pins and needles, of swelling of a limb, sensations suggesting that tight strings or bands are tied around a part of the body, or as if water were trickling over the skin. Sensory experiences of this type result from disordered function in the pathways conducting the finer and discriminative aspects of sensibility. Thus tingling or pins and needles can result from ischaemia of peripheral nerves, from polyneuropathy, from transient ischaemia of the sensory cortex, or they may be a feature of sensory Jacksonian epilepsy resulting from irritation of the sensory cortex. Similar symptoms are experienced by patients with lesions of the posterior columns of the cord and it is usually in such individuals that the 'tight, constricting band' or the 'trickling' type of sensation is felt. If there is a lesion of the posterior columns of the cord in the cervical region, sudden flexion or extension of the neck may give an 'electric shock' sensation which travels rapidly to the hands and feet; this sign (Lhermitte's sign) is commonly observed in disseminated sclerosis and in cervical spondylosis. Similarly, tapping over the trunk of an ischaemic nerve (as in patients with median nerve compression in the carpal tunnel) or over a sensory nerve which has been injured in some other way, will often give paraesthesiae which shoot along the peripheral course of the nerve concerned. A comparable sign produced by tapping a nerve in which regeneration is occuring is known as Tinel's sign.

As well as spontaneous paraesthesiae, patients with disordered function of the posterior columns of the cord or of the sensory cortex often observe that the affected part has become clumsy or even useless. If a hand is affected, they may be unable to use it except under the most careful visual supervision and cannot recognise objects felt in a pocket or handbag, unless they can be taken out and examined visually. Fine movements such as fastening buttons or threading needles are grossly impaired. If both lower limbs are affected then the patient is unsteady; he feels as if he were walking on cotton wool, and appreciates that he is worse in the dark. When the eyes are covered while washing the face, he will tend to fall forwards into the washbasin.

Turning now to the sensory abnormalities which are discovered on physical examination, **anaesthesia** is generally used to describe a cutaneous area in which the sensation of touch is totally lost, while **hypaesthesia** implies impaired touch appreciation. Similarly, **analgesia** refers to absence and **hypalgesia** to diminution of the appreciation of painful sensations. When thermal sensations cannot be appreciated the term **thermoanaesthesia** is sometimes utilised, but this very rarely occurs unless hypalgesia is also present. **Hyperalgesia** is allegedly an increased sensitivity to painful stimuli and **hyperaesthesia** a heightened perception of touch. In fact, however, careful examination will generally reveal that in the one case the pain threshold, and in the other the touch threshold, is actually raised above normal, owing to a disorder of the pain or touch pathways. The apparent over-reaction is due to some abnormal and often unpleasant additional quality added to the primary sensation which is in itself impaired; for this reason the term **hyperpathia** (Head's protopathic pain) is generally preferred to hyperalgesia which is semantically incorrect.

Romberg's sign is an important physical sign of impaired position and joint sense in the lower limbs. The preservation of the upright position depends upon labyrinthine, cerebellar and visual postural reflexes as well as upon those reflexes whose afferent pathway is from the proprioceptors of the lower limbs. So long as the eyes are open, and even if the conduction of proprioceptive stimuli from the lower limbs is grossly impaired, the patient is able to maintain his position, but once the eyes are closed he will sway or fall. Cerebellar or labyrinthine disease will also cause the patient to sway excessively, but severe instability and a tendency to fall under these circumstances results only from a severe impairment of position and joint sense in the lower limbs. The same patient will show **sensory ataxia** when he walks; being unsure of the position of his feet in relation to the ground, he lifts them unusually high and then bangs them down heavily (the steppage gait). He is also unsteady, and owing to loss of visual control of posture, is much more so in the dark.

Ataxia of sensory type is also apparent in the upper limbs if they are affected by similar lesions. The hands are clumsy, and fine movements cannot be performed, particularly when the hands are out of sight (e.g. inserting a collar-stud). If the affected arm is held outstretched with the eyes closed, it tends to 'wander' in space, upwards or sideways or indeed in any direction, unlike the downward drift of the limb showing motor weakness from pyramidal tract disease. At the same time there are also purposeless movements of the fingers, of which the patient is quite unaware, and these may have a 'writing' character (**pseudoathetosis**).

Abnormalities of the finer and discriminative aspects of sensibility are more difficult to assess, although in a patient with a lesion of the sensory cortex, the threshold for two-point discrimination is much greater on the abnormal than on the normal side, and there may be a total inability to recognise figures or letters drawn on the skin. Sensory stimuli are also incorrectly localised on the affected side. Lesions of the parietal lobe of less severity can be demonstrated by the phenomenon of so-called **sensory inattention.** The patient is well able to appreciate stimuli when applied independently to the two sides of the body, but when two similar stimuli are applied simultaneously to homologous points on the skin of the two sides, one may then be ignored, a finding which implies a disturbance in function of the sensory area of the contralateral cerebral cortex. It is well-appreciated that following amputation of a limb or of some other part of the body, it takes some time, in a sense, for the brain to realise that the limb is no longer there, and there is generally a clear-cut 'phantom' sensation as if the amputated part were still present and were able to move; sometimes the phantom is painful. It is of interest that a phantom limb can be abolished by a lesion of the contralateral sensory cortex.

Another defect which can be observed in patients with lesions of the arm area of the opposite sensory cortex is an inability to appreciate the form and texture of objects placed in the hand. Correctly this abnormality should be entitled **stereoanaesthesia,** but the term

astereognosis is more often used. Strictly speaking the latter term should be reserved for a failure to recognise the nature of objects when the primary sensory modalities are intact. This is an agnosic defect, due to a disorder of sensory association and akin to the other more complex disorders of parietal lobe function which have been described in Chapter 5.

THE CLINICAL SIGNIFICANCE OF SENSORY ABNORMALITIES

In order to localise the situation of the lesion responsible for an abnormality of sensation, it must be asked whether the sensory changes which have been demonstrated could be due to a lesion of one or several peripheral nerves, to one of sensory roots, of the spinal cord, of the brain stem, of the thalamus, or of the sensory cortex.

Identification of the sensory abnormalities which result from **peripheral nerve lesions** or from lesions of the brachial and lumbo-sacral plexuses can only stem from a knowledge of the cutaneous distribution of the various peripheral nerves and of the components of the plexuses (Fig. 9). If a nerve is sectioned, and it is one with an extensive cutaneous area of supply, there will be a central area of sensory loss to all forms of sensation and a surrounding zone in which tactile loss is more extensive than that for pain and tempera-ture sensation. There is considerable overlap in the cutaneous supply of the individual peripheral nerves so that section of a small cutaneous nerve may produce no definable sensory abnormality. This fact is even more true of the dermatomes innervated by the individual **sensory roots**; these have a strictly segmental distribution (Fig. 10) but if a single root is sectioned it may be virtually impossible to distinguish any area of sensory impairment, in view of the overlap in the supply of neighbouring roots. When more than one root is interrupted, however, there is generally some cutaneous sensory loss whose distribution will clearly indicate which roots are involved. A working knowledge of the dermatome distribution of the individual sensory roots is essential in clinical neurology. With this information it is relatively easy to distinguish on clinical grounds the sensory loss resulting from a root lesion from that due to abnormality of a peripheral nerve. Associated signs of a lower motor neurone lesion can be of the greatest value in confirming the distinction.

In clinical practice, for instance, the sensory loss resulting from an ulnar nerve lesion affects mainly the little finger and the ulnar half of the ring finger, while that due to a disorder of the median nerve involves chiefly the thumb, the first two fingers and the radial half of the ring finger. The ulnar nerve lesion will also give rise to wasting of

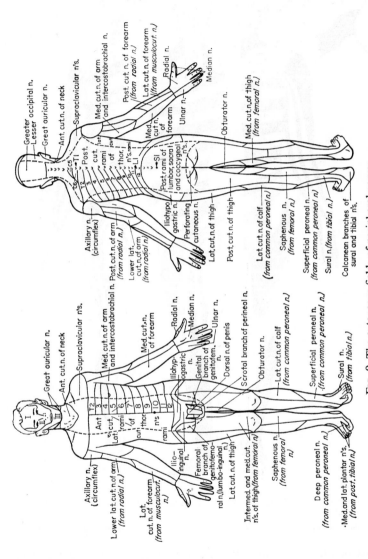

Fig. 9. The cutaneous fields of peripheral nerves

From *Peripheral Nerve Injuries*, by W. Haymaker and B. Woodhall, Saunders, Philadelphia and London, 1945.

G*

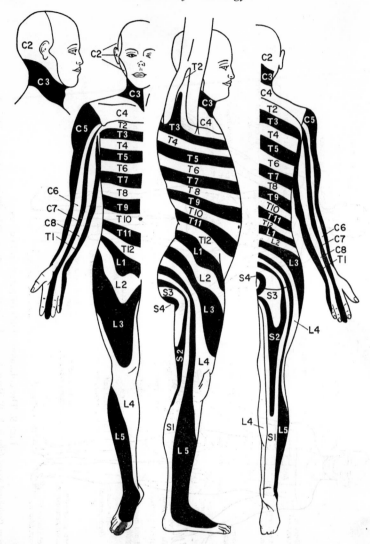

FIG. 10. A diagram of the distribution of the sensory spinal roots on the surface of the body.

(From *Introduction to Clinical Neurology*, by G. Holmes, Livingstone, Edinburgh. 1946.)

most of the small hand muscles, while median nerve damage will affect only those in the lateral part of the thenar eminence. In contradistinction, compression of the lower cord of the brachial plexus, which can also give rise to wasting and weakness of the small hand muscles, will produce sensory impairment in the medial aspect of the upper arm and forearm and not in the fingers.

When multiple peripheral nerves are symmetrically involved, as in **polyneuropathy,** it is the longest sensory fibres which tend to be most severely affected. Hence sensory impairment, which generally affects all forms of sensation, but may affect one more severely than the others, is most severe in the periphery of the limbs. Although this type of sensory impairment is often described as of 'glove and stocking' distribution, the borderline between normal and abnormal areas of sensory perception is not usually abrupt, but there is a gradual transition between the two. When there is widespread disease of posterior spinal roots (as in the Guillain–Barré syndrome of post-infective polyneuropathy) there is often an ascending level of sensory loss which eventually involves the entire trunk and all four limbs, but the disease can cease to progress at any stage. The condition may mimic a transverse lesion of the spinal cord, as motor paralysis is often severe. Indeed in some cases motor weakness predominates and sensory impairment is slight. A rare variety of hereditary sensory neuropathy exists in which pain fibres are affected almost exclusively and there is a peripheral insensitivity to pain, often resulting in perforating ulcers of the feet and in extensive destruction of bones and joints (Morvan's syndrome).

Sensory abnormalities resulting from **spinal cord disease** depend upon which sensory pathways are principally affected. Total transection of the spinal cord will give rise to a total loss of all forms of sensation below the segmental level on the trunk at which the cord transection took place. Often there is a zone of 'hyperaesthesia' in the skin area supplied by the segment of spinal cord immediately above the lesion. In hemisection of the spinal cord (**the Brown–Séquard syndrome**) there is loss of tactile discrimination, impaired touch perception and loss of position and joint sense on the same side of the body as that on which the cord has been divided, and these sensory faculties are impaired on the trunk up to the dermatome of the cord segment at which the lesion is present. There are also signs of pyramidal tract dysfunction on the same side. On the opposite side of the body there is loss of pain and temperature sensation, but the sensory level for these modalities is a few segments lower, in view of the fact that pain fibres ascend in the posterior horn for a few segments before crossing to the spinothalamic tract on the opposite side. A Brown–Séquard syndrome can result from trauma or from cord compression by a neoplasm and is occasionally an initial manifestation of disseminated sclerosis.

The principal lesion of **tabes dorsalis** is in the root entry zone of the posterior nerve roots and there is ascending degeneration of the posterior columns. Hence patients with this disease show severe sensory ataxia and there is often pain loss, and impairment of deep pressure sensation, over the bridge of nose, centre of sternum, perineum and tendons of Achilles, while position and joint sense and vibration sense are greatly impaired in the lower limbs. The tendon reflexes are lost owing to a break on the sensory side of the reflex arc. Similar impairment of deep reflexes in the lower limbs may be seen in **subacute combined degeneration of the cord,** in which disease sensory ataxia is also usual and vibration and position sense are commonly lost in the lower limbs. Signs of pyramidal tract disease are also present as a rule in this disease. The degenerative changes of **syringomyelia** usually occur in the central grey matter of the spinal cord in the cervical region; hence the decussating pain and temperature fibres are interrupted, resulting in dissociated anaesthesia, i.e. loss of pain and temperature sensation but preservation of touch and of position and joint sense. Commonly this sensory loss is unilateral, affecting the whole of one upper limb and shoulder and ending on the trunk at the mid-line and with a sharp lower level like the edge of a cape. As the anterior horns of the cord and the pyramidal tracts may also be compressed there is often wasting of upper limb muscles and a spastic paraplegia. The sensory changes of **disseminated sclerosis** are usually due to lesions of the posterior columns, giving impaired tactile discrimination, vibration sense and sense of position, sometimes in one arm, in both lower limbs, or even in all four limbs. Occasionally, however, a plaque of demyelination affects one trigeminal nucleus to give facial hemianaesthesia and sometimes, though rarely, there is a unilateral lesion of the cord involving the spinothalamic tract and giving loss of pain and temperature sensation in one lower limb.

Lesions of the brain stem may give sensory abnormalities which can easily be interpreted on an anatomical basis. Dissociated sensory loss in the face can result from syringobulbia, due to involvement of the descending root of the trigeminal nerve, while lesions of the pons and medulla can give facial sensory impairment on one side (due to a lesion of the trigeminal nucleus) with hemianaesthesia and/or hemianalgesia of the trunk and limbs on the opposite side due to involvement of the ascending sensory tracts. A lesion of the upper pons or mid-brain, however, may give a complete contralateral hemianaesthesia. More often such unilateral sensory loss is dissociated, involving only pain and temperature sensation owing to selective involvement of the spinothalamic tract.

A patchy contralateral hemianaesthesia and hemianalgesia can also result from a **thalamic lesion** and there will often be in addition spontaneous pain of a peculiarly unpleasant and disturbing nature on the anaesthetic side. Fortunately this **thalamic syndrome,** which usually results from cerebral infarction, is rare. The pain most commonly affects the face, arm and foot.

Lesions of the **sensory cortex,** if irritative in nature, give rise to sensory Jacksonian epilepsy, often taking the form of spreading paraesthesiae whose 'march' corresponds closely to the anatomical 'representation' of the parts of the body in the sensory cortex. This symptom is easy to confuse with the paraesthesiae which often occur during the aura of migraine, and result from transient cortical ischaemia. When there is destruction of a part of the postcentral gyrus, then in the corresponding part of the opposite half of the body there is no impairment of pain sensibility and comparatively little of touch, but the appreciation of position, of tactile discrimination and localisation and of form and texture is profoundly impaired. Figures written upon the skin cannot be recognised, and the threshold for two-point discrimination is greatly raised. In a less severe cortical lesion, there will simply be tactile inattention on the affected side. Defects of recognition and interpretation of sense data which may be noted in lesions of the parietal lobe have already been discussed in Chapter 5.

One final diagnosis which must be considered as a possible cause of sensory abnormalities discovered on clinical examination is **hysteria.** In a suggestible patient it is only too easy to discover areas of spurious sensory loss. A total hemianaesthesia affecting all modalities of sensation and even vibration sense over one half of the skull, is a common hysterical manifestation, as is anaesthesia of the palate or of the limbs in 'glove and stocking' distribution. In the latter case, unlike the findings in polyneuropathy, there is an abrupt line of demarcation between the area of complete sensory loss and that where all sensation is normal. In a patient with hysterical sensory loss it may be possible to 'find' (with suggestion) a small area within the anaesthetic region (impossible to explain on an anatomical basis) where a pin-prick is felt acutely. Another useful pointer is that the patient, though claiming that all forms of sensation are impaired in the affected part, is yet able to localise in space one finger or toe, say, quite accurately with his eyes closed, indicating that the sense of position is in fact well preserved.

Sensory examination is a technique which can only be learned by experience and which even so is full of pitfalls, particularly in an anxious and suggestible patient. Nevertheless consistent and clear-cut sensory abnormalities can be of the greatest value in achieving accurate anatomical localisation of a lesion within the nervous system, while the precise nature of the changes may give invaluable aid in determining the character of the lesion.

REFERENCES

BICKERSTAFF, E. R., *Neurological Examination in Clinical Practice* (Oxford, Blackwell, 1963).

HAYMAKER, W. and WOODHALL, B., *Peripheral Nerve Injuries*, 2nd ed. (Philadelphia and London, Saunders, 1953).

HEAD, H., *Studies in Neurology* (London, Oxford University Press, 1920).

HOLMES, G., *Introduction to Clinical Neurology*, 2nd. ed., Chapters 8 and 9 (Edinburgh, Livingstone, 1952).

MATTHEWS, W. B., *Practical Neurology* (Oxford, Blackwell, 1963).

MAYO CLINIC, SECTION OF NEUROLOGY, *Clinical Examinations in Neurology*, Chapter 9 (New York, Saunders, 1956).

VICTOR, M. and ADAMS, R. D., 'Disorders of sensation', in *Principles of Internal Medicine*, Ed. Harrison, T. R., 4th ed., Chapter 28 (New York, McGraw-Hill, 1962).

WALSHE, F. M. R., *Critical Studies in Neurology* (Edinburgh, Livingstone, 1948).

CHAPTER 11

THE AUTONOMIC NERVOUS SYSTEM

THE activity of the autonomic nervous system is largely concerned with the control of visceral activity; its influences are widespread, affecting the cardiac rhythm and output, respiration, blood-vessel tone and the behaviour of the hollow viscera of the alimentary and urogenital systems, as well as the secretion of the ducted and ductless glands. It is probably as well that these activities are in a sense automatic and reflexly controlled, and that they are but little influenced by the will, for many of them are too vital to allow of any interference from the capricious behaviour of the mind. It is the combined activities of the autonomic nerves and of the endocrine glands which are concerned in maintaining the constant internal thermal and biochemical environment of the body, a function which Cannon entitled homeostasis. Although many of the visceral functions of the autonomic nervous system and particularly its control of the heart, lungs and abdominal viscera are beyond the scope of this volume, there are many ways in which disease of the central or peripheral nervous system can affect autonomic activity, and accurate interpretation of the abnormalities so produced may be invaluable in diagnosis. Owing to the complex and apparently illogical arrangement of the autonomic pathways it is easy to fail to appreciate some of the general principles upon which the interpretation of autonomic disorders depends. However, a basic knowledge of the distribution of these nerves within the body, and of their function, is necessary for these principles to be rationally applied.

ANATOMY AND PHYSIOLOGY

The autonomic nervous system can be divided into two principal components, namely the **sympathetic** system and the **parasympathetic** system (Fig. 11). These two systems are in a sense antagonistic in their effects for where one excites the other inhibits. Thus activity of the sympathetic system produces dilatation of the pupil and slight protrusion of the eye, an increased cardiac output with tachycardia, dilatation of the bronchioles, vasoconstriction of skin vessels but dilatation of the coronary and intramuscular arteries, sweating, inhibition of intestinal movement, and probably closure of vesical and rectal sphincters, and erection of hairs (the pilomotor

187

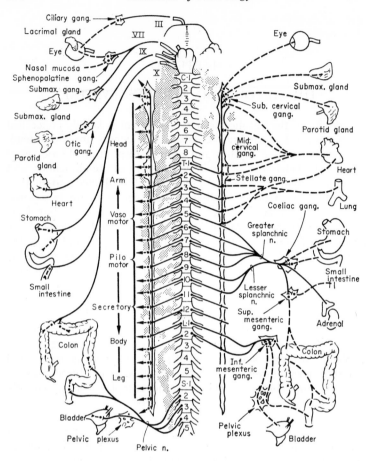

FIG. 11. A diagram of the spinal cord and brain stem showing thoracolumbar or sympathetic nerves and ganglia on the right, and craniosacral or parasympathetic nerves and ganglia on the left. The dual autonomic supply of the viscera is demonstrated.

(By courtesy of Dr Eaton and W. B. Saunders Co.)

effect) on the skin. In other words the animal is prepared for immediate action in response to any emergency. Most sympathetic fibres are adrenergic, i.e. they produce their effects upon plain muscle or other tissues by secreting adrenaline at their nerve-endings, and their effects can be reproduced by an increase in the amount of circulating adrenaline in the blood. Some few sympathetic fibres, however, and particularly those which innervate the sweat glands (sudomotor fibres) are cholinergic, i.e. they produce their effects by secreting acetylcholine at the effector organ. Parasympathetic fibres are, on the contrary, mainly cholinergic, and stimulation of the parasympathetic system gives constriction of the pupil, slowing of the heart and a diminished cardiac output, constriction of the bronchioles, increased intestinal peristalsis and evacuation of the bladder and bowels, and increased secretory activity of the salivary and lacrimal glands. The parasympathetic system also plays a principal role in sexual activity, including erection of the penis and ejaculation in the male, and orgasm in the female.

Unquestionably there are areas of the **cerebral cortex** which exercise a controlling influence upon autonomic activity but, as yet, the exact areas of the cerebrum concerned and the mechanisms by which they produce their influence are not fully defined. However, it is apparent that certain areas of the prefrontal cortex, and particularly the cingulate gyrus, are of importance, as lesions of the cingulate area may dull the emotions, a fact which is sometimes made use of in the operation of cingulectomy. Stimulation of the prefrontal cortex may also provoke sweating in the opposite arm and leg. Furthermore, the voluntary act of evacuation of the bladder and bowels appears to be initiated in the paracentral lobule of the hemisphere; probably motor impulses from this area, which are destined to activate the appropriate parasympathetic nerves, travel downwards with the pyramidal tract. Evidence has also been obtained from recent experiments that certain areas of cortex in the temporal lobe and insula, and particularly the hippocampal gyrus, may, with the amygdaloid nucleus, exercise important control over visceral as well as emotional activity.

It is apparent, however, that although the cerebrum influences the autonomic nervous system, the most important cell stations from which visceral and other autonomic activity is finally controlled lie in the **hypothalamus.** Nuclei in this area receive fibres from the 'visceral' areas of cerebral cortex mentioned above and in turn they give rise to descending pathways which enter the brain stem and spinal cord. It is also clear that the hypothalamic nuclei, being closely related anatomically to the pituitary gland, are in a position to influence powerfully the endocrine system. In general it can be said that the anterior nuclei of the hypothalamus are particularly concerned with parasympathetic activity and, via the tuber cinereum, with controlling the secretions of the pituitary gland. The posterior nuclei, by contrast, influence sympathetic activity; it is lesions of this area which can give rise to emotional disturbances such as 'sham rage' in animals or to lethargy and hypersomnia. Temperature regulation, control of the emotions and of sleep are also mediated through hypothalamic nuclei. The corpora mamillaria, too, which form a part of the hypothalamic system, are clearly of importance in memory regulation, as lesions in this area may prevent the patient from recording new impressions, a feature which is seen typically in the Korsakoff syndrome (*see* Chapter 6).

Though they are not clearly defined, there are unquestionably descending pathways from the hypothalamus which control both sympathetic and parasympathetic activity. These travel downwards, in the case of the sympathetic fibres, to the dorsal portion of the spinal cord to end in relation to the cells in the lateral horn of grey matter, while the parasympathetic fibres end in the nuclei of the oculomotor, facial, glossopharyngeal and vagus nerves, or in the sacral region of the spinal cord. No peripheral autonomic fibres travel directly to any viscus, but in each case a ganglion lying outside the central nervous system is interposed, so that there are always preganglionic fibres arising within the central nervous system and postganglionic fibres arising in the ganglia. In the case of the sympathetic nerves the ganglia lie lateral to the vertebral bodies and with connecting fibres form the sympathetic chain. Many of the parasympathetic ganglia are situated close to the effector organ so that in this case the preganglionic fibres are long.

The Sympathetic Nervous System

Preganglionic medullated sympathetic fibres (white rami) take origin from the lateral horn of grey matter in each segment of the spinal cord from the first thoracic to the second lumbar. These then pass laterally to the sympathetic chain in which there are ganglia corresponding to each of those segments of the cord from which sympathetic fibres arise; from these ganglia non-medullated post-ganglionic fibres (grey rami) join the corresponding somatic spinal nerve, to be distributed to the blood vessels and skin of the appropriate dermatome. However, fibres also run up and down in the chain to three cervical ganglia (superior, middle and inferior or stellate) and to four lumbar ganglia; these are necessary in view of the fact that there is no sympathetic outflow from the spinal cord in these regions. The thoracic and abdominal viscera receive a sympathetic supply through postganglionic fibres of the thoracic ganglia; these fibres form the splanchnic nerves and the coeliac, mesenteric and hypogastric plexuses. The sympathetic innervation of the cranium and of the upper limbs comes from the cervical ganglia and that of the lower limbs from the lumbar ganglia. Fibres travelling to the cranium traverse the inferior and middle cervical ganglia to synapse with nerve cells in the superior cervical ganglion, whence post-ganglionic fibres arise which enter or overlie the cranium in the coats of the internal and external carotid arteries and are then distributed to the blood vessels, smooth muscle, sweat glands, lacrimal and salivary glands.

Many workers believe that there are afferent sympathetic fibres which are concerned with the transmission of visceral sensation, but others regard the autonomic nervous system as entirely motor and insist that afferent fibres accompanying sympathetic efferents are not themselves sympathetic. Whatever their exact nature, these fibres enter the posterior nerve roots, and visceral sensation is thereafter conveyed centrally along with somatic sensation.

The Parasympathetic Nervous System

This part of the autonomic system is often called the craniosacral outflow as its function is motor and its fibres only leave the central nervous system in the cranial nerves and in the sacral region. Fibres arising in the oculomotor nucleus (its parasympathetic portion known as the Edinger–Westphal nucleus) travel with the oculomotor nerve to enter the ciliary ganglion in the orbit, whence long and short ciliary nerves to the ciliary and pupillary muscles arise. The superior salivary nucleus in the brain stem gives origin to fibres which travel with the facial nerve, but in the geniculate ganglion some of these leave to form the greater superficial petrosal nerve. This nerve enters the sphenopalatine ganglion which gives origin to secretomotor fibres to the lacrimal gland. Other fibres from the superior salivary nucleus are conveyed by the chorda tympani to the submaxillary ganglion and give rise to fibres which innervate the submaxillary and sublingual glands. The axons of the inferior salivary nucleus, on the other hand, travel with the glossopharyngeal nerve; they form the lesser superficial petrosal nerve, enter the otic ganglion, and postganglionic fibres of this ganglion promote secretion by the parotid gland. Finally, so far as the cranial outflow is concerned, the preganglionic fibres which arise in the dorsal nucleus of the vagus nerve end in a great many ganglia which lie in the walls of the numerous viscera which this nerve innervates.

The sacral outflow of the parasympathetic system leaves the spinal cord in the second, third and fourth sacral nerves, the so-called nervi erigentes. These preganglionic fibres pass to the vesical plexus and to numerous ganglia in the walls of the bladder, rectum and other pelvic organs, and from these ganglia postganglionic fibres arise.

The Bladder and Bowel

The wall of the bladder consists of unstriped muscle, which forms the detrusor; it and the internal sphincter are both supplied by parasympathetic nerves arising from the nervi erigentes. Stimulation of these parasympathetic fibres gives rise to contraction of the detrusor and to relaxation of the internal sphincter. Evacuation of the bladder cannot, however, occur until the external sphincter relaxes and this consists of striped muscle, being supplied by the pudendal nerve and thus being under voluntary control. Normally the tone of the detrusor keeps the bladder contracted upon its contents, but when the intravesical pressure rises to a certain level rhythmical contractions of the bladder wall develop and after a time there is reflex relaxation of the internal sphincter; evacuation can then be resisted only by voluntary contraction of the external sphincter. When the sphincter is relaxed and micturition occurs, the abdominal muscles also contract.

Sympathetic fibres from the hypogastric nerves also supply the bladder wall and, if stimulated, may inhibit bladder contraction. In fact, however, section of these nerves has little practical effect upon bladder function. Some of the afferent fibres concerned in the vesical reflexes travel with these fibres but others travel with the pelvic nerves.

The physiological stimulus for bladder evacuation is an increase in the intravesical pressure which gives rise to the desire to micturate. If this desire is unfulfilled, repeated contractions eventually follow. As previously mentioned there are also higher centres in the para-central lobule of the cerebral cortex and also very probably in the mid-brain which exercise some control over micturition; these produce their influence through fibres which descend with the pyramidal tracts. Hence disease of the spinal cord, as we shall see below, can profoundly influence bladder function. Disordered function is often assessed by measuring with a manometer the changes in intravesical pressure which follow the introduction of a standard volume of fluid into the bladder via a catheter. Normally this **cystometrogram** reveals a sudden rise in pressure as the fluid is introduced, followed by a gradual fall and thereafter by rhythmical contractions of the bladder wall. But if the bladder is hypotonic as a result of nervous disease these reflex contractions fail to occur.

In many respects the innervation of the rectum is very similar to that of the bladder. Stimulation of the parasympathetic nerves gives contraction of the rectal musculature but relaxation of the internal sphincter, as both consist of unstriped muscle. The external sphincter of the anus, however, which is striated muscle, is supplied by the pudendal nerve and can resist evacuation. As with the bladder, distension with faeces gives reflex contraction of the rectum and the desire to defaecate.

Sexual Activity

Sexual function in the male can be divided into first, desire or libido which is essentially an emotional function; secondly, erection of the penis due to tumescence of the corpora cavernosa, and thirdly, ejaculation of semen. The second and third functions are mediated through the activity of parasympathetic nerves, while closure of the internal sphincter through the action of the sympathetic is also necessary during ejaculation. Loss of libido may be due to disease of the mind or of the endocrine glands, while impotence (retention of desire but inability to achieve an effective penile erection) can also be psychologically determined. However, impotence can also result from disease of the spinal cord or cauda equina, and is then due to a lesion of the parasympathetic motor pathway or of the afferent sensory pathways; in such a case the ability to ejaculate is also absent. However, since the sexual act is a function which, once initiated, is subsequently controlled reflexly to a large extent, erection and ejaculation can occur despite a severe transverse lesion of the cord. Indeed in some cases of severe spinal cord injury persistent erection of the penis (priapism) is seen. Disorders of sexual function in the female are less well understood. Lack of desire (frigidity) is relatively common in otherwise normal females and is usually of psychogenic origin. Disease of the cauda equina or of the lower spinal cord may abolish the ability to achieve orgasm, but the effects of nervous disease upon female sexuality are much less apparent than in the male.

Precocious sexual development is generally the result of over-activity of the adrenals or ovaries but can occasionally be seen in patients with hypothalamic or mid-brain neoplasms or in male patients with pinealomas. Excessive sexuality is generally a constitutional disorder, which is of psychic rather than physical origin, and usually shows some affinities with psychopathy.

Some Autonomic Reflexes

In addition to the visceral reflexes referred to above, certain cutaneous reflexes dependent upon autonomic pathways are of value in neurological diagnosis. Thus local warming of a limb will initially give rise to vasodilatation and flushing of the skin, followed by sweating in the part that is warmed. Subsequently general vasodilatation and sweating occur in other parts of the body; this occurs even when all nervous connexions between the stimulated limb and the remainder of the body have been divided and must therefore depend upon stimulation of the hypothalamus by the warmed blood. The converse effects (vasoconstriction, pilomotor responses) follow cooling of a limb. Sweating and pilomotor activity may, however, be lost in a part of the body which has lost its sympathetic nerve supply, whether it be the postganglionic or preganglionic fibres which have been divided. The absence of sweating in a localised area of skin can be demonstrated by dusting the skin with either quinizarin powder or a starch and iodine mixture; sweat turns quinizarin purple and starch and iodine blue.

The 'flare' reaction is another important reflex which occurs independently of the central nervous system. It is an axon reflex; in other words the afferent stimulus travels centrally along a fibre, but then spreads to other branches of the same fibre, in which stimuli travelling peripherally are evoked; these produce a peripheral effect. If the skin is scratched firmly there is temporary blanching along the scratch-line due to local injury to capillaries, but this is soon followed by a spreading vasodilatation or 'flare', resulting from the axon reflex. A central weal will also occur due to local histamine release, but the 'flare', and the pilomotor response which may also occur in the same area, are reflexly determined. Since this axon reflex does not traverse the spinal cord it remains intact in spinal cord lesions and in lesions lying central to the posterior root ganglia; it is only impaired when the afferent sensory fibres or the ganglia themselves are diseased. Hence an absence of the 'flare' can be a valuable physical sign of a lesion of the somatic sensory nerves.

We may therefore conclude that in disease of the efferent sympathetic pathways, whether preganglionic or postganglionic, reflex vasodilatation (flushing of the skin) and sweating are abolished but a 'flare' will develop. When the sensory nerves from an area of skin are diseased, vasodilatation and sweating may occur, but the 'flare' is abolished.

SOME COMMON DISORDERS OF THE AUTONOMIC
NERVOUS SYSTEM

Horner's Syndrome

A lesion of the cervical sympathetic chain or ganglia will cause constriction of the pupil on the same side due to unopposed action of the parasympathetic; drooping of the eyelid, due to paralysis of that part of the levator palpebrae superioris which is composed of smooth muscle and is innervated by sympathetic nerves; slight retraction of the globe of the eye into the orbit because of paralysis of smooth orbital muscle which is similarly innervated; and loss of sweating on the affected side of the head and neck. Hence the features of Horner's syndrome are myosis, ptosis, enophthalmos and anhidrosis of head and neck, all on the same side as the lesion. This condition can result from a lesion of the sympathetic ganglia in the neck, whether due to disease or operation; it can rarely be congenital or may result from any lesion of the cervical and upper dorsal spinal cord (such as syringomyelia), which destroys the lateral horn of grey matter. Sometimes, too, it is due to a lesion of the lateral part of the medulla, as in infarction due to thrombosis of the posterior inferior cerebellar artery, causing division of the descending sympathetic pathway from the hypothalamus. Finally, in a small number of patients a Horner's syndrome can appear for which no cause is ever determined.

Cranial Nerve Syndromes

A lesion of one oculomotor nerve will give rise to a fixed dilated pupil on the affected side, owing to paralysis of the parasympathetic fibres and unopposed action of the sympathetic. Diseases of the glossopharyngeal and vagus nerves rarely produce any recognisable evidence of autonomic disturbance, but following a facial palsy, misdirection of regenerating parasympathetic fibres can result in fibres intended for the salivary glands reaching the lacrimal gland so that lacrimation occurs when the patient eats (the syndrome of crocodile tears). Facial sweating during meals (gustatory sweating) is another reflex phenomenon which is occasionally seen in apparently normal individuals.

Lesions of the Cauda Equina and Spinal Cord

A severe lesion of the cauda equina will have profound effects upon bladder and bowel function as a result of damage to the sacral parasympathetic outflow. The bladder becomes toneless and reflex contraction can no longer occur as it distends, so that retention of urine develops. As distension increases so the elasticity of the bladder wall forces urine into the urethra, and as the external sphincter is generally paralysed as well, dribbling incontinence or retention with overflow occurs. If the lesion of the cauda equina is permanent, reflex bladder activity cannot be re-established and owing to enforced catheterisation and stasis of urine within the bladder, severe urinary infection supervenes. In some such cases permanent suprapubic drainage of the bladder is necessary but eventually in many cases evacuation by manual compression is achieved. Similarly, retention of faeces occurs, sometimes with incontinence, and regular enemas may be required to empty the bowel.

The initial effects of an acute transverse lesion of the spinal cord are similar; there is retention of urine with overflow and also faecal retention. As the stage of spinal shock wears off, reflex bladder and bowel evacuation are gradually established, occurring solely in response to increasing intravesical and intrarectal pressure and independently of the will. Thus automatic bladder and bowel activity are developed; micturition and defaecation can be evoked by anything which increases intravesical pressure, including pressure upon the abdomen, or straining. They can also occur as a result of any stimuli applied to the lower limbs, as a part of the 'mass reflex' which includes flexor withdrawal of the limbs. The patient with a total transverse lesion of the cord may become aware that his bladder is full through sensations of headache, sweating or abdominal fullness and may then be able to initiate micturition by pressure upon the lower abdomen.

Retention of urine can also result from lesions in the parasagittal region affecting both paracentral lobules of the cerebral hemispheres, while incomplete lesions of the spinal cord affecting the pyramidal tracts, in relation to which the descending fibres controlling micturition are believed to travel, can also affect bladder function. Sometimes, in such a case, there is delay in the ability to initiate micturition and even incomplete retention with overflow. More often, in the patient with a spastic paraplegia, say, as a result of disseminated sclerosis, there is heightened reflex activity of the bladder and precipitancy or urgency of micturition results. The patient is unable to resist the desire to micturate and precipitate evacuation of the bladder occurs. Incontinence of urine also occurs in some patients with bilateral lesions of the medial aspect of the frontal lobes, as in some elderly atherosclerotic individuals or occasionally as a result of aneurysms of the anterior communicating or anterior cerebral arteries.

Apart from their effect upon bladder and bowel function, lesions of the spinal cord can influence other autonomic activities. Thus following an acute transverse lesion, and during the stage of spinal shock or diaschisis, the skin of the body below the level of the lesion is dry, pale and cool, but subsequently when reflex activity is established, profuse sweating in the affected area is common and can be provoked by a variety of cutaneous and other stimuli. It should also be remembered that local disease of the dorsal region of the spinal cord may damage the lateral horn of grey matter and will give sympathetic denervation of the affected segments with physical signs corresponding to those produced by division of preganglionic fibres.

Referred Pain

The afferent pathway for visceral sensation is initially along afferent fibres which accompany autonomic nerves, and particularly those of the sympathetic. These fibres enter posterior nerve roots and then travel centrally with somatic afferents. It is well recognised that pain of visceral origin can be felt in skin areas which are not at first sight anatomically related to the viscus concerned; thus cardiac pain may be referred to the substernal region, but also to the left arm, to both arms or to the jaw. It is not clear whether referred pain results from a spread of excitation to somatic afferent fibres with which the 'sympathetic' afferents are travelling in the posterior roots, or whether this spread occurs between sensory neurones within the spinal cord; the latter mechanism seems the more probable of the two.

Peripheral Nerve Lesions

Whereas section of a sensory nerve peripheral to its posterior root ganglion will generally abolish the 'flare' response in the anaesthetic area of the skin, a lesion of the lower motor neurone usually produces no recognisable autonomic effects. However, as a result of disuse the skin of the affected part may become smooth, shiny and inelastic, while subcutaneous tissue and even bone, as well as the denervated muscle, will atrophy. Owing to loss of the 'pumping' action of the muscles upon the veins, the affected part, especially a hand or foot, often becomes cyanosed and oedematous. These so-called trophic changes are due to disuse and not to a lesion of autonomic nerves; the autonomic reflexes are intact. The sequelae of a sensory nerve lesion are often more serious, particularly if pain fibres are severely involved, since if the part is analgesic, injury to the insensitive skin and joints will readily occur, giving rise to indolent or perforating ulcers and gross disorganisation of joints (Charcot's arthropathy). Other trophic changes, such as loss of sweating and of the pilomotor response, only follow a lesion of preganglionic or postganglionic sympathetic efferents and do not always result therefore from lesions of peripheral somatic nerves, unless these contain sympathetic fibres.

After an incomplete lesion of a peripheral nerve, particularly in the region of the forearm and wrist, it is not uncommon for a curiously unpleasant type of pain to occur in the affected hand, with excessive sweating and excessive sensitivity to touch and pain. This syndrome is known as **causalgia** and it seems that the stimuli responsible for the pain are carried with autonomic nerves and not along somatic afferents, as total division of somatic sensory nerves may fail to relieve the pain, while sympathectomy does so. The exact mechanism which gives rise to causalgia is not understood. Similarly, the mechanism by which painful swelling of the hand, often giving rise eventually to atrophy of muscles and even of bone (Sudeck's atrophy) develops in some cases of pericapsulitis of the shoulder joint or 'frozen' shoulder (**the 'shoulder-hand' syndrome**) is obscure, but this condition too is often relieved by cervical sympathectomy.

Hyperhidrosis

Though excessive sweating, particularly of the hands and feet, can be due to emotional disturbances or to endocrine disorders such as thyrotoxicosis, it may also be a congenital condition which, if intolerable, can be alleviated by sympathectomy. It is also seen sometimes in Parkinson's disease. Localised cutaneous areas of increased sweating can occur following peripheral nerve lesions, as in causalgia, while excessive perspiration in response to any peripheral stimulus is seen below the level of a transverse lesion of the spinal cord.

Hypothalamic Syndromes

That **disorders of sleep,** taking the form of either hypersomnia or wakefulness with reversal of the sleep rhythm, may result from hypothalamic lesions has been mentioned in Chapter 6. **Excessive appetite** can also occur, and in the so-called Kleine–Levin syndrome, which usually occurs in adolescent males, hypersomnia and macrophagia occur, but may resolve spontaneously after some weeks in which the patient does little but sleep and eat. Conversely, some hypothalamic lesions can produce **anorexia** leading to extreme **cachexia;** a syndrome of this nature also results from a hypothalamic lesion of unknown aetiology which occurs in infancy and early childhood.

That **disorders of memory,** and Korsakoff's syndrome in particular, can result from lesions of the corpora mamillaria is well known. Actual **visual hallucinations** (the so-called peduncular hallucinations) can also be produced by lesions in this neighbourhood, while numerous **emotional** and **personality disorders,** including excessive anger and irritability on the one hand, and apathy leading to akinetic stupor on the other, have been attributed to lesions of the hypothalamus. The importance of this region in regulation of the **body temperature** is also well-recognised, and irritation of hypothalamic nuclei, say as a result of sudden distension of the third ventricle owing to haemorrhage, or of some other condition causing a sudden increase in the intracranial pressure, may give rise to hyperpyrexia. A similar mechanism is probably responsible for the **hyperglycaemia** and **glycosuria, albuminuria,** and acute **gastric ulceration** with haemorrhage, which sometimes occur in patients with brain disease; basal neoplasms and subarachnoid haemorrhage are particularly liable to produce these effects.

Diabetes insipidus, a condition in which the patient passes very large quantities of dilute urine and consequently has polydipsia or excessive thirst, may also be the result of an anterior hypothalamic lesion. It appears that hypothalamic nuclei control the output of antidiuretic hormone from the posterior lobe of the pituitary gland and a reduced output of this hormone, resulting in diabetes insipidus, may follow a lesion of the hypothalamus or of the posterior pituitary, or even of the pathway joining the two in the tuber cinereum.

Obesity and sexual underdevelopment are other signs which are sometimes due to disease of the hypothalamus or pituitary or both. In idiopathic adiposogenital dystrophy (Frohlich's syndrome) the obesity is present from birth, is greatest around the shoulders and hips, and there is marked genital hypoplasia and immaturity. The condition is more common in males, but when females are affected sexual function is more often normal.

The Laurence–Moon–Biedl syndrome is another congenital disorder of the hypothalamic–pituitary axis and is almost certainly genetically determined. Like Frohlich's syndrome it is characterised by obesity and hypogonadism but in addition there is mental retardation, polydactyly (usually there are six fingers and toes) and retinitis pigmentosa, giving rise to progressive visual impairment.

CONCLUSIONS

It is apparent that disease or disordered function of the hypothalamus, which is in essence the control centre from which autonomic activities are regulated, can give rise to a bewildering variety of clinical manifestations, but from an understanding of some simple principles concerning the behaviour of this part of the nervous system, it may be possible to interpret the significance of a great many important symptoms and physical signs. Similarly, a knowledge of the structure and function of the more peripheral components of the autonomic nervous system is necessary in order to interpret those symptoms and signs of autonomic dysfunction, and particularly those of abnormal bladder and bowel activity, which may occur in patients with nervous disease.

REFERENCES

ADAMS, R. D., 'Disturbances of autonomic function', in *Principles of Internal Medicine*, Ed. Harrison, T. R., 4th ed. Chapter 29 (New York, McGraw-Hill, 1962).

BRAIN, W. R., *Diseases of the Nervous System*, 6th ed., Chapter 20, (London, Oxford University Press, 1962).

HOLMES, G., *Introduction to Clinical Neurology*, 2nd ed., Chapters 16 and 17 (Edinburgh, Livingstone, 1952).

WHITE, J. C. and SMITHWICK, R. H., *The Autonomic Nervous System* (New York, Macmillan, 1941).

CHAPTER 12

DEVELOPMENTAL, HEREDITARY AND DEGENERATIVE DISORDERS

AMONG the many disorders of the nervous system which receive consideration in this volume there exist a group of syndromes or diseases which are particularly difficult to classify according to rational criteria. Some are clearly inherited but we do not know how the gene or genes responsible for these conditions produce their effect upon the nervous system. Nor do we know in the case of many of them whether they constitute a number of separate diseases or merely variants of a single disease process. Others are clearly due to some abnormality of unknown cause which has afflicted the developing nervous system of the affected individual *in utero*, while others which are normally grouped together for convenience on account of clinical similarities are probably due to a variety of causes, some well-recognised and others obscure. And in yet another group of conditions there is evidence of a pathological process involving some part of the central or peripheral nervous system, a process which is so inexplicable in our present state of knowledge that we can only classify it as being degenerative in type. In this chapter an outline of some of the commoner nervous disorders which fall into these categories will be given and their interrelationship will be considered. Many uncommon developmental defects, such as the microcephalies, macrocephalies and ageneses of portions of the brain will not be considered, in view of their rarity. These are described in some of the larger textbooks to which reference is made at the end of the chapter.

CEREBRAL PALSY

The term cerebral palsy is generally used to identify a group of nervous disorders which are apparent from the time of birth, which are very variable in their clinical manifestations and severity, and probably also in their aetiology. Although abnormalities of movement are generally the most prominent clinical features in such cases there are often associated defects of intellect, of emotional development, of speech in the broadest sense, and of sensation. Between one and two of every thousand school-children are victims of some form of cerebral palsy. In most of the children which fall into this category the limbs are stiff and spastic and this is why the entire group of cases are often referred to, particularly by the lay public, as spastic children. In fact, in as many as 10 per cent of cases it is involuntary movements of an athetoid type and not spasticity which constitute the principal disability, while in about 5 per cent of cases, the limbs are actually hypotonic and the child may be ataxic rather than spastic.

The aetiology of cerebral palsy has been a fertile source of dispute. Some have claimed that virtually all cases are due to **birth injury** with meningeal haemorrhage, a view which is now clearly untenable, while others have suggested that an encephalitis, or some degenerative cerebral process of unknown aetiology, occurring *in utero*, is the cause. The truth appears to be that the pathological changes seen in such cases are so diverse that no single cause can be implicated. It seems that a **genetic factor** is probably responsible for the condition in up to 15 per cent of cases, as other members of the family, particularly sibs, are afflicted, either with cerebral palsy or with mental defect or epilepsy. Probably in a proportion of cases, **intra-uterine cerebral anoxia** due to placental insufficiency is responsible, and there is certainly a high incidence of threatened abortion or accidental haemorrhage in pregnancies resulting in the birth of spastic children. Very possibly, too, the anoxia resulting from a prolonged convulsion in early infancy can give rise to similar changes, as may anoxia or direct trauma to the brain during the course of a breech or forceps delivery or any prolonged labour. Certainly 50 per cent of spastic children have abnormal deliveries and many are born prematurely. **Kernicterus,** the degeneration and bilirubin-staining of the basal ganglia which frequently results from Rh-incompatibility (icterus gravis neonatorum) often gives rise to a variety of cerebral palsy in which mental defect, deafness and athetosis are prominent features.

Although all varieties of cerebral palsy usually reveal themselves through a delay in development, and a failure to pass the so-called intellectual and physical milestones at the appropriate age, most cases fall into a number of distinctive clinical syndromes. The age at which the parents are aware that their child is abnormal varies depending upon the severity of the condition, but it is usually within the first twelve to eighteen months of life; in a number, delay and difficulty in walking are not apparent until late in the second year.

The condition can result simply in **mental backwardness,** but more often there is associated clumsiness and spasticity of the limbs in addition. The diagnosis of mental defect in early life, depending as it does upon a failure to achieve new milestones of intellectual development (smiling, following lights, groping for objects, forming syllables and words, etc.) at the normal age, is a matter which requires great skill and experience in assessing the infant's behaviour against a background of known variations in intellectual development. It is important to remember that certain children with cerebral palsy have specific defects of motor function (**apraxia**), of sensory function (**agnosia**), of the special senses (**nerve deafness**) or of speech (**aphasia, articulatory apraxia, dyslexia**) which can give a false impression of mental defect if one's clinical appraisal is too superficial or limited. In some cases developmental disorders of execution and cognition (learning defects) are present in isolation without any accompanying manifestations of spasticity or ataxia. Congenital reading defect (developmental dyslexia) is a good example, but apraxic and agnosic disorders ('clumsy children') also occur and may be difficult to recognise in the early stages, though a discrepancy between verbal and performance scores in an I.Q. test may be a useful pointer. These and other forms of so-called minimal cerebral dysfunction have often been overlooked in the past.

The commonest variety of cerebral palsy is **spastic diplegia** (Little's disease) which may or may not be associated with a degree of mental defect. In its mildest form it presents with little more than a delay of a few months in learning to walk, with some clumsiness and unsteadiness of gait, symmetrical exaggeration of the lower limb reflexes and extensor plantar responses. In a very severe case, walking never becomes possible, all four limbs are spastic and there is also severe spastic dysarthria and/or dysphagia. More often the patient is unable to walk until the fifth or sixth year and then does so with the characteristic 'scissors gait', and contractures develop in the tendons of Achilles and posterior thigh muscles.

In patients with **athetosis,** which is usually bilateral and symmetrical, there may also be facial grimacing and an intermittently explosive kind of dysarthria. Voluntary movements of the limbs sometimes abolish the abnormal movements but are slowly and clumsily performed. Often the involuntary movements are not clearly apparent until the second year of life or even later, and at an earlier stage the limbs are hypotonic and movement is inco-ordinate while the plantar responses are flexor. Some cases, however, have associated spasticity. More rarely the patients with a hypotonic or flaccid variety of diplegia do not develop involuntary movements but are seen to have nystagmus and asymmetrical **ataxia** of all four limbs, which is usually due to an abnormality of the cerebellum (**cerebellar diplegia**).

The prognosis of cerebral palsy clearly varies, depending upon the severity of the intellectual and motor deficit. In the presence of severe mental defect, little can be done and this is unfortunately true of certain cases in which the motor abnormality is gross. Sometimes abnormal movements can be alleviated by surgical methods (*see* Chap. 20), while many patients can with appropriate training be helped to lead useful lives. Children with specific disorders of language and reading, though requiring patient individual training, are particularly profitable subjects.

Infantile hemiplegia is another condition which is commonly classified with the varieties of cerebral palsy, although it clearly differs considerably from the diffuse and symmetrical cerebral disorders mentioned above. It can occur bilaterally (double hemiplegia) and is then distinguished from cerebral diplegia through the fact that the upper limbs are more severely affected than the lower. The condition can be present from birth (congenital hemiplegia), when it may be due to a congenital cystic deformity of one cerebral hemisphere (porencephaly) or possibly to infarction occurring *in utero*. More commonly it develops acutely in infancy or early childhood, often during the course of an acute infection such as whooping cough or an exanthem, or following a so-called 'febrile convulsion'. Probably the most common pathological cause is infarction due to either arterial or venous occlusion, resulting in scarring and atrophy of the hemisphere and localised dilatation of the lateral ventricle (secondary porencephaly). There is evidence to suggest that it may in some cases be due to an inflammatory process of unknown cause in the wall of the internal carotid artery. Characteristically the arm on the affected side is severely paralysed, finger and hand movement being virtually abolished, and the hand and forearm assume a typically flexed posture, lying across the front of the chest. The leg, though spastic with exaggerated deep reflexes and an extensor plantar response, is less severely affected, and all patients are eventually able to walk, often with surprisingly little difficulty. If the dominant hemisphere is involved, aphasia results; the earlier the age at which the hemiplegia develops, the more complete and rapid is the recovery of speech function. Indeed if the patient is a young infant, the development of speech is not perceptibly delayed and this function appears to become established in the contralateral hemisphere. The residual neurological deficit can be of all grades of severity and occasionally the resulting disability is trivial. In the more severe cases, however, epilepsy is a common complication, as the scar in the affected hemisphere acts as a focus of epileptic discharge. Particularly in those cases in which epileptic seizures are frequent and severe, intellectual impairment and behaviour disorders are common.

HYDROCEPHALUS

Hydrocephalus can be defined as an increase in the volume of cerebrospinal fluid within the cranial cavity. This may occur as a compensatory phenomenon when the brain or any part of it is atrophic through disease, but no symptoms then result from the presence of excessive fluid. It is when the increase in fluid results in a rise in the intracranial pressure that clinical effects become apparent. This variety of hydrocephalus results from increased formation of cerebrospinal fluid (possible due to hyperaemia of the choroid plexuses as in meningitis), from obstruction to the circulation of the fluid, or from impaired absorption (as in thrombosis of the superior longitudinal sinus).

When hydrocephalus is due to an obstruction to circulation of the fluid through some part of the ventricular system (lateral ventricle, third ventricle, aqueduct, fourth ventricle), this condition is known as **obstructive hydrocephalus** and there is then enlargement of those ventricles which lie between the choroid plexuses and the block. An obstruction to the free flow of fluid throughout the subarachnoid space gives rise to **communicating hydrocephalus** and there is then dilatation of all the cerebral ventricles.

Obstructive hydrocephalus may be **congenital** or acquired. The commonest congenital cause is stenosis or malformation of the aqueduct of Sylvius, but less commonly there is a congenital membranous occlusion of the foramina of Magendie and Luschka. Another cause is the Arnold–Chiari malformation which is usually, but not always, associated with a spinal meningomyelocele. The medulla oblongata is elongated and a tongue of cerebellar tissue protrudes downwards through the foramen magnum; in this condition, and in basilar impression (*vide infra*) there may be an obstruction to the outlet of fluid from the fourth ventricle into the basal cisterns. In most cases of congenital hydrocephalus there is conspicuous enlargement of the head, present sometimes at birth, but usually developing subsequently. The head may be excessively translucent, it yields a typical 'cracked-pot' note on percussion and the eyes tend to be pushed forwards and downwards. Convulsions, mental impairment, optic atrophy and spastic weakness of the limbs commonly develop, and many patients die within the first four years of life, but there is evidence that the condition becomes arrested in a considerable proportion of cases, who then survive with a variable degree of disability for many years. **Acquired** obstructive hydrocephalus can result from any lesion, whether inflammatory or neoplastic, which distorts intracranial hydrodynamics in such a way as to cause an obstruction in a cerebral ventricle or in the aqueduct. This is why a cerebral tumour often presents with the clinical features (headache, vomiting, papilloedema) which are the characteristic results of hydrocephalus occurring in adult life.

The clinical effects of **communicating hydrocephalus** are similar to those of the obstructive variety, but except in severe cases this is frequently a self-limiting disorder. It generally follows conditions such as meningitis (or rarely subarachnoid haemorrhage) which lead to the formation of inflammatory adhesions in the subarachnoid space; sometimes these absorb with the passage of time. The syndrome of **otitic hydrocephalus** is one of headache and severe papilloedema which commonly complicates middle-ear disease and is generally due to aseptic thrombosis of the lateral and/or superior longitudinal sinuses, giving impaired absorption of cerebrospinal fluid. This condition is also self-limiting, and complete recovery generally occurs provided vision can be preserved; a similar disorder may follow trauma; it can complicate pregnancy or any wasting disease, or else it can occur apparently spontaneously, when it has been variously entitled 'toxic hydrocephalus', 'pseudotumour cerebri' or **'benign intracranial hypertension'.** Although in some such cases venous sinus thrombosis is the cause, many are unexplained and the fact that the lateral ventricles are often shown by ventriculography to be small or normal in size suggests that swelling of the brain tissue itself may be responsible for the increased intracranial pressure and that there is in fact no true hydrocephalus.

PRESENILE DEMENTIA

This condition has been considered in Chapter 7. Whereas a syndrome of progressive intellectual deterioration in late middle-life (the presenium) can be due to a variety of causes (general paresis, frontal neoplasm, cerebral atherosclerosis, liver disease, vitamin B_{12} deficiency, myxoedema), some of which are remediable, there exist a group of progressive degenerative cerebral diseases which give dementia as their principal presenting feature. The pathological changes (atrophy of gyri with senile plaques of argyrophilic glial fibres in the cortex) are identical with those of senile dementia and the presenile group of cases demonstrates many features of premature senility. **Alzheimer's disease,** in addition to progressive dementia, often gives rise to aphasic and apraxic defects and convulsions; it occurs sporadically, while **Pick's disease** may affect more than one member of a sibship and tends to give focal atrophy of localised cerebral areas, particularly the frontal lobes, so that euphoria and volubility often precede florid dementia. A variety of degenerative cerebral disease of undetermined aetiology in which a rapidly progressive dementia is associated with Parkinsonian features, signs of pyramidal tract disease, and muscular wasting in the periphery of the limbs due to degeneration of anterior horn cells in the spinal cord, is sometimes referred to as the **Jakob–Creutzfeld disease,** though it is more correctly described as 'the Parkinsonism-

H

dementia complex' and pathological observations suggest that a rare form of rapidly progressive presenile dementia accompanied by an irregular spike and wave pattern in the EEG and resulting from a subacute spongiform degenerative change in the brain comes much closer to the original description of Jakob and Creutzfeld.

HUNTINGTON'S CHOREA

This genetically-determined degenerative disorder, in which pathological changes are particularly apparent in the frontal and temporal cortex and caudate nuclei, is inherited as an autosomal dominant character and usually becomes apparent first in late middle-life. The characteristic features are progressive dementia, facial grimacing and uncontrollable choreiform movements of the limbs. Air encephalography in such cases often demonstrates atrophy of the caudate nuclei.

TUBEROUS SCLEROSIS (EPILOIA)

This degenerative disorder, which occasionally affects more than one member of a sibship, is characterised pathologically by the development of sclerotic masses of glial overgrowth in the cerebral cortex and by a hyperplasia of sebaceous glands upon the face, affecting the cheeks and lower lip, but often sparing the upper lip (adenoma sebaceum). Most sufferers are mentally defective and all are epileptic. Convulsions usually begin early in life and are intractable. The disorder can sometimes be recognised in infancy or early childhood if the characteristic yellowish plaques or phakomata are seen in the retina. Cerebral gliomas commonly develop in such cases and few survive beyond the third decade.

CEREBRAL LIPIDOSIS

A number of diseases exist which are characterised by disorders of lipid metabolism, resulting in the accumulation of abnormal lipids within cells, often including those of the central nervous system. In **Niemann–Pick's disease** the cortical nerve cells may contain sphingomyelin, as do reticuloendothelial cells in many other parts of the body, but nervous symptoms are usually unobtrusive, while splenomegaly and hepatomegaly are striking. Neurological involvement may also be seen in **Gaucher's** disease in which kerasin accumulates, particularly in the cells of the spleen and liver; occasionally neurological symptoms and signs (paresis of the limbs, fits, and intellectual deterioration) occur. In **Hand–Schuller–Christian** disease the accumulation of cholesterol gives xanthomatous deposits, particularly in the bones of the skull and pelvis. The disease is commonest in childhood and usually gives rise to diabetes insipidus and exophthalmos. The commonest lipidosis to affect the central nervous system, however, is the so-called **cerebromacular degeneration** in which gangliosides are deposited in the cells of the central nervous system and these become enormously ballooned. The infantile variety of this disorder, which often affects more than one member of a family, is usually called **Tay–Sachs disease** or **amaurotic family idiocy** and is confined to the Jewish race. Other varieties of the disorder, to which many eponymous titles have been given, may develop in later childhood and even in early adult life. The characteristic features of all varieties of the disease are progressive dementia and paralysis and epilepsy of myoclonic type; the myoclonic jerks are frequently evoked by startle, while major convulsions also occur. In infancy and early childhood, blindness frequently develops and there is a typical cherry-red spot at the macula. The EEG often reveals almost continuous irregular spike-and-wave discharges which some regard as almost diagnostic of this disease. The condition in all its forms is invariably progressive to a fatal termination, usually in from one to ten years, the course being shorter in younger patients.

PROGRESSIVE MYOCLONIC EPILEPSY

In this familial disorder, first described by Unverricht, repeated myoclonic jerking of the face, trunk and limbs of increasing and uncontrollable severity is associated with progressive dementia; this disease, too, is eventually fatal. Pathologically there is particularly striking degeneration of the dentate nuclei of the cerebellum. In many such cases abnormal mucopolysaccharides can be found in the serum and inclusion bodies may be found in affected cells in the cerebellum.

NEUROFIBROMATOSIS

This disorder, which is genetically determined, and inherited as an autosomal dominant character, is characterised by the development of widespread benign tumours which grow from the neurolemmal sheaths of nerves. **Cutaneous pigmentation** in the form of *café-au-lait* spots and/or larger areas of diffuse pigmentation with an irregular edge, is an almost invariable association. Cutaneous fibromata are often widespread throughout the body as sessile or pedunculated soft pink swellings, while firmer beady nodules may be found attached to peripheral nerves. Sometimes plexiform neuromatous enlargement of peripheral nerves occurs and is associated with an overgrowth of skin and subcutaneous tissue to give an appearance resembling localised elephantiasis. Bone involvement can produce hyperostosis of the facial or long bones while small plaques or phakomata may be seen in the retina. Neurofibromas sometimes cause painful compression of peripheral nerves; they may grow on spinal roots, giving rise to root pain and spinal cord compression; and they can develop intracranially on cranial nerve sheaths (e.g. acoustic neuroma, trigeminal neuroma) to give clinical features indicating intracranial neoplasia. Intracranial meningiomas and gliomas also occur in these patients more often than could be accounted for by coincidence, and a glioma of an optic nerve is particularly common. Sarcomatous change in a fibroma is an occasional complication. In severe cases a series of neurosurgical operations may sometimes be required for the relief of symptoms as neurofibromas in different situations produce their effects, but many cases run a relatively benign course and the patients survive to a normal age. It is remarkable to find that in some patients in whom radiographs clearly demonstrate the presence of several large intraspinal neurofibromas, signs and symptoms of spinal cord compression remain slight for a great many years and pain is the most prominent symptom. Surgery is best avoided in such cases unless increasing limb weakness or severe sphincter disturbance appear.

THE HEREDITARY ATAXIAS AND RELATED DISORDERS

Among the degenerative disorders of the nervous system there exist a large group of comparatively rare progressive disorders or syndromes, many of which are identified by eponymous titles, and which have in common the fact that their appearance seems to depend entirely upon genetic factors. In some families these diseases, if distinctive diseases they be, appear to be inherited as autosomal dominant characters, in others, despite similar clinical features, as autosomal recessives. Only in one condition which may provisionally be included in this group, namely **Leber's optic atrophy,** does a sex-linked recessive mechanism hold. This inherited disorder is characterised by sudden bilateral visual impairment developing, usually in males, in early adult life, and bilateral central scotomas are found in the visual fields. It can be regarded as an inherited form of retrobulbar neuritis; its relationship to neuromyelitis optica (*see* Chap. 14) is uncertain.

The remaining clinical features which can appear alone or in combination in the diseases of the hereditary ataxia group include progressive dementia, insidiously progressive optic atrophy, pigmentary retinal degeneration, agenesis or degeneration of cranial nerve nuclei, including those of the oculomotor, facial and auditory nerves, cerebellar ataxia, sensory ataxia and/or peripheral loss of pain sensation, due either to lesions in the posterior root ganglia or in the posterior columns of the spinal cord, spastic paraplegia or quadriplegia, wasting and weakness of peripheral limb muscles, hypertrophy of peripheral nerves, and skeletal deformities. A bewildering variety of individual syndromes have been described within the confines of this group. It is now apparent that, whereas there are a number of disorders which appear repeatedly in different families with reasonably stereotyped clinical manifestations, a very large number of different combinations of the clinical features outlined above has been reported occasionally in individual families, and many of these rare combinations have received distinctive names.

RETINITIS PIGMENTOSA. This condition is characterised in the beginning by night blindness but later by progressive visual deterioration and constriction of the visual fields. Epilepsy and nerve deafness are commonly associated. The optic disk is pale, the retinal vessels are attentuated and there is a typical arborisation of dark pigment in the retina, particularly towards the periphery.

AGENESIS OR DEGENERATION OF CRANIAL NERVE NUCLEI. A condition which gives rise to progressive bilateral ptosis and impairment of ocular movement in all directions was once referred to as progressive nuclear ophthalmoplegia, but it is now apparent that in most such cases the condition is one of muscular dystrophy of the external ocular muscles. However, a similar syndrome is sometimes seen in association with cerebellar ataxia and retinal pigmentation and it seems possible that in some such cases the lesion may indeed be nuclear. Bilateral facial paralysis present from birth (facial diplegia–Möbius's syndrome), is probably due to an agenesis of the facial nerve nuclei. Progressive nerve deafness can also be an inherited disorder, occurring either alone or in combination with other neurological manifestations.

HEREDITARY SPASTIC PARAPLEGIA is a genetically determined disorder in which spastic weakness of the lower limbs generally develops in early adult life and progresses slowly over many years, eventually involving the upper limbs and even the bulbar muscles. Pes cavus is commonly present.

FRIEDREICH'S ATAXIA is probably the most common and stereotyped of the hereditary ataxias. In addition to a spastic paraplegia, there are usually signs of cerebellar ataxia in all four limbs and also of impairment of sensation mediated through the posterior columns of the cord (absent vibration sense, impaired position and joint sense). Scoliosis and pes cavus are usually present in addition, while there is often an associated myocardial degeneration. Owing to the degeneration of the root entry zones of the posterior nerve roots, it is not unusual for deep tendon reflexes to be absent, even when the plantar responses are clearly extensor. There is often dysarthria of 'cerebellar' type and nystagmus is common. The condition is slowly progressive, beginning usually in adolescence—often the patient is able to walk for many years but death is usual, often from heart failure, in middle-life. It is not uncommon for apparently unaffected relatives of patients with Friedreich's disease to show mild stigmata of the disease (pes cavus, scoliosis) without neurological signs, and benign varieties (formes frustes) of the syndrome are also seen occasionally, in which signs of spinal cord disease are few and the pathological process appears to become arrested.

HEREDITARY CEREBELLAR ATAXIA is a term applied to a group of inherited disorders which are mainly characterised by a progressive and symmetrical cerebellar ataxia. In most families symptoms first appear in early adult life but sometimes the condition develops in late middle-age (late-life cerebellar ataxia). When the neurological signs indicate that the disease process is virtually limited to the cerebellum and its connexions, the condition is often referred to as *Marie's ataxia*, but when there is associated optic atrophy, external ophthalmoplegia and spastic paraparesis, without skeletal deformity, a diagnosis of the *Sanger–Brown variety* is often made. If, in addition to cerebellar ataxia, there are also dementia, a titubating tremor of the head, static tremor of the limbs and a spastic paraplegia, then this clinical picture is typical of *olivopontocerebellar atrophy*. *Refsum's syndrome (heredopathia atactica polyneuritiformis)* includes cerebellar ataxia, nerve deafness and a peripheral neuropathy of predominantly sensory type, while the *Roussy–Levy* syndrome is a name given to a syndrome of hereditary areflexia which is sometimes accompanied by cerebellar ataxia and pes cavus or by peripheral amyotrophy. Yet another variety of familial cerebellar ataxia may be associated with consistent amino-aciduria, and may well be due to some specific but as yet unidentified metabolic disorder (*Hartnup disease*). Recent evidence suggests that Refsum's syndrome is almost certainly a disorder of lipid metabolism.

HEREDITARY SENSORY NEUROPATHY. While symptoms and signs of dysfunction of the posterior columns of the spinal cord are common in Friedreich's ataxia, there is a much more severe inherited disorder of sensory pathways in which the principal pathological change is one of degeneration in posterior root ganglia. The appreciation of pain and temperature sense as well as touch and position are greatly impaired, particularly in the lower limbs, so that perforating ulcers of the feet, disorganisation of joints (Charcot-type arthropathy) and eventually destruction of terminal phalanges (Morvan's syndrome) are common. The condition bears a superficial resemblance to syringomyelia, in which disease, however, sensory loss of dissociated type (*vide infra*) is generally confined to the upper limbs.

PERONEAL MUSCULAR ATROPHY (CHARCOT – MARIE – TOOTH DISEASE). This is in many ways the most benign of the hereditary degenerative nervous diseases, for despite the gross muscular atrophy and weakness which affect particularly the muscles of the foot and leg below the knee, and later, as a rule, the small muscles of the hands, sufferers generally remain active despite this disease for a great many years and even into late adult life. The condition is due to a chronic degenerative change in nerve roots and peripheral nerves, so that it is properly regarded as a neuropathy. Yet the involvement is curiously localised, for in the upper limb the muscular atrophy never advances beyond the forearm, while in the lower limbs it affects the legs and distal one-third of the thighs but spreads no further (the inverted champagne-bottle leg). Bilateral foot drop and claw hands are characteristic and the appreciation of vibration is generally absent at the ankles, but there is remarkably little else to find, as a rule, on sensory examination.

PROGRESSIVE HYPERTROPHIC INTERSTITIAL POLYNEUROPATHY (Dejerine–Sottas) is another hereditary disease in which the distribution of the muscular involvement is virtually identical with that seen in peroneal muscular atrophy, though there may be more extensive peripheral sensory impairment. Furthermore, the peripheral nerves (the ulnar and the external popliteal are easiest to feel) are greatly enlarged, due apparently to a proliferation of the neurolemmal sheath, which forms additional layers around the nerve fibres in an 'onion-skin' manner. From the prognostic standpoint this condition is similar to peroneal muscular atrophy.

In this short account of the so-called hereditary ataxia group, no attempt has been made to cover the ground comprehensively, but it is important to realise that although some such conditions breed true, a remarkable variety of atypical and transitional forms appear; there are many sporadic cases which do not at first sight appear to fit any single category of neurological disease. Prognosis and management become much more straightforward once it is found that such a case in reality belongs to the hereditary ataxia group.

PARKINSONISM

Parkinsonism, or 'the shaking palsy', as first described by James Parkinson in 1817, is a common degenerative nervous disorder. It occurs in two principal forms, namely **paralysis agitans,** and **post-encephalitic** Parkinsonism which develops as a sequel of encephalitis lethargica. Similar clinical manifestations can result from cerebral atherosclerosis, from head injury (as in the punch-drunk boxer), from neurosyphilis and from poisoning with carbon monoxide or manganese, but in such cases the resemblance to typical Parkinson's disease is generally superficial. The syndrome of so-called **atherosclerotic Parkinsonism** usually occurs in elderly hypertensive patients; facial masking and progressive stiffness of the limbs may develop but tremor is not seen, the plantar responses often become extensor, dementia commonly supervenes and many patients eventually develop signs of 'pseudobulbar palsy' due to progressive cerebral and brain-stem softening. In both paralysis agitans and the post-encephalitic variety, the maximal site of pathological change is in the substantia nigra of the mid-brain. The clinical features of the two varieties of the disease are broadly similar, differing only in detail. For instance, the age of onset is generally earlier and the rate of progress of the disorder is much more rapid in post-encephalitic Parkinsonism; in this variety, too, rigidity is often more striking than tremor, while in paralysis agitans the reverse is usually the case. Oculogyric crises (*vide infra*) occur only in the post-encephalitic variety, while in this type mental changes, taking the form of emotional lability, dementia, or even psychotic manifestations including paranoia and delusions, are more common. Paralysis agitans is more common in men than in women, and develops usually after the age of fifty, while in post-encephalitic cases an onset in early adult life and even in childhood or adolescence has been quite frequent, following almost immediately upon the acute encephalitic illness. New cases of the post-encephalitic type are becoming increasingly rare with the virtual disappearance of encephalitis lethargica, but it cannot be denied that a small number of cases of Parkinsonism which have developed in recent years may nevertheless be the sequel of a mild encephalitis occurring many years ago, or of an unrecognised, more recent, sporadic outbreak of the disease.

The characteristic clinical features of Parkinsonism include disorders of facial expression, posture, gait, attitude and movement, and also muscular rigidity and tremor. The recognition of an early case of paralysis agitans can be a matter of extreme difficulty, even for the most skilled clinician. It has been wisely said that in certain cases the diagnosis will almost certainly be missed despite meticulous examination unless it is made as the patient enters the room. It must be remembered that the condition not uncommonly begins unilaterally with clumsiness of one hand and slight dragging of one leg. When tremor is inconspicuous it is easy to overlook the correct diagnosis in such a case, unless one remembers that Parkinsonism frequently gives a slowly progressive hemiparetic syndrome in late middle-age.

The immobile, unblinking **facial expression** of the established case is characteristic; if the disorder is more severe there may be a trickle of saliva from the corner of the mouth and tapping above the bridge of the nose gives a rhythmical blinking which continues indefinitely in time with the taps (glabellar tap sign.) The speech is often slow, quiet and monotonous. Usually, too, the patient is slightly stooped; he walks with quick, shuffling steps as if constantly about to fall forwards while chasing his own centre of gravity **(the festinant gait).** Typically there is a deficiency of associated movements; swinging of the arms, in particular, is greatly impaired. Characteristically the patient will say that he has become greatly slowed in all his activities and that fine movements carried out with the affected hand or hands have become increasingly clumsy; usually the handwriting has become much smaller (micrographia).

The **muscular rigidity** of Parkinson's disease varies greatly in distribution and severity. In one case it may be mild and localised, affecting only one arm and leg, in another profound and generalised, rendering the patient mute and virtually immobile. Typically it affects flexor and extensor muscles to an equal extent, unlike spasticity, and it can be of the plastic or 'lead-pipe' variety or else 'cog-wheel' in type. One of the earliest signs in the limbs may be a reduced range and amplitude of movement, well demonstrated on asking the patient to carry out repeated opposition of the thumb and individual fingers of an affected hand. Often the tendon reflexes are increased in moderately rigid limbs; contractures of the fingers and feet may occur in advanced cases.

Tremor, of the static type, is the typical involuntary movement of Parkinsonism. It is most apparent in one or both hands and/or feet but occasionally involves the head and other midline structures. Usually it is abolished by voluntary movement, but may persist while the movement is performed (action tremor). It is typically rhythmical and sometimes of pill-rolling type, occurring four to eight times a second and generally being accentuated by emotional stress and excitement.

The **oculogyric crises** of the post-encephalitic form of the disease consist of attacks of involuntary conjugate movement of the eyes, usually in an upward direction, with retraction of the upper lids. These are a most distressing symptom and are often difficult to control.

Sensory disorders are not a feature of the Parkinsonian syndrome, but **autonomic disturbances** (excess sweating, retention of urine) occasionally occur. The disease is progressive but varies greatly in clinical course from case to case. The more severe of the post-encephalitic cases can be almost totally disabled and bed-ridden within a few years from the onset, but, with few exceptions, paralysis agitans is much more benign and patients may live reasonably active lives, but with increasing restrictions, for many years. The lot of the patient with Parkinson's disease, has, however, been greatly alleviated by the many new drugs and surgical procedures which have been introduced in recent years (*see* Chapter 20).

SYRINGOMYELIA

Syringomyelia is a slowly progressive degenerative disorder in which cavitation develops within the central grey matter of the spinal cord and sometimes extends into the lower brain stem (**syringobulbia**). This cavitation usually occurs in the cervical cord and may extend over many segments from the lower medulla into the upper dorsal region. Similar changes in the lumbar region have been known to occur but are rare. The disorder is usually sporadic, though rare familial cases have been described; it is more common in males than in females and is generally first apparent clinically between the ages of twenty and forty years. The aetiology is unknown, but maldevelopment or incomplete closure of the central canal of the cord are believed by many to be responsible. As a rule, however, the syringomyelic cavity is separate from the central canal; it is occupied by clear gelatinous material, is not lined by ependyma, and is surrounded by an area of gliosis. Occasionally a true dilatation of the central canal or hydromyelia, with clinical effects similar to those of syringomyelia, develops in a patient with a tumour compressing the cervical cord, or in cases of the Arnold-Chiari malformation, in which the clinical picture of syringomyelia may be mimicked, particularly if hydrocephalus and spina bifida are absent.

Since the centrally-situated cavity interrupts the decussating sensory fibres carrying pain and temperature sensation which are destined to ascend in the spinothalamic tract, the most prominent clinical feature of syringomyelia is dissociated anaesthesia (loss or impairment of pain and temperature sensation with preservation of light touch, position and joint sense and tactile discrimination). The cavity may also extend anteriorly to destroy anterior horn cells and laterally to compress the pyramidal and spinothalamic tracts. The posterior columns are affected late in the course of the disease if at all. In the brain stem the motor nuclei of the lower cranial nerves and the spinal tract and nucleus of the trigeminal nerve are commonly involved.

The onset of the disease is typically insidious. The first symptoms are usually sensory in type; the patient may notice numbness of a part of one hand or becomes aware that injuries to the hand are no longer painful. Sometimes aching or burning pain in the limb is experienced. Less commonly the earliest manifestations are those of progressive weakness of a hand, with inability to extend the fingers, and flexion contracture soon develops. Often the symptoms and physical signs are unilateral for some time.

Dissociated anaesthesia is often found initially in a part of the hand or forearm, or else it may form a 'half-cape' over the shoulder and upper arm with a sharp line of demarcation at the midline and horizontally across the upper chest wall. Eventually the whole of one arm and a 'cape' area is affected and later still the sensory loss may become bilateral. Not infrequently the upper cervical segments are also involved to give hypalgesia and thermoanaesthesia over the neck and scalp; the forehead may then become analgesic or else the sensory loss shows a 'balaclava helmet' distribution, with only the more central portions of the face being sensitive. Similar sensory impairment is uncommon in the lower parts of the trunk and in the lower limbs; when it does occur it is generally more patchy in distribution and usually results from compression of the spinothalamic tract in the cervical region. Only rarely is it due to a syrinx in the lumbar cord. Destruction of anterior horn cells gives rise to **wasting and weakness of upper limb muscles,** often with some fasciculation. Usually the small muscles of the hands are first involved, but later the upper arm and shoulder girdle are affected. Extension of the disease process to the brain stem results in nystagmus, atrophy of the tongue and of the sternomastoids, weakness of palatal, pharyngeal and laryngeal muscles, and occasionally a Horner's syndrome develops. Compression of the pyramidal tracts in the cervical region eventually leads to **spastic weakness of the lower limbs** with increased deep reflexes and extensor plantar responses; impaired vibration sense and position and joint sense in the lower limbs are uncommon, but occasionally appear in the more advanced cases.

Trophic changes, resulting in the main from impaired pain sensation, are generally striking. The affected hand is often brawny and swollen with multiple scars resulting from previous trauma; indolent ulcers frequently follow minor injury. Disorganisation of joints (Charcot's arthropathy) often occurs particularly in the shoulder or elbow and swelling of the joint with gross but painless crepitus on movement will then be apparent. In severe cases, actual necrosis of terminal phalanges is seen (Morvan's syndrome).

In general, syringomyelia is a relatively benign disorder. Progression is usually very slow and the disease process may appear to become arrested for periods of many years, although occasional cases deteriorate more quickly. Death usually results in the end from an unrelated disease, though bulbar paralysis may be responsible for fatal bronchopneumonia. Treatment is largely symptomatic, as radiotherapy, though it may sometimes relieve pain, appears to have no definite influence upon the progression of the disease process. In very occasional cases, surgical decompression of the spinal cord with aspiration of the syringomyelic cavity is helpful if a block is demonstrated on myelography.

SPINA BIFIDA

Incomplete closure of the vertebral canal can be associated with a variety of abnormalities in the underlying spinal cord and in the roots of the cauda equina. In severe cases there is a protruding sac containing the meninges and the termination of the spinal cord and cauda equina (meningomyelocele). Under such circumstances there is a soft swelling over the lumbosacral area, the legs are generally paralysed from birth, there may be associated cerebral abnormalities (hydrocephalus, the Arnold–Chiari malformation) and the condition may be incompatible with prolonged survival.

In spina bifida occulta, however, there is generally no palpable swelling and the bony defect is only apparent on X-ray. Many individuals with such a congenital defect in a mild form are symptom-free throughout life, but others are late in walking. Subsequently a variety of neurological abnormalities may develop, varying from mild pes cavus and some precipitancy of micturition on the one hand to severe disorders of urinary, faecal and sexual function with muscular weakness, wasting and sensory loss in the legs and perineal area of variable degree on the other. These symptoms are due to disordered function of the nerve roots of the cauda equina; in many such cases treatment can only be symptomatic, but in some it is possible to divide surgically a fibrocartilaginous band constricting roots within the spinal canal or to remove an associated intraspinal cyst of congenital origin. Hence in such a case, clinical deterioration is generally an indication for investigation, including myelography.

It has become increasingly apparent in recent years that in some children with atrophy or deformity of one foot with or without localised reflex changes and/or sensory loss, minor forms of **spinal dysraphism** may be found and these are always associated with some degree of spina bifida though this may be occult. In many such cases surgical treatment (division of constricting fibrous bands or removal of an intradural lipoma) is helpful. Occasionally the condition first becomes apparent in adolescence or early adult life.

MYELODYSPLASIA

This developmental anomaly of the lower part of the spinal cord, which is probably due to an incomplete closure of the neural tube in the embryo, gives symptoms which are generally similar to those of spina bifida occulta, with which it may be associated. The clinical picture is in some respects like that of lumbar syringomyelia, but the condition is non-progressive. Pes cavus, muscular weakness and wasting and sensory loss in the lower limbs of variable extent are generally combined with sphincter disturbances (intermittent incontinence of urine and faeces).

BASILAR IMPRESSION OF THE SKULL

A congenital malformation of the occipital condyles of the skull can lead to the partial invagination of the first cervical vertebra into the foramen magnum. This generally results in an upward movement of the odontoid process of the axis with consequent compression of the lower cranial nerves, cerebellar tonsils, upper cervical nerve roots and the upper part of the spinal cord. In such individuals the neck is unusually short and characteristic radiological appearances are found. The clinical features are variable in degree and severity, but include hydrocephalus (due to partial obstruction of cerebrospinal fluid circulation through exit foramina of the fourth ventricle and basal cisterns), cerebellar ataxia in the limbs, and a spastic quadri-paresis. A characteristic feature can be severe loss of position and joint sense in both hands. Once symptoms and signs have appeared they tend to progress, but the condition can sometimes be alleviated by surgical decompression, involving removal of the posterior border of the foramen magnum. The syndrome is often referred to as platybasia, as the base of the skull is flattened, but there are other causes of radiological platybasia which do not give rise to neuro-logical signs. Basilar impression may be associated with congenital anomalies of the cervical spine (e.g. fusion of multiple cervical vertebrae—the Klippel–Feil syndrome), while such anomalies in turn can give rise to neurological symptoms and signs suggestive of a lesion in the neighbourhood of the foramen magnum, even when no significant degree of basilar impression is present.

PAGET'S DISEASE AND OTHER SKELETAL ABNORMALITIES

The progressive thickening and distortion of bone which occurs in Paget's disease of the skull can give rise to neurological symptoms and signs. Thus optic atrophy may result from compression of the optic nerves in their exit foramina and other cranial nerves can be similarly involved. As a result of the platybasia which results from this disease, it is possible for a clinical picture resembling that of basilar impression to develop. Paget's disease of the vertebral column is occasionally responsible for a progressive paraplegia due to spinal cord compression and a similar syndrome is known to occur infrequently in **achondroplasia.**

VASCULAR MALFORMATIONS

A remarkable variety of vascular anomalies of the nervous system have been described. The intracranial **arteriovenous angioma,** which is one of the commonest, will be considered in Chapter 17. A similar anomaly is occasionally found in the spinal cord; here too, malformation and dilatations of the smaller blood vessels (**telangiectases**) are sometimes seen, and may give rise to intramedullary haemorrhage with consequent clinical symptoms.

One unusual but stereotyped cerebral vascular malformation is the **Sturge–Weber syndrome.** In this condition a subcortical angiomatosis of precapillaries, a lesion which eventually becomes calcified after a few years of life to give a characteristic radiological pattern outlining the gyri of the posterior part of one cerebral hemisphere, is associated with a port-wine naevus of the face on the same side. Often the eye on this side is also enlarged (buphthalmos or ox-eye). Usually these patients show a contralateral infantile hemiplegia and suffer from recurrent epileptiform convulsions. Some cases can be greatly benefited by removal of the affected cerebral hemisphere.

NEUROMUSCULAR AND MUSCULAR DISORDERS

In addition to the conditions which have received consideration in this chapter, there exist a group of neuromuscular and muscular disorders which are clearly genetically-determined. This group of conditions, which includes the muscular dystrophies, will be considered in Chapter 18.

REFERENCES

BRAIN, W. R., *Diseases of the Nervous System*, 6th ed., Chapters 3, 12 and 13 (London, Oxford University Press, 1962).
CRITCHLEY, M., *Developmental Dyslexia* (London, Heinemann, 1964).
DODGE, P. R. and ADAMS, R. D., 'Developmental abnormalities of the nervous system', in *Principles of Internal Medicine*, Ed. Harrison, T. R., 4th ed., Chapter 283 (New York, McGraw-Hill, 1962).

FORD, F. R., *Diseases of the Nervous System in Infancy, Childhood and Adolescence*, 3rd ed., Chapters 3 and 4 (Springfield, Ill., Thomas, 1952).

INGRAM, T. T. S., *Paediatric Aspects of Cerebral Palsy* (Edinburgh, Livingstone, 1964).

MORIARTY, J. A. and KLINGMAN, W. O., 'Congenital and prenatal diseases', in *Clinical Neurology*, 2nd ed., Ed. Baker, A. B. (New York, Hoeber-Harper, 1962).

RICHARDSON, E. P., JR. and TORUK, A., 'Degenerative diseases of the nervous system', in *Principles of Internal Medicine*, Ed. Harrison, T. R., 4th ed., Chapter 290 (New York, McGraw-Hill, 1962).

CHAPTER 13

TRAUMA AND THE NERVOUS SYSTEM

THE functioning of the various parts of the central and peripheral nervous system can be gravely disturbed as a result of physical injury. Although penetrating wounds of the brain, spinal cord and peripheral nerves are commonly encountered in war-time, these are relatively uncommon in civil practice. Nevertheless, closed head injuries (in which the skull is not penetrated), resulting in the main from road and industrial accidents, constitute a major problem. Although the finer points of diagnosis and management in cases of severe craniocerebral injury are largely a matter for the specialist neurosurgeon, every physician and general practitioner requires a working knowledge of the nosology of the different types of head injury, of their usual clinical course and of their sequelae. To refer all patients with relatively minor head injuries for neurosurgical advice would at present place an impossible load upon these special units and it is therefore essential that the physician or general surgeon who may care for these cases initially should be on the look-out for possible complications. It should also be remembered that it is occasionally very difficult to decide in an individual case whether neurological symptoms and signs which are present have resulted from a head injury or whether the initial event had been a cerebral vascular accident, say, following upon which the patient had fallen and injured the head. The clinical syndromes produced by injury to or compression of the spinal cord and peripheral nerves can also present difficult problems in diagnosis and management. This chapter will therefore deal first with head injuries, their effects, complications and sequelae, secondly with injury to the spinal cord, and thirdly with peripheral nerve lesions.

HEAD INJURIES

The immediate effects of head injury may be classified into three principal groups which are first, concussion, a temporary and reversible disorder of brain function which is not apparently associated with any recognisable pathological change in the brain; secondly, cerebral contusion or laceration, in which there is direct bruising or tearing of brain tissue; and thirdly, intracranial haemorrhage, either from tearing of the middle meningeal artery or its branches following skull fracture (extradural haemorrhage), subdural haematoma, which results from an injury to veins traversing the subdural space, or traumatic subarachnoid haemorrhage which is a common accompaniment of cerebral contusion or laceration.

Concussion

There have been many attempts to explain the phenomenon of concussion; this produces the syndrome of impaired consciousness which follows upon a closed head injury. Probably it is due to a transitory disturbance of function in the brain stem reticular substance. The patient who recovers from concussion is usually unable to recall the actual moment of injury and indeed his memory may be blank for several preceding seconds or even minutes. The duration of this **retrograde amnesia** may be a guide to the severity of the injury, but much more valuable in this respect is the duration of the **post-traumatic amnesia** (i.e. the period for which memory was lost after the accident, corresponding to the duration of severe concussion). After a relatively severe injury the patient may be comatose with shallow slow respiration, a feeble pulse, and widely dilated pupils; during recovery, after minutes or even several hours the pupils react, the pulse becomes stronger and the patient responsive. For some time, however, he is restless, confused and irritable, complains of headache and may vomit repeatedly. When coma is complete for more than a few hours it is probable that the injury has been more serious than simple concussion. Following upon a less severe injury the patient may merely be dazed for some minutes or hours and may undertake purposive activities of which he subsequently has no recollection; generalised headache and vomiting are usual at this stage. Most patients recover satisfactorily from concussion within two to three days, but headaches and other symptoms of the post-traumatic syndrome (*vide infra*) sometimes persist for weeks or months and occasionally for several years.

Contusion and Laceration

Cerebral contusion may take the form of localised bruising of the brain directly beneath the point of impact in a case of closed head injury. Alternatively, a contusion, or a laceration, which can be similarly produced, though it can, of course, result from a penetrating wound, may occur on the side of the brain away from the site of injury, due possibly to a sudden thrust of the relatively mobile brain against the inner table of the skull (contrecoup injury). The term contusion has also been applied to a generalised cerebral disturbance more severe than concussion in which there are multiple small intracerebral haemorrhages as well as diffuse cerebral oedema, changes which result at least in part from a sudden violent movement of cerebrospinal fluid along those perivascular cuffs of the meninges which penetrate the brain along the blood vessels.

The patient with a very severe cerebral contusion is usually unconscious immediately, but becomes progressively more deeply comatose until he dies from medullary compression. Some few cases remain unconscious and unresponsive but can nevertheless be kept alive for many weeks or months by means of careful nursing. Usually in patients who show no significant recovery of awareness within a week from the time of injury there has been a degree of damage to the cerebral white matter or to the brain stem reticular substance which is incompatible with recovery; in very rare instances, however, patients have recovered, though with considerable intellectual impairment, after months of unconsciousness. In less severely injured cases, there is often a period of several days during which the patient is comatose or semicomatose. There may be signs indicating damage to the brain stem (decerebrate posture and spasms, cranial nerve palsies) or to one or other cerebral hemisphere (focal convulsions, or hemiplegia), though these are often difficult to identify while the patient is unconscious. With some degree of returning awareness comes the stage of so-called traumatic delirium, in which the patient may be noisy, unco-operative, confused and even violent. It is at this stage that symptoms or signs of focal contusion or laceration often become apparent. Gradually, as improvement continues, the patient becomes more rational and orientated, though headache commonly persists, and symptoms of the post-traumatic syndrome are often particularly severe in such cases. There may also be persisting aphasia, paralysis or cranial nerve palsies if the local injury has been sufficiently severe. If the cranial nerve injuries have been due to tearing of the nerve trunks owing to a fracture of the skull involving their exit foramina (as may occur particularly with the facial, auditory, abducent and optic nerves) the injury is often permanent. A sixth nerve paralysis can occur, however, as a transient phenomenon following upon a relatively mild head injury, being a false localising sign due to cerebral oedema and raised pressure. Occasionally during the stage of recovery, a characteristic Korsakoff syndrome (*see* Chapter 7) develops, but this generally recovers. In other cases the initial injury has been so severe, and damage so widespread, that permanent impairment of the intellect, or traumatic dementia, results. The so-called traumatic encephalopathy or **punch-drunk syndrome** of professional boxers, in which there is usually deterioration of memory and intellect, with tremor and slowness or poverty of movement resembling that of Parkinson's disease, is probably due to the cumulative effect of many comparatively minor episodes of cerebral contusion. In such cases air encephalography usually demonstrates absence of the septum pellucidum.

Intracranial Haemorrhage

Multiple small intracerebral haemorrhages may result, as already mentioned, from cerebral contusion, and on occasion more extensive and localised bleeding into brain tissue follows injury. It is also very common for some degree of bleeding into the subarachnoid space to be present following upon a closed head injury, particularly if the skull has been fractured. It is, however, the types of haemorrhage which occur in the extradural and subdural spaces, and in which bleeding can continue for some time after injury, that are particularly important to recognise, as these require specific treatment.

An acute **extradural haematoma** can follow upon any head injury in which there has been a fracture of the skull vault involving one of the channels on the inner table in which lies the middle meningeal artery or one of its branches. Characteristically in such a case there will have occurred a head injury of moderate severity with concussion but with recovery of consciousness within a few minutes or hours. For an hour or two the patient may then have been reasonably alert and conscious, but subsequently he became increasingly drowsy and lapsed into semicoma or coma. In some such cases, signs of compression of one cerebral hemisphere (contralateral hemiparesis, homolateral fixed dilated pupil or third nerve palsy, due to compression of the third nerve at the edge of the tentorium cerebelli) may develop. There are certain cases in which no lucid interval occurs following injury, and in which diagnosis of this condition must depend upon progressive deepening of unconsciousness following the injury. Early diagnosis is imperative as operation is usually curative; otherwise death soon results from brain stem compression and infarction.

An acute **subdural haematoma** is another complication of head injury, resulting from rupture of veins which traverse the subdural space. When this condition develops acutely, as it may after severe trauma at any age, the clinical picture differs little from that of extradural haemorrhage. It is cases of subacute or chronic subdural haematoma which more often present baffling diagnostic problems, but their recognition is equally important as the condition may readily be treated neurosurgically; if unrecognised it is soon fatal. Chronic subdural bleeding generally occurs in elderly patients in whom the subdural veins are particularly fragile; it can follow a trivial injury, such as jarring the head on a low beam, and sometimes it seems to occur spontaneously. 'Spontaneous' subdural bleeding is particularly liable to occur in patients receiving long-term anti-coagulant therapy or in those with chronic liver damage. Typically the injury has no immediate ill-effects, but over the succeeding days or even weeks the patient complains of vague headache, intermittent drowsiness and lapses of memory. There may be episodes of confusion, a lack of attention to detail, failure of concentration, and long periods spent alone in the bathroom. Drowsiness, headache and sometimes vomiting become progressively more severe, and the patient eventually lapses into a state of stupor or intermittent mutism or eventually semicoma. Commonly there is fluctuation in the conscious level, lucid intervals alternating with periods of confusion or stupor. Focal neurological signs, Jacksonian epilepsy, dilatation of the homolateral pupil and papilloedema can result from increased intracranial pressure, and eventually respiration and cardiac function are impaired. The cerebrospinal fluid is often xanthochromic but contains no blood. The electroencephalogram may be helpful, revealing a unilateral suppression of the alpha rhythm or else unilateral slow activity, while radiographs of the skull will sometimes demonstrate a shift of the pineal gland. Carotid arteriography gives diagnostic appearances, but more often when this diagnosis is suspected, exploratory burr-holes are indicated, since evacuation of the clot generally results in complete recovery.

Complications and Sequelae

Infection is an important complication of head injury. When a fracture of the skull is accompanied by wounds of the scalp, cranial osteomyelitis, which can in turn lead to extradural suppuration, is clearly an important complication, while penetrating wounds carry with them the possibility of infection of the meninges (meningitis) or of the brain tissue itself (suppurative encephalitis, cerebral abscess). Even when there is no wound of the scalp it is not uncommon for a fracture of the skull to enter the paranasal sinuses or middle ear. Organisms can then pass through a tear in the dura mater, giving rise to meningitis; this complication should always be borne in mind if there has been bleeding or leakage of cerebrospinal fluid from the ears or nose and there may then be an indication for antibiotic therapy, followed later by surgical repair of the tear in the dura. It is not uncommon in such cases for air to enter the cranial cavity and even the cerebral substance, giving rise to an encysted collection or **aerocele.** This can be responsible for recurrent infection if a communication with the sinus or middle ear persists, or for Jacksonian epilepsy or symptoms and signs indicating the presence of an intracranial space-occupying lesion.

The commonest cause of **post-traumatic epilepsy** is, however, a focal cerebral contusion or laceration which, having healed by the formation of a scar, is often adherent to the inner surface of the dura mater. If the scar is large it may produce an evagination of the lateral ventricle, in the form of a cyst (traumatic porencephaly). The incidence of epilepsy is clearly greater following upon penetrating wounds of the skull; between 25 and 35 per cent of such patients develop fits as a result of the injury (these figures, however, are derived from cases of gunshot wound, and in civil practice the incidence is probably lower). After closed head injuries in which there has been no clinical evidence of localised injury to the brain, upwards of 2 per cent of cases have seizures, but after severe contusion the proportion is probably higher. These usually begin between six months and one year after the injury, but occasionally they do not develop for several years. Commonly the fits are focal or of Jacksonian type, and then the clinical features will depend upon which area of the brain has been injured; in other cases in which, presumably, the epileptic discharge spreads rapidly throughout the brain, major epileptiform convulsions are the rule. Usually treatment with anticonvulsant drugs is indicated, but from time to time surgical excision of a cortical scar can be considered. It is a good general rule to assume that, except in childhood, when fits may occasionally follow a relatively minor head injury, no brain injury giving rise to post-traumatic amnesia of less than 24 hours' duration will be followed by genuine post-traumatic epilepsy.

The post-traumatic syndrome is a name which has been applied to a constellation of disabling symptoms which may follow head injury. It is most common and persistent following cases of severe cerebral contusion and in these it may sometimes accompany some degree of post-traumatic dementia. Following simple concussion it is generally mild and of brief duration, but much depends upon the individual's premorbid personality. Whereas it is clear that the condition has an organic basis, emotional factors may be responsible for its exaggeration and perpetuation. Patients of good personality may quickly recover even after severe trauma, while those of less stable constitution are often considerably disabled for some time following a relatively trivial injury. The problem of financial compensation is one which may greatly complicate prognosis and management and it is uncommon for a post-traumatic syndrome to improve as long as a medicolegal action is pending. The characteristic features of the condition are first, headache, which is often persistent or paroxysmally severe; it is generally felt in the frontal and/or occipital regions, is most severe in the mornings, and is accentuated by coughing or by movement. Secondly, defects of memory and concentration and lack of interest are usual, as are periods of depression or anxiety and episodes of fear, panic or depersonalisation. Commonly, too, there is a complaint of giddiness or instability, which is not always true vertigo though the latter may occur, particularly after sudden changes in the position of the head. Syncopal attacks, accompanied by hysterical manifestations in some cases, are also frequent and may sometimes be difficult to distinguish from post-traumatic epilepsy. These symptoms can persist for many weeks or months, and may even in occasional cases be permanent in some degree, but many patients recover completely in from six months to two years following upon the injury. The symptoms are nevertheless distressing and many patients show considerable personality change from their premorbid state; appropriate management is often a matter of great complexity, but reassurance and confident predictions of eventual recovery are all-important.

THE SPINAL CORD

The effects of a sudden penetrating injury to the spinal cord and those of cord compression are broadly similar, though certain clinical differences in effect stem from the fact that in the one case the lesion is sudden and in the other it is often more gradual.

Cord Injuries

The spinal cord may be damaged by penetrating wounds resulting from missiles but more often it is injured as a result of indirect violence. Thus severe flexion or hyperextension injuries of the neck can injure the cord, particularly when fracture-dislocation of the spine results. Even without a fracture, however, the cord may be contused. Falls from a height on to the feet or buttocks can similarly injure the lower spinal column and secondarily the cord. Sudden compression of the cord will also result from collapse and angulation of a vertebral body due either to tuberculosis or to a spinal metastasis.

The broad pathological varieties of spinal cord injury are similar to those which affect the brain. Thus **spinal concussion** is generally a temporary but reversible disorder of function which in the beginning can be remarkably complete. In **spinal contusion** or bruising, there are actual pathological changes including oedema and small focal haemorrhages, and the degree of eventual recovery is less complete as ascending and descending degeneration of spinal tracts takes place. **Laceration of the cord** implies an actual break in continuity which is irremediable, and symptoms resulting from such an injury show no improvement; furthermore, since penetrating wounds are often responsible for laceration, there is the additional complication of possible infection, which may give meningitis or myelitis.

A spinal cord injury generally produces an immediate flaccid paralysis and sensory loss in the limbs and trunk below the level of the lesion, with retention of urine and faeces. As the period of spinal shock wears off, movement and sensation will gradually return if the lesion was reversible, but if more severe, the patient will remain paraplegic and the upper level of sensory impairment will fail to recede. In such a case, reflex activity is eventually restored below the level of the lesion, the tendon reflexes become exaggerated, the plantar responses are extensor and automatic bladder and bowel activity are gradually established. Usually contractures of the hamstrings develop and there is a **paraplegia-in-flexion,** as tone is excessive in the flexor muscles. Minimal cutaneous stimulation of the lower limbs will often evoke painful flexor spasms which are a part of the primitive withdrawal reflex, and these may occasionally be accompanied by the so-called mass reflex of autonomic activity with profuse sweating below the lesion and evacuation of the bladder and bowels. Paraplegia-in-flexion usually develops after a complete or almost complete cord transection, since the pathways joining the spinal cord to the brain stem reticular substance, pathways which are responsible for an extensor hypertonus corresponding to that seen in the decerebrate posture, are interrupted. In partial lesions, however, in which the injury involves predominantly the pyramidal or corticospinal tracts, this extensor hypertonus is predominant, to give **paraplegia-in-extension,** and the flexor withdrawal reflex, which depends entirely upon short spinal reflex arcs, is partially suppressed. Many other clinical syndromes may result from incomplete spinal injuries. Of these, the Brown–Séquard syndrome, resulting from hemisection of cord, is an example (*see* Chapter 10). The prognosis of spinal cord injuries must of course depend upon the severity of the injury; reversal of the symptoms of spinal concussion generally occurs within at the most four weeks after the injury. Thereafter comparatively little further recovery of function is to be expected, but remarkable degrees of adaptation are sometimes possible.

Injuries of the **cauda equina** (the spinal roots below the termination of the spinal cord) are comparatively uncommon. These generally give rise to total paralysis of the bladder and bowels and of sexual function, with flaccid paralysis of the lower limbs; the actual distribution of muscular paralysis will depend upon which roots are involved. Since regeneration of these roots can occur, the prognosis of cauda equina injuries is somewhat better than that of cord injury, provided the continuity of their neurolemmal sheaths has not been destroyed.

Haematomyelia

Haematomyelia is a condition in which bleeding occurs within the

substance of the spinal cord. It can occur spontaneously in patients
with bleeding disorders, or may result from small vascular malformations or telangiectases within the cord, while it is rarely the result of
haemorrhage into a syringomyelic cavity. More often it is due to
relatively minor injury to the spine. It almost always develops in the
cervical region and there is good evidence that it often complicates
cervical spondylosis, a condition in which there are multiple chronic
central protrusions of intervertebral disks. This results in a narrowing of the cervical spinal canal, so that a sudden movement of
hyperextension of the neck, as may occur following a sudden blow
upon the forehead, produces sharp but transient compression of the
spinal cord, and this in turn gives rise to haematomyelia. The
haemorrhage as a rule takes place in or around the central canal of
the cord and can extend over several segments. Recent evidence
suggests that in some such cases there is central softening of the cord
without haemorrhage, but the clinical effects are similar.

As a rule, the patient with cervical haematomyelia experiences a
sudden weakness or total paralysis of all four limbs; this phase of
spinal shock may pass off in a day or two, but spastic weakness of the
lower limbs persists, sometimes affecting one leg more than the
other if the bleeding is not entirely central and if one pyramidal tract
is selectively compressed. As the bleeding in the cervical cord extends
into the anterior and posterior horns of the cord there is loss of the
spinal reflexes innervated by the affected segments of the cord as well
as atrophy and weakness of lower motor neurone type in the muscles
innervated by the affected roots. Wasting of small hand muscles is
particularly common. Furthermore, as in syringomyelia, decussating
sensory fibres travelling to the spinothalamic tracts are interrupted
so that there is generally some dissociated sensory loss in the upper
limbs. If the lesion is extensive there will also be compression of the
posterior columns of the cord to give impairment of position and
joint sense and of vibration sense, particularly in the lower limbs.

In considering prognosis, much depends upon the severity and
extent of the injury; considerable recovery of function can occur in
the three months following upon the acute episode but some lower
motor neurone weakness and dissociated sensory loss in the upper
limbs commonly persists, with residual spasticity in the legs. And if
the cervical spinal canal remains narrowed as a result of cervical
spondylosis, the spinal cord is clearly vulnerable and may be injured
further following relatively minor trauma.

Spinal Cord Compression

Compression of the spinal cord can result from disease in the
vertebral column or in the spinal canal itself. Apart from the injuries

of the vertebral column which may cause compression of the cord
and to which reference has already been made, the commonest
skeletal disorders to have this effect are intervertebral disk protrusions, either acute or chronic, tuberculous osteitis of the spine
(Pott's disease) and primary or secondary neoplasms of the vertebral
bodies. The commonest situation in which central disk prolapse can
compress the cord is in the cervical region; a sudden soft protrusion
of the nucleus pulposus may be responsible, but more often there
are one or several chronic protrusions which have become calcified
to produce bony hard ridges between the vertebrae (cervical spondylosis) and the clinical picture is one of slowly progressive spinal cord
disease (**cervical myelopathy**). In patients with Pott's disease, most
common in children and young people, a paraplegia often develops
abruptly; this often occurs in older patients when a metastasis in a
vertebral body causes a pathological fracture with sudden collapse
and angulation. Primary neoplasms of the vertebrae (osteoma,
haemangioma, myeloma) and Paget's disease (osteitis deformans)
give a more slowly progressive clinical picture. Diseases within the
spinal theca which may compress the cord, include spinal extradural
abscess (*see* Chap. 14), arachnoiditis due to syphilis or to chronic
trauma, extra- and intra-medullary neoplasms (*see* Chap. 16), meningeal deposits of neoplastic tissue or of a reticulosis, and exceptionally,
congenital fibrous bands or cysts of developmental origin (which are
usually associated with spina bifida) or parasitic cysts.

The **clinical features** of compression of the spinal cord depend
upon the level of the lesion and the rapidity of its development. Not
only must one take into account the direct effects of pressure but also
those which can result from a secondary alteration in blood supply.
In general, however, the symptoms and physical signs so produced
can be classified into two principal groups which are first, those
resulting from compression of nerve roots at the level of the lesion
and secondly, those due to interference with the functioning of long
ascending or descending tracts. The principal symptom of root compression is pain, which is generally aching in character, and radiates
into the cutaneous area from which the root or roots concerned
receive sensory impulses. If the motor roots are also involved there
will be weakness, wasting, and sometimes fasciculation of the
muscles which they supply. Interruption of the spinal reflex arc will
produce absence of spinal reflexes, if any, which are innervated by
the segment which is being compressed. If the pressure is developing
asymmetrically, these phenomena can occur unilaterally in the first
instance. Compression of long tracts may give weakness and dragging of a leg and/or clumsiness of one arm and hand, again depending
upon the situation of the lesion, and eventually a spastic paraplegia

or quadriplegia will result. When there is involvement of the spino-thalamic tract, the patient often experiences an unpleasant burning pain in a limb or on the trunk and some hypalgesia will generally be found on examination. Similarly, involvement of the posterior columns will give rise to characteristic paraesthesiae below the level of the lesion, often with typical 'electric shocks' radiating downwards on movement of the neck, if the lesion is cervical; there will also be impairment of position and joint sense, sometimes of light touch, and generally of vibration sense in the lower limbs. These so-called 'long-tract' symptoms and signs develop particu-larly early when the lesion is intramedullary. As a general rule, the pyramidal tract is the most sensitive to pressure, possibly because of the comparative vulnerability of its blood supply, while the spino-thalamic tracts are most resistant. Hence a slowly progressive lesion will generally give signs initially of pyramidal tract dysfunction, next sensory phenomena of 'posterior column' type, and lastly those indicating a spinothalamic tract lesion.

Sphincter disturbances tend to develop comparatively late but precipitancy or difficulty in initiating micturition may eventually be experienced. When a severe paraplegia has developed there is commonly excessive sweating below the level of the lesion. Distur-bances of sphincter control appear early as a result of lesions com-pressing the cauda equina, in which pain in the lower back is usual and there are also symptoms and signs indicating muscular weakness of 'lower motor neurone' type in the lower limbs. Cutaneous sensory loss is also apparent, its distribution varying depending upon the roots which are involved; compression of lower sacral roots, for instance, often produces perianal and perineal anaesthesia. Some of the most difficult lesions to localise accurately on clinical grounds are those which compress both the lower part of the spinal cord (the conus medullaris) and several roots of the cauda equina; under these circumstances, there are generally severe disorders of sphincter control, along with a combination of 'upper motor neurone' and 'lower motor neurone' signs in the lower limbs.

Accurate **clinical localisation** of the site of spinal cord compression can be greatly assisted by the presence of certain specific symptoms and physical signs. The distribution of root pain, or the situation of local spinal pain and tenderness may be very valuable, while a 'sensory level' on the trunk, below which the appreciation of sensation is impaired, is also of the greatest value. It should, how-ever, be remembered that the actual site of the lesion may be several segments higher than that suggested by this sensory 'level'. Weak-ness of lower abdominal muscles, too, or selective absence of the lower abdominal reflexes will localise the lesion to approximately the tenth dorsal segment of the cord. Reflex changes are also useful; thus absence or inversion of the biceps and radial jerks with exaggeration of the triceps jerk indicates a lesion of the fifth and sixth cervical segments, while absence of the knee jerks and retention or exaggeration of the ankle jerks indicates usually that the third or fourth lumbar segment is involved. In the lower limbs, too, the distribution of sensory impairment or muscular weakness may clearly indicate disease of one or more motor or sensory roots. Thus perianal anaesthesia is diagnostic of lower sacral root involvement. In determining localisation on the basis of these clinical features it must always be remembered that the spinal cord is very much shorter than the spinal column and that it ends at the lower border of the first lumbar vertebra. Thus the seventh cervical segment of the cord lies beneath the arch of the sixth cervical vertebra, the sixth dorsal segment beneath the fourth dorsal arch; under the tenth dorsal arch are the first and second lumbar segments, under the twelfth the fifth, while the sacral and coccygeal segments are opposite the body of the first lumbar vertebra.

Although these clinical features are a valuable guide to localisation of a spinal lesion, they are usually insufficient for the surgeon, should operative intervention be deemed necessary. Often, however, when compression has occurred acutely, irreversible damage has taken place before the surgeon can operate. The results of removal of extramedullary tumours are nevertheless uniformly good, if done sufficiently early. Although there are certain causes of cord compression in which the results of surgical decompression are variable (e.g. cervical spondylosis), this is the only effective treatment in some patients. Examination of the cerebrospinal fluid can be of great value in diagnosis since usually Queckenstedt's test will indicate a complete or partial block and the protein content of the fluid will be raised (*see* Chap. 3). Radiography of the spine may indicate the cause of the compression, but usually myelography is needed for accurate localisation.

Injuries to Peripheral Nerves and Plexuses

A detailed description of the many clinical phenomena which can result from injury to or compression of peripheral nerves or plexuses is outside the scope of this volume, but an attempt will be made to describe briefly the salient features of some of the lesions which most commonly occur in clinical practice. It should be remembered that there are two principal types of lesion which may affect nerve trunks. These are first, neuropraxia, a temporary and completely reversible block of nervous conduction which can last for days or even weeks without permanent pathological change; and secondly, neuronotmesis, in which there is actual interruption in continuity of nerve fibres with subsequent Wallerian degeneration, so that regeneration of nerve fibres is required before recovery can occur. In the early stages these two types of lesion may be indistinguishable, save by highly specialised methods of investigation (*see* Chap. 3). Bearing this fact in mind it should next be remembered that a total lesion of a mixed motor and sensory peripheral nerve gives flaccid paralysis and eventually atrophy of the muscles which it supplies. There is also cutaneous sensory loss, though the area of anaesthesia and analgesia is often less than would be expected, as a result of 'overlap' from nerves supplying adjacent cutaneous areas. Trophic changes (shiny skin, loss of sweating, indolent sores) may be seen in the extremities after complete peripheral nerve lesions. It will be important now to consider the clinical phenomena which result from lesions of some of the more important nerve plexuses and peripheral nerves. Direct trauma, pressure or irritation are usually responsible, and inflammatory lesions of the nerves are comparatively uncommon. The condition which has often been referred to as an interstitial neuritis of individual peripheral nerves is generally due to pressure upon or ischaemia of the nerve trunk, although allergic or hypersensitivity neuropathies do occur.

The **phrenic nerve** is derived from the third, fourth and fifth cervical anterior roots; compression or irritation of the nerve can give rise to an irritating, unproductive cough or hiccup, while a complete lesion results in paralysis of the diaphragm on the affected side. The nerve is usually paralysed as a result of lesions affecting the anterior horn cells of the cord or the anterior roots, as in poliomyelitis, the Guillain–Barré syndrome and spinal neoplasms, but it may be injured in its peripheral course by penetrating wounds, malignant disease in the chest, or an aortic aneurysm.

The **brachial plexus** is formed from the anterior primary divisions of the fifth to eighth cervical nerves and of the first dorsal nerve. Sometimes the plexus is prefixed, receiving contributions from the fourth cervical, or postfixed, with fibres from the second dorsal segment. The divisions split into anterior and posterior trunks which again unite to form three cords. The outer cord is formed from the anterior trunks of the fifth to seventh cervical nerves, the inner or lower cord from the anterior trunk of the eighth cervical and the entire contribution from the first dorsal, while the posterior cord is formed from all the posterior trunks. The lateral head of the median nerve and the musculocutaneous nerve come from the outer cord, the medial head of the median nerve and the ulnar from the inner cord and the circumflex and radial nerves from the posterior cord. The long thoracic nerve, which supplies the serratus anterior and is derived from the fifth to seventh cervical roots as well as the supra-scapular nerve which innervates the spinati, and comes from the fifth and sixth segments, are formed proximal to the brachial plexus.

The brachial plexus can be injured or compressed by penetrating wounds, by dislocation of the head of the humerus, by tumours in the root of the neck or by lesions causing compression at the thoracic outlet. Even more commonly it is damaged by traction injuries of the arm, perhaps in an infant during delivery, or on an operating table while the patient is anaesthetised. A common injury is one of the inner cord of the plexus due to hyperabduction of the arm at the shoulder; or alternatively downward compression of the point of the shoulder or a violent pull downward on the arm may tear the outer cord. Injury to the outer cord gives rise to paralysis of the biceps brachii and also of the radial flexors of the wrist and fingers. An inner cord lesion, often resulting from dislocation of the shoulder, gives paralysis of all the small muscles of the hand with sensory loss along the ulnar border of the hand and forearm. The posterior cord is rarely injured. The two common varieties of *birth injury to the plexus* are first, Erb's paralysis, in which the contribution from the fifth cervical nerve is torn; and secondly, Klumpke's paralysis in which the first dorsal nerve is damaged. In Erb's paralysis there is paralysis of the deltoid, spinati, biceps and brachioradialis so that the arm hangs limply by the side, internally rotated with the forearm pronated. Klumpke's paralysis give a 'claw' hand due to paralysis of small hand muscles with some sensory loss down the inner side of the forearm. Whereas about 50 per cent of cases of the Erb type recover, the prognosis of the Klumpke type is less good. Surgical treatment is of no value, but splinting of the arm to prevent over-stretching of paralysed muscles can allow some degree of recovery to take place.

A syndrome with clinical features indicating an inner cord injury can result from compression or angulation of the cord as it crosses a *cervical rib* which joins the transverse process of the seventh cervical vertebra to the first rib; a fibrous or cartilaginous band in the same situation may have a similar effect. Commonly in such a case there is aching pain down the inner side of the arm and forearm, and this is accentuated by carrying heavy weights in the hand, while muscular weakness and wasting in the hand and sensory loss on the ulnar side of the hand and forearm develop slowly over a period of months or years. An ipsilateral Horner's syndrome due to pressure on the stellate ganglion is occasionally seen. This so-called cervical rib syndrome, which is uncommon (many individuals have cervical ribs which are visible radiologically but do not give rise to symptoms) is one variety of the so-called *thoracic outlet or costoclavicular outlet* syndrome. It is widely believed that similar compression of the inner cord of the brachial plexus and sometimes of the subclavian artery can be the result of narrowing of the space between a prominent first rib and the clavicle through which the neurovascular bundle to the upper limb must pass. Alternatively, distortion resulting from angulation of the cord as it crosses the scalenus anterior has been implicated. The syndrome has been generally attributed to drooping of the shoulders, particularly in middle-aged female patients who are accustomed to carrying heavy shopping bags in their hands. While it is true that the characteristic cervical rib syndrome as outlined above can occasionally result from other causes of compression in the costoclavicular outlet, the syndrome has lost much of its former respectability since it has become apparent that many of the symptoms previously attributed to this cause are due to other lesions, including cervical spondylosis, and, in the case of acroparaesthesiae (*vide infra*), a common syndrome in middle-aged women, compression of the median nerve in the carpal tunnel.

Isolated lesions of the **long thoracic nerve** are not uncommon and often result from an inflammatory lesion of the nerve which is presumed to be allergic in aetiology. The result is 'winging' of the scapula due to paralysis of the serratus anterior. When the patient pushes forward with the arm outstretched horizontally the scapula protrudes backwards from the chest wall like an 'angel's wing'.

When the **circumflex nerve** is injured, as it may be by direct trauma, shoulder dislocation or 'allergic' neuritis, the deltoid muscle is paralysed and there is often a patch of sensory loss over the belly and insertion of the deltoid.

The **radial nerve** innervates the triceps, brachioradialis, the radial extensor of the wrist and most of the long extensors of the fingers. Hence a lesion of this nerve high up in the spiral groove in the humerus will result in paralysis of extension of the elbow together with wrist-drop and finger-drop. If the lesion is lower down the triceps is generally spared. Often sensory loss is remarkably slight and is confined to a small area on the dorsum of the hand between the thumb and index finger, even though the nerve innervates a much more extensive skin area. The nerve is frequently damaged in its spiral groove when the humerus is fractured, or by pressure, as when the upper arm rests for a long period over the back of a chair (Saturday-night paralysis).

The **musculocutaneous nerve** is rarely injured alone but a lesion will result in paralysis of flexion of the elbow (biceps brachii and brachialis).

A lesion of the **median nerve** at the elbow gives paralysis of the radial flexors of the wrist and also of most of the long flexors of the fingers, except for those which move the ring and little fingers. There is also weakness and wasting of the muscles which form the outer half of the thenar eminence (abductor pollicis brevis and opponens pollicis). There is sensory loss over the radial part of the hand and on the palmar aspect of the thumb, index, middle, and half the ring finger. The distal part of the extensor aspect of these fingers may also be anaesthetic. A lesion at the wrist gives a similar distribution of sensory loss, but the only muscles involved are those of the thenar eminence. Lesions of the median nerve generally result from direct trauma, and causalgia is a particularly common sequel. *Compression of the median nerve in the carpal tunnel* is a syndrome which is much more common than is generally realised. It usually results from excessive use of the fingers (as in housewives, women who knit a great deal and pianists) and is probably the result of a tenosynovitis of the flexor tendons, causing swelling of their sheaths and increased pressure beneath the carpal ligament. Local injuries of the wrist, rheumatoid arthritis, acromegaly and disorders which give rise to soft tissue swelling (pregnancy, myxoedema, nephrotic syndrome) can have a similar result. The condition is most common in middle-aged women, though it may occur in men. It is often bilateral but worse in the hand which is used more often (usually the right). The most typical symptoms are burning pain, aching or tingling and pins and needles in the fingers (acroparaesthesiae) which are worse in bed at night or in warm surroundings (due to vasodilatation and increased nerve compression). Often the patient will say that the symptoms affect all the fingers until asked to take particular note of this question, when she will admit that the little finger is spared. Not infrequently aching pain and paraesthesiae spread far up the arm. Percussion of the median nerve at the wrist will sometimes evoke tingling in the affected fingers, while the application of a tourniquet to the arm at above arterial blood pressure gives rise to ischaemic paraesthesiae in the fingers within one to three minutes (an abnormally short period). Often there is some sensory impairment over the tips of the thumb and radial three fingers, while the muscles of the lateral half of the thenar eminence may be weak or even greatly wasted in advanced cases. The symptoms, which are disabling and can last for a great many years, are sometimes relieved by rest or by injection of hydrocortisone into the carpal tunnel; operative section of the carpal ligament will afford a permanent cure.

The **ulnar nerve** at the elbow lies behind the medial epicondyle of the humerus; a lesion at this level results in paralysis of the flexor carpi ulnaris, of the ulnar portion of the flexor digitorum and of most of the small muscles of the hand with the exception of the lateral half of the thenar eminence and the two most lateral lumbricals. In such a case the hand is deviated radially, there is inability to flex the ring and little fingers completely and a 'claw-hand' results from paralysis of the small hand muscles and from unopposed action of their antagonists. On testing it will be found that there is inability to abduct the little finger, to adduct the thumb and to separate or oppose the fingers, while lumbrical weakness means that the terminal phalanges of the affected fingers cannot be fully extended. Sensory impairment is apparent over the palmar and dorsal aspects of the little finger and the ulnar half of the ring finger and sometimes spreads up the palm and medial aspect of the forearm. The nerve can be damaged at the elbow by penetrating injuries or fractures of the humerus or it may be subjected to repeated irritation in its groove behind the humerus in patients who have an unusually wide 'carrying angle' or arthritic osteophytes in this area. In some such cases the nerve trunk becomes swollen, tender and fibrotic and surgical transposition, so that it is brought to lie in front of the epicondyle, is necessary. The nerve can also be temporarily damaged by pressure after leaning on the elbow for a long period, or after 'sleeping on the arm'. In the region of the wrist the nerve may be injured by penetrating injuries particularly, and it is not uncommon for the median and ulnar nerves and several tendons to be severed, particularly when a hand is thrust through a glass door or window. Atrophy and weakness of the interossei, lumbricals and adductor pollicis, with sparing of the hypothenar eminence, can result from continuous or repetitive pressure on the medial side of the palm, a hazard of certain occupations, and is due to repeated trauma to the deep palmar branch of the nerve. A similar syndrome occasionally develops spontaneously without any history of trauma and may be found to be due to the presence of a ganglion compressing this branch of the nerve. Conduction velocity studies are of considerable value in the diagnosis of many of these syndromes.

The **lumbar plexus** is formed from the twelfth dorsal and first to fourth lumbar nerves, the **sacral plexus** from the fourth and fifth lumbar and first to third sacral nerves. The principal nerves arising from the lumbar plexus are the femoral and obturator, while the greater part of the sacral plexus forms the sciatic nerve. Injuries of the lumbar and sacral plexuses are relatively uncommon, but they may be damaged by undue pressure of the foetal head during delivery; a syndrome which commonly results from this cause is unilateral paralysis of the anterior tibial and peroneal muscles due to a lesion of one lumbosacral cord.

A common clinical syndrome, known as **meralgia paraesthetica,** results from compression of the lateral cutaneous nerve of the thigh as it passes beneath the lateral part of the inguinal ligament or as it traverses the fascia lata to reach its cutaneous distribution. It usually occurs in the obese, and in middle-age, but not invariably so, and can be unilateral or bilateral. The principal symptoms are an unpleasant burning ache, with superadded tingling or pins and needles, which are accentuated by standing for long periods, and occur over a considerable part of the lateral aspect of the thigh. In this area there is often some hypalgesia and anaesthesia on testing. The condition, though benign, is often very troublesome, and surgical decompression or division of the nerve may be necessary, but is not always completely effective in relieving symptoms. Repeated injections of local anaesthetic around the nerve occasionally afford relief.

Lesions of the **obturator nerve** are uncommon but can follow hip dislocation or a difficult labour. The adductor muscles of the thigh are paralysed, but as a rule there is no sensory loss.

The principal effect of a lesion of the **femoral nerve,** which generally results from penetrating wounds, compression by pelvic neoplasms, or a so-called 'interstitial neuritis' of unknown aetiology, is paralysis of the quadriceps muscle with inability to extend the knee and loss of the knee jerk. There may also be some weakness of hip flexion owing to involvement of the iliacus and sensory impairment is usual over the medial and anterior aspects of the lower two-thirds of the thigh; if the saphenous nerve, a branch of the femoral, is also affected, the analgesia and anaesthesia will also extend down the inner side of the leg and foot. In some cases of so-called *'diabetic amyotrophy'* it is believed that painful wasting of one quadriceps results from a localised femoral neuropathy.

The **sciatic nerve** has two principal divisions which are destined to form the medial and lateral popliteal nerves, respectively, and it divides at a variable point in the back of the thigh. It enters the buttock via the sciatic notch and then passes into the thigh mid-way between the greater trochanter of the femur and the ischial tuberosity. A complete lesion of the nerve will produce paralysis of the hamstring group of muscles, resulting in an inability to flex the knee, as well as paralysis of all muscles below the knee. The foot becomes flail, it cannot be dorsiflexed or plantarflexed and the toes are immobile. The patient can walk but does so with a drop-foot and is unable to stand on his toes. There is sensory loss over virtually the whole of the foot, except for a small area on the medial surface near the heel, and also over the lateral and posterior aspect of the leg below the knee. The ankle jerk and the plantar response cannot be elicited. Damage to the sciatic nerve is generally the result of gunshot wounds or other penetrating injuries of the buttock or thigh, though it may also be injured as a result of pelvic or femoral fracture or a misplaced

I

injection. Its constituent roots are frequently compressed by prolapse of an intervertebral disk, giving rise to the syndrome of sciatica.

Lesions of the **lateral popliteal nerve** are relatively common in civil practice and usually result from repeated trauma to the nerve as it curls around the neck of the fibula; in this situation it lies just beneath the skin and is particularly vulnerable. Compression by a tight garter or bandage, as a result of repeated crossing of the legs, or in workers who habitually sit with one leg folded beneath them (as when working on roofs) are common aetiological factors. A complete lesion results in paralysis of the dorsiflexors of the foot and toes and of the peroneal muscles, giving foot drop with some degree of inversion. There is generally sensory impairment over the antero-lateral aspect of the leg and foot, extending medially to the cleft between the fourth and fifth toes.

When the **medial popliteal nerve** is injured, an uncommon event which is for practical purposes seen only after a penetrating wound, the muscles of the calf and of the sole of the foot are paralysed and the foot is partially dorsiflexed and everted. Sensory loss is usually noted on the sole of the foot and the plantar surface of the toes.

In this chapter an attempt has been made to give an outline of the effects of trauma upon the central and peripheral nervous system. For more detailed information concerning the effects of injury to the skull, vertebral column and spinal cord, the reader is referred to textbooks of neurosurgery and orthopaedic surgery. In a case of peripheral nerve injury, a working knowledge of the anatomical relationship of the nerves and plexuses and of the innervation of the skeletal muscles and dermatomes is necessary for accurate diagnosis and localisation of the responsible lesion; in this connexion help can be obtained from the standard anatomical texts.

REFERENCES

BOWDEN, R. E. M., *Peripheral Nerve Injuries* (London, Lewis, 1958).

BRAIN, W. R., *Diseases of the Nervous System*, 5th ed., Chapters 5 and 18 (London, Oxford University Press, 1962).

BROCK, S., *Injuries of the Brain and Spinal Cord*, 4th ed. (New York, Springer, 1960).

GURDJIAN, E. S. and WEBSTER, J. E., *Head Injuries* (London, Churchill, 1958).

GUTTMANN, L., 'Injuries of the spinal cord', in *The History of the Second World War, U.K. Medical Series: Surgery*, Ed. Sir Zachary Cope, Chapter 10 (ii), p. 422 (London, H.M.S.O., 1953).

MEDICAL RESEARCH COUNCIL, *Aids to the Investigation of Peripheral Nerve Injuries*, War Memorandum No. 7 (London, H.M.S.O., 1943).

ROWBOTHAM, G. F., *Acute Injuries of the Head*, 4th ed. (Edinburgh, Livingstone, 1964).

CHAPTER 14

INFECTION AND ALLERGY AND THE NERVOUS SYSTEM

IN common with the other structures of the human body, the central nervous system, its meningeal coverings and its peripheral ramifications may be invaded by infective agents, of which bacteria, viruses, spirochaetes and parasites of various types are examples. Sometimes a bacterial infection of the nervous system, for instance, is but one part of a more widespread disease process affecting the human organism; some viruses, on the other hand, the so-called neurotropic group, have a particular predilection for nervous tissue. In general it can be said that infective agents produce an inflammatory response; inflammatory changes in the nervous system and particularly in and around its blood vessels can also be the result of an allergic or hypersensitivity response to an infective agent or foreign protein (e.g. serum) which is present elsewhere in the body but which has not in fact invaded nervous tissue. Many of the nervous complications of general infections are probably due to pathological mechanisms of this nature, while others are the direct result of circulating toxins which are produced by the infecting agent.

BACTERIAL INFECTIONS

Bacteria may enter the nervous system as a result of direct spread from an infective focus in the cranial bones or vertebrae, as in patients with suppuration in the middle ear or paranasal sinuses, or osteomyelitis of a vertebra. This spread can be facilitated by injury which has produced a penetrating wound, or a fracture of the cranial vault with a tear of the adherent dura mater. Alternatively the organisms arrive via the blood stream, being derived from a focus of infection elsewhere in the body; commonly this spread is via the arterial system, when it can be assumed that invasion of the nervous system is preceded by a phase of bacteraemia or pyaemia, but an alternative route is through the profuse anastomosis of vertebral veins by means of which infection may spread directly from the thorax or abdomen to the cranial cavity. The common bacterial infections of the nervous system produced by these mechanisms are meningitis, septic venous sinus thrombosis, intracranial abscess and spinal extradural abscess.

239

Meningitis

If one excludes meningitis of virus or parasitic origin, most cases of meningitis are due either to pyogenic infection or to tuberculosis, although traumatic or aseptic meningitis can result from intracranial haemorrhage and some meningeal inflammatory changes are found in spirochaetal infections and in patients with carcinomatosis.

PYOGENIC MENINGITIS

The commonest variety of pyogenic meningitis is **meningococcal meningitis** or cerebrospinal fever. The disease can occur in epidemic form and the organism is believed to enter the body via the nasopharynx. During epidemics the incidence of apparently unaffected individuals who carry the organism in the nasopharynx is high. There is a preliminary phase of bacteraemia or even septicaemia before meningeal manifestations appear, and in a few cases acute meningococcal septicaemia is rapidly fatal due to adrenal haemorrhage (Friedrichsen–Waterhouse syndrome). More often the first phase is asymptomatic but is followed by frontal and occipital headache of mounting severity with high fever. Occasionally at this stage there are rose-red or purple spots on the skin of the trunk, but these are infrequent in sporadic cases. As the headache worsens and becomes generalised, so drowsiness and confusion supervene and the patient may lapse into semicoma within twelve to twenty-four hours. Vomiting is frequent and often projectile in character. On examination the patient tends to lie on one side with his eyes away from the light and the knees pulled up towards the chin; he is irritable and resents interference, pulling back the bedclothes when an attempt is made to remove them. Generally the pulse rate is slow. Neck stiffness is invariable and in severe and established cases there may even be neck retraction. Kernig's sign is usually positive (restriction of straight-leg raising). Paralysis of one or other sixth cranial nerve is sometimes observed and the patient who is sufficiently conscious will then complain of diplopia. Usually the deep tendon reflexes are depressed, but focal neurological signs are rare. Although the inflammatory process affects principally the leptomeninges (arachnoid and pia mater), so that suppuration is mainly confined to the subarachnoid space, there are secondary degenerative changes in the superficial areas of the cerebral cortex, brain stem and cranial nerves in some cases. Hence fits occasionally occur, particularly in childhood; in cases treated late or ineffectively, there may be residual diplopia or nerve deafness, while sometimes there is a communicating hydrocephalus giving rise to papilloedema and residual mental backwardness. Other rare complications include spread of infection to the brain or subdural space to give abscess formation.

The cerebrospinal fluid is typically under greatly increased pressure and is cloudy or frankly purulent. There are large numbers of pus cells present, the protein content of the fluid is increased but sugar is absent. Scanty meningococci may be found on a direct smear of the fluid stained by Gram's stain, and the organisms can be cultured, though they are very difficult to grow. If no organisms are isolated in a case of pyogenic meningitis, the infection is probably meningococcal.

The clinical picture of pyogenic meningitis due to other bacteria is similar. That due to the **pneumococcus** can also be due to a blood-borne infection, without clear evidence of an infective focus elsewhere, and the same is true of **haemophilus influenzae** meningitis. In pneumococcal meningitis the organisms are seen in profusion in direct smears of the cerebrospinal fluid. Most cases of meningococcal meningitis now survive with antibiotic and sulphonamide therapy, but the prognosis of pneumococcal meningitis is much less favourable despite treatment, and the mortality rate remains substantial; influenzal meningitis, which is particularly common in childhood, is less ominous, but can run a long smouldering course for some weeks even after the initial acute phase has been satisfactorily controlled. Meningitis due to the **streptococcus** or **staphylococcus** is usually due to a spread of infection from the middle ear or elsewhere, although there is a curiously localised variety of spinal staphylococcal meningitis in which the exact method of bacterial entry has not yet been determined. In neonates, a purulent meningitis is often found to be due to infection with **Listeria monocytogenes.**

TUBERCULOUS MENINGITIS

Tuberculous meningitis can arise as a complication of miliary tuberculosis and meningeal inflammation may smoulder for some weeks before it becomes clinically apparent. It is therefore wise to examine the cerebrospinal fluid in cases of miliary tubercle in order to determine whether subclinical meningitis is present. The disease can also develop in children with primary tuberculosis or in adults with pulmonary disease and in most such instances it is due to an acute or subacute exudative reaction in the meninges following upon the rupture of a small cerebral or cerebellar tuberculoma into the subarachnoid space. Cerebral tuberculomas are as a rule small, although very rarely one is of sufficient size to present as a space-occupying lesion.

The symptoms of tuberculous meningitis are similar in character but as a rule different in tempo from those of the pyogenic variety, although there are occasional cases in which the onset is equally abrupt and progression just as rapid. In children and young adults who have previously been vaccinated with BCG the illness is rare, but when it does occur it is often comparatively mild initially and is easily mistaken for a benign lymphocytic meningitis. More often, however, there is a period of several days or even weeks of fluctuating premonitory malaise, anorexia, vomiting, vague headache and disinterest, before sustained fever, persistent headache and signs of meningeal irritation become clearly evident. When present, retinal miliary tubercles, which are yellowish nodules about half the size of an optic disk, are of great value in diagnosis. It is important to recognise the disease as early as possible, since the longer it is in existence before treatment, the more probable are complications such as diplopia, communicating hydrocephalus and focal neurological signs (monoparesis or hemiparesis), which can be the result of cerebral infarction due to an associated tuberculous arteritis. Adhesions in the spinal subarachnoid space may cause considerable difficulty in treating the condition with intrathecal streptomycin, and an actual spinal block sometimes develops; similar adhesions around the brain stem can be responsible for attacks of decerebrate rigidity, which generally imply a gloomy prognosis. The complications and sequelae of tuberculous meningitis are more severe than those of any other variety.

Sarcoidosis

The relationship of Boeck's sarcoid to tuberculosis remains a matter of dispute, but many believe that this condition is an atypical or modified response to tuberculous infection. While lymphadenopathy in the mediastinum or elsewhere, iridocyclitis and hepatic involvement are the more common manifestations of this syndrome, the nervous system is sometimes involved, and the result is usually a combination of chronic meningitis on the one hand with multiple cranial nerve palsies, a pleocytosis and increased protein in the cerebrospinal fluid, and sometimes a peripheral neuropathy on the other.

Intracranial Thrombophlebitis

Suppurative thrombophlebitis of intracranial venous sinuses most often affects the lateral, cavernous and superior longitudinal sinuses, due to centripetal spread of infection from the middle ear, skin of the face and frontal sinus, respectively. In all three conditions the patients have pyaemia and are acutely ill with a high remittent fever. Lateral sinus thrombosis must be suspected in patients with otitis media who present such a clinical picture without signs of meningitis or intracerebral spread of infection, while septic thrombosis of the cavernous sinus generally gives unilateral proptosis, chemosis of the conjunctiva and oculomotor paresis. In superior longitudinal sinus thrombosis there may be oedema and tenderness of the scalp over the vertex and spastic weakness of one or both lower limbs; a subdural abscess not uncommonly results. Aseptic thrombosis of the lateral or sagittal sinuses may also complicate middle-ear disease but then gives rise to the syndrome of so-called 'benign intracranial hypertension', 'pseudotumour cerebri', or 'otitic hydrocephalus' (*see* Chapter 18).

Intracranial Abscess

Localised suppuration within the cranial cavity can occur outside the dura mater, when an **extradural abscess** results. This condition is invariably the result of a cranial osteomyelitis which in turn is usually the result of otitis media or paranasal sinusitis. Generally there is a remittent fever and some tenderness over the overlying scalp, but symptoms and signs of increased intracranial pressure are rare and cerebrospinal fluid changes, if present at all, are minimal.

A **subdural abscess** or **empyema** is almost always a sequel of frontal sinusitis but rarely results from middle ear disease; often the layer of pus extends over the whole of one cerebral hemisphere. Initially there is headache and tenderness over the affected frontal sinus or mastoid bone but subsequently the patient becomes drowsy or stuporose, his fever mounts and neck stiffness develops, Jacksonian seizures are frequent in the contralateral limbs and a hemiparesis or hemiplegia is invariably present eventually. Usually there is a polymorphonuclear pleocytosis in the cerebrospinal fluid with a marked rise in protein content. If not treated within a few days by surgical evacuation this condition is rapidly fatal.

Abscess formation in the subarachnoid space is very rare indeed and in fact the commonest site for intracranial suppuration is within the brain substance itself, a **brain abscess.** In about 40 per cent of cases this is due to a direct spread of infection through adherent meninges from the bones of the middle ear, when the principal sites are the temporal lobe (upward spread) or one cerebellar hemisphere (lateral spread); another 10 per cent are due to frontal sinusitis, when the frontal lobe is usually involved. Of the remaining 50 per cent, a few are due to penetrating injuries, but the majority are metastatic; in many of these the primary focus of infection is in the lung (bronchiectasis, empyema, lung abscess) but it may lie anywhere in the body. Brain abscesses are particularly liable to develop in patients with cyanotic congenital heart disease, even without bacterial endocarditis. The cocci are the organisms usually responsible. Pathologically there is an initial stage of focal necrosis and liquefaction, or suppurative encephalitis, but this is followed by the formation of a capsule from glial and fibrous elements, with eventual localisation of the abscess.

When a patient with otitis media or sinusitis notes the suppression of a previously profuse discharge and this is followed by headache, vomiting and confusion, it is reasonable to suppose that inflammation has spread intracranially. Often, however, the patient seems to recover from an attack of otitis, say, but remains unwell, with attacks of depression or irritability, vague intermittent headache and nausea, anorexia, weight loss and mild fever. Even in haematogenous cases, though the onset can occasionally be acute, with focal seizures and neurological signs, there may be minimal headache and progressive personality change and if the signs and symptoms of infection have been masked by antibiotic therapy, the patient may be considered to be suffering from an intracranial tumour.

Usually, however, there is some degree of intermittent pyrexia, and symptoms and signs of increased intracranial pressure (headache, vomiting, papilloedema, bradycardia) develop steadily. Other manifestations depend upon the localisation of the abscess. There will be aphasia if a frontal or temporal lobe abscess involves the dominant hemisphere; a temporal lobe lesion often gives a quadrantic visual field defect and minimal weakness of the contralateral face and hand, while in frontal lobe abscess, impairment of memory and intellectual function are particularly prominent and a contralateral hemiparesis is common. When the cerebellum is involved, headache is often suboccipital in distribution, nystagmus is seen and signs of cerebellar dysfunction (ataxia, intention tremor, etc.) are present in the ipsilateral arm and leg.

In the early stages, examination of the cerebrospinal fluid can be very helpful but this test is of course not without risk, particularly if the intracranial pressure is greatly raised. Usually the pressure of the fluid is raised and it contains up to 100 white cells/mm³, of which many are lymphocytes, though a proportion are usually polymorphonuclear; there is a moderate rise in protein, while the sugar content of the fluid is normal. The EEG may be almost diagnostic, revealing a striking focus of delta activity over the affected cerebral hemisphere. Accurate localisation can only be achieved by ventriculography; treatment, apart from systemic antibiotic therapy, is then neurosurgical. Where possible the abscess is excised; in other instances it is aspirated and antibiotic solutions are instilled into the cavity. About 30 per cent of cases die; many of the survivors suffer from headaches, epilepsy (up to 50 per cent) and residual limb weakness or ataxia according to the situation of the lesion.

Intraspinal Suppuration

An **intramedullary spinal abscess** is a very rare condition of metastatic origin; it usually presents with initial paraesthesiae in the lower limbs followed by a flaccid paraplegia of rapid progression. Generally there is an evident site of suppuration elsewhere in the body, but few cases are diagnosed during life, and the condition is difficult to distinguish from other varieties of acute myelopathy and from rapidly-growing intramedullary neoplasms. It should be borne in mind as a possible diagnosis in patients presenting with signs of an acute lesion of the spinal cord, as some cases improve following surgical drainage.

Much more common and particularly important to diagnose is **spinal extradural abscess.** This can be of tuberculous origin in a patient with tuberculous caries of the spine (Pott's disease), but a staphylococcal aetiology is more common nowadays. In about a third of all cases the condition is secondary to osteomyelitis of a vertebral body but in the remainder the infection, of metastatic origin, appears to develop primarily within the extradural space. Suppuration and exuberant granulation tissue may extend over several segments of the spinal cord and eventually spread into the spinal muscles and soft tissues of the back. Compression of the spinal cord and interference with its circulation are the most important complications.

The initial symptom of the condition is usually an ache in the affected area of the spine, followed by root pain and by fever. Intense spinal tenderness follows, particularly in the osteomyelitic cases, and paraesthesiae in the lower limbs followed by ascending paralysis subsequently develops. The diagnosis must be made as early as possible as paralysis, once present, may be irreversible, while surgical exploration and drainage of the abscess, combined with appropriate antibiotic therapy, can be curative. Lumbar puncture (which usually demonstrates a complete spinal block) and myelography are usually essential for diagnosis and localisation, but should be carefully performed in view of the danger of introducing organisms into the subarachnoid space. Even in the osteomyelitic cases, radiographs of the spine are often normal initially.

Leprosy

Leprosy, an infectious disease due to the mycobacterium leprae, is endemic in certain tropical countries, particularly Africa and India. It is characterised by a very long incubation period, a prolonged remittent course and involvement of the skin, mucous membranes and peripheral nerves. The more acute and infectious or lepromatous form affects particularly the nasal mucosa and the skin; it is the

I*

chronic tuberculoid form in which the peripheral nerves are generally involved. In the beginning there are generally thickened, pigmented and anaesthetic areas of skin; later the areas of numbness increase in size, many peripheral nerves are thickened and tender and eventually there is destruction of the distal phalanges in the hands and feet with painless ulcers of the extremities.

VIRUS INFECTIONS OF THE NERVOUS SYSTEM

The neurotropic viruses have in common the fact that they are visible only under the electron microscope, that they generally pass through filter candles and that they are intracellular parasites. They attack principally nerve cells and hence the main brunt of the pathological changes which they produce falls upon the grey matter of the central nervous system. Viruses are certainly responsible for acute anterior poliomyelitis, various forms of encephalitis and encephalomyelitis, rabies, lymphocytic meningitis, herpes zoster and probably also for encephalitis lethargica. Occasionally certain viruses which are not normally neurotropic, such as those of mumps and glandular fever (infectious mononucleosis) may attack the nervous system, giving rise to an encephalitic or meningitic illness.

Acute Anterior Poliomyelitis

Three principal strains of poliomyelitis virus have been identified and are known as the Brunhilde, Lansing and Leon strains, of which the Lansing is probably the most virulent. The virus attacks particularly the anterior horn cells of the spinal cord, around which collections of inflammatory cells are generally found in fatal cases, but the cells of motor brain stem nuclei and even those of the cerebral cortex may be invaded. The virus appears to enter the nervous system by travelling along peripheral and autonomic nerves. It is generally believed that the usual portal of entry into the body is the alimentary tract, although it is possible that in some cases it may be via the nasopharynx, particularly after recent tonsillectomy. In cases of the latter type there is a particular tendency for the bulbar nuclei to be involved.

As alimentary infection is derived from contaminated water or food, and flies are a common vector of the disease, epidemics are particularly liable to occur in late summer and early autumn, though sporadic cases occur all the year round. The disease was once almost completely confined to young children (hence the name 'infantile paralysis'), but in recent years, particularly in countries such as the United States, Britain and Scandinavia, in which standards of hygiene have been steadily improving, there has been a tendency for more older children and young adults to be afflicted. It is believed that this change can be accounted for by the fact that fewer children now acquire immunity as a result of subclinical infections in early life. The pattern is now changing even further as most children and young people have been effectively protected by inoculation.

The incubation period of the illness is usually between seven and fourteen days. There is much evidence that during epidemics many individuals are infected with the virus and acquire immunity without developing clinical symptoms of infection (**subclinical cases**). A second group of patients experience a mild febrile illness without clinical evidence that the nervous system is involved (**abortive cases**); in a third group there is a meningitic illness with headache, fever, neck stiffness and a pleocytosis in the cerebrospinal fluid but no muscular paralysis ensues (**non-paralytic cases**). The fourth group of patients in whom paralysis develops (**paralytic cases**) constitute a relatively small proportion of the whole. It is now apparent that excessive physical exertion or localised trauma to a limb (e.g. a prophylactic inoculation) during the pre-paralytic phase of the illness can promote paralysis of the affected member.

In non-paralytic cases and in the pre-paralytic phase of the more severely ill cases, headache, fever, neck stiffness and Kernig's sign are usually present and there may be abdominal pain and widespread muscular pain and tenderness. Attempted spinal flexion is often particularly painful. Sometimes after two or three days of fever there is apparent improvement for from twenty-four to forty-eight hours followed by a recrudescence of fever and the onset of paralysis, with severe muscular pain and tenderness. The distribution of muscular weakness is very variable from case to case. Typically it is asymmetrical, affecting perhaps one arm and the opposite leg, but any muscle group may be involved. Occasionally the weakness increases in an ascending manner with considerable danger to life, owing to respiratory paralysis. In a small but growing group of cases the main brunt of the disease falls upon the brain stem (polioencephalitis), and there may be paralysis of the facial, pharyngeal and laryngeal muscles. The combination of pharyngeal and respiratory paralysis which occurs in some such bulbar cases is particularly sinister because of the danger of inhalation of secretions or vomit and in such patients tracheotomy and assisted respiration are usually required. Once paralysis has appeared, it usually reaches its maximum distribution within twenty-four hours, but in a few cases it continues to progress for two or three days. Fortunately the extent of the muscular weakness at the height of the illness is not always clearly related to the degree of permanent paralysis which will remain; some anterior horn cells are only temporarily affected, recovery occurring subsequently. This is the principal justification for the use of mechanically assisted respiration in cases of this disease. Nevertheless there is nearly always some degree of residual paralysis, followed by muscular wasting and often fasciculation, contractures of paralysed muscles, bony deformity and failure of growth in the affected member. Rarely it seems that progressive muscular weakness and atrophy can develop some years later to give a clinical picture like that of progressive muscular atrophy (*see* Chap. 18).

It is very difficult indeed to assess with any degree of accuracy the mortality of the disease, in view of the large number of subclinical and abortive cases which occur. Furthermore, the mortality varies from epidemic to epidemic, having been as high as 25 per cent of the paralytic cases in some, but this is an exceptionally high figure and 10 per cent is more usual. Respiratory paralysis and/or infection is generally the cause of death.

The cerebrospinal fluid in the first two to three days of the illness generally shows an increase of polymorphonuclear leucocytes, but these are soon replaced by a lymphocytic pleocytosis, up to 200 or more cells per mm^3. A substantial rise in the protein content of the fluid persists much longer than the pleocytosis.

Prevention of this disease is, of course, more satisfactory than any form of treatment. Passive immunisation with γ-globulin will give temporary protection during an epidemic, but permanent immunity can only be achieved either by acquiring a natural infection or by active immunisation. The Salk and British vaccines have been shown to be partially effective, particularly in reducing the incidence of paralytic cases; these are now being supplanted by a Sabin type oral vaccine, utilising live but attenuated virus.

Encephalitis Lethargica

This disease is probably due to a neurotropic virus, although no organism has yet been isolated. The principal site of pathological change is in the grey matter of the mid-brain, and particularly in the substantia nigra. The disease appeared in Europe in 1915 and occurred in epidemic proportions up to the early 1920's, when its frequency began to wane. No epidemics have occurred subsequently, but it is believed that sporadic cases still occur from time to time. It seems that thirty years ago the illness was usually acute, beginning with headache, vomiting, convulsions and confusion; nowadays the condition probably presents in a more subacute or chronic form, with the manifestations of post-encephalitic Parkinsonism (*see* Chap. 12).

In the more acute cases, there was a characteristic lethargy and somnolence, sometimes amounting to stupor, during the day, but the patient was often awake, though confused and perhaps delirious, at night (reversal of sleep rhythm). Ocular palsies and pupillary changes were always present, giving rise to blurring of vision and diplopia. Choreiform movements of the limbs, tremor and tics involving the facial and respiratory muscles were also seen. Sometimes Parkinsonian features (mask-like face, festinant gait, tremor, oculogyric crises) were observed in the early stages of the illness, but more often they did not become clearly apparent until several years after the acute illness. Nevertheless, it is probable that in such cases, even after an interval of many years, the causal organism is persisting in the central nervous system. Indeed in many patients with the post-encephalitic type of Parkinsonism, there is no history of a previous recognisable encephalitic illness. Not only are physical abnormalities of this type common sequelae; in children particularly there may be severe behaviour disturbances following the illness, including cruelty, violence and moral and intellectual degeneracy. Many such individuals require permanent institutional treatment.

Only about 25 per cent of patients afflicted by this disease in its acute form seemed to recover completely. About one-third of the cases died within four weeks of the onset, but the remaining patients were usually disabled in the end by Parkinsonism.

The cerebrospinal fluid in this disease is frequently normal, but there may sometimes be a minimal pleocytosis and increase in protein.

Other Forms of Virus Encephalitis and Encephalomyelitis

A number of specific varieties of encephalitis have been discovered in various parts of the world and have been found to be due to neurotropic viruses. In this group are the Japanese type B and St Louis varieties, in which infection is transmitted by the mosquito. Equine encephalomyelitis, which occurs in the U.S.A., is transmitted by the mosquito from a reservoir of virus in birds or in the wood-tick. Louping-ill, a virus disease of sheep, has also been known to give rise to an encephalitic illness in man in Great Britain. Although all of these varieties of encephalitis show differences from one another in clinical presentation, course and mortality, each gives rise to an encephalitic illness characterised by headache, fever, a period of confusion, stupor or semicoma and/or rigidity or tremor of the limbs. In equine encephalomyelitis particularly there may be spastic paresis of the limbs, fits and permanent mental deterioration. Each one of these conditions (and there are probably many more varieties as yet unrecognised) is likely, after an acute onset, to result in a relatively protracted illness, with fluctuating levels of consciousness; and the mortality can be as much as 60 per cent in certain epidemics. Though some patients recover completely, a proportion show intellectual and physical residua which persist when the acute illness is over. In each variety of encephalitis the cerebrospinal fluid is abnormal; there is a lymphocytic pleocytosis in the Japanese B and St Louis type, and in louping-ill, but polymorphonuclears predominate, often in large number, in the early stages of the equine variety.

Similar, though generally less severe, encephalitic illnesses occur in Great Britain and only rarely is the causal virus identified except perhaps in the small proportion of cases of infectious mononucleosis in which an encephalitic illness develops. Probably in Western Europe post-infective encephalitis (*see* Chapter 15) is more common than the viral variety, although a transient encephalitic illness does sometimes occur in influenza.

Benign Myalgic Encephalomyelitis

This name has been given to a variety of encephalomyelitic illness which has occurred in Britain, in continental Europe and in the United States of America in recent years. It has also been called 'epidemic neuromyasthenia'. It is probably a virus infection, but no organism has yet been isolated, even from the large number of cases which occurred in the Royal Free Hospital, London, in 1955. The illness usually begins with lassitude and malaise, headache and neck stiffness and generalised muscular pain. Vertigo, vomiting and diplopia are common, as are disorders of concentration and behaviour and many cases are initially regarded as suffering from hysteria. Paraesthesiae are frequent and there is variable paralysis and sensory loss in the limbs with, however, preservation of deep reflexes. In some cases there is an associated hepatitis. There is little or no fever and the cerebrospinal fluid is always normal. The illness may run a prolonged relapsing course of many weeks or months, and during the period of recovery an inordinate degree of fatigue with persistent depression is common.

Subacute Encephalitis

This subacute variety of encephalitis which has been variously entitled subacute inclusion body encephalitis (Dawson) and subacute sclerosing leuco-encephalitis (van Bogaert) is believed to be a virus infection, possibly due to invasion of the nervous system by the virus of herpes simplex. The disease is commonest in infancy and childhood; nerve cell degeneration, gliosis and inflammatory changes occur in the cerebral cortex and many nerve cells and astrocytes contain pink inclusion bodies. The disease is characterised clinically by progressive dementia, spastic paralysis of the limbs and myoclonus, and runs a fatal course, usually within nine to twelve months.

The EEG is virtually diagnostic, revealing bizarre generalised repetitive slow wave complexes separated by periods of comparative electrical silence.

Rabies

Rabies in man follows a bite from an infected animal, usually a dog, which excretes the virus in its saliva. The virus enters the nervous system along the peripheral nerves and attacks nerve cells in which the characteristic acidophilic inclusions (Negri bodies) may eventually be demonstrated. Rabies in animals is characterised first by a change in behaviour with perversion of appetite, excessive excitement, salivation and progressive paralysis with muscular spasms. The incubation period in man is from twenty-eight to sixty days or even more; during this asymptomatic period, protective inoculation can prevent the development of the disease. The first symptom of the disease is usually apprehension, depression and restless sleep. This is followed by pharyngeal spasm (hydrophobia) which soon extends to the muscles of respiration and then to those of the trunk and limbs, producing opisthotonus. Any attempt to drink will bring on the spasms which are accompanied by profuse salivation and are succeeded by profound paralysis. Death may occur during the spasms or subsequently, and is usually due to respiratory or cardiac failure.

Lymphocytic Meningitis

This benign disorder is due to a virus which also afflicts mice, and the house mouse may be the source of the human disease which can occur sporadically or in small epidemics. The condition is commonest in childhood but also affects adults. The prodromal symptoms are those of fever and are rapidly succeeded by headache, drowsiness and neck stiffness. Severe disturbances of consciousness are uncommon and many patients remain alert throughout; diplopia is an infrequent complication. The illness usually persists for about a week but complete recovery is the rule. The cerebrospinal fluid is usually under increased pressure and may contain 1,000 or more cells per mm³, of which the great majority are mononuclear, though an occasional polymorphonuclear leucocyte is seen; the protein content of the fluid is raised and a 'cobweb clot' may form on standing. The sugar content of the fluid is generally normal and a bromide test (*see* Chap. 3) is normal; these are valuable points in differential diagnosis from tuberculous meningitis with which the condition is most often confused. It is sometimes impossible clinically to distinguish this condition from a non-paralytic case of poliomyelitis or from the meningeal illness which can complicate mumps or infectious mononucleosis (glandular fever). A similar picture is also seen in some cases of canicola fever (*vide infra*) and as a result of infection with one of the Coxsackie viruses; another form of Coxsackie virus infection gives rise to epidemic myalgia (Bornholm disease).

Herpes Zoster

In herpes zoster or shingles, the principal sites of pathological change are the posterior root ganglia and the sensory ganglia of the cranial nerves, but occasionally the grey matter of the spinal cord and brain stem can be damaged. Intranuclear inclusions have been demonstrated in cases of this disease and the causal virus is larger than many of the others in the neurotropic group; it resembles closely, and may indeed be identical with, that of varicella (chicken-pox). The condition can develop without apparent precipitating cause, and does so usually in elderly people, but it may appear following upon trauma to the spinal cord, in patients with inter-vertebral disk prolapse, spinal tumour or subarachnoid haemor-rhage, and often follows radiotherapy to the nervous system. The course of events in such cases suggests some excitation by the patho-logical condition concerned of a virus which was previously lying dormant in the nervous system.

The incubation period of the illness is about fourteen days; the first symptom is usually a continuous dull burning pain in the dis-tribution of the affected nerve root or roots, and this mounts in severity. There is often cutaneous hyperaesthesia. Within three to four days an erythematous rash appears in the affected region and is followed by a vesicular eruption which dries within a few days leaving pigmented scars which may itch for a time. The pain and skin eruption are always unilateral. Persistent severe pain is often present for some weeks, months or even years after the initial illness, particularly in elderly people (post-herpetic neuralgia). Often the skin area affected is rendered permanently anaesthetic and in certain cases the anterior horn cells of the same segment of the spinal cord are also damaged, giving rise to muscular weakness and wasting. Rarely there is evidence of damage to long tracts (pyramidal and spinothalamic), indicating a 'zoster myelitis'. Zoster of the oph-thalmic division of the fifth cranial nerve is a particularly unpleasant variety of the disease; the vesicles which are present in the supra-orbital region may spread to the cornea, leaving permanent scars. Oculomotor paresis can also occur. Herpes of the geniculate ganglion produces vesicles on the tympanic membrane with a watery or sanguineous discharge from the ear, homolateral deafness and facial paralysis and loss of taste on the anterior two-thirds of the tongue (the Ramsay Hunt syndrome). Sometimes there is sensory loss on the affected side of the face. Rarely in severe cases of herpes zoster there is some headache and neck stiffness indicating meningeal inflammation, and a herpes zoster encephalitis has been described but is very uncommon.

SPIROCHAETAL INFECTIONS OF THE NERVOUS SYSTEM

The principal spirochaetal agents which may invade the central nervous system are first, and most important, the treponema pallidum of syphilis, and secondly the leptospirae of Weil's disease and of canicola fever.

Neurosyphilis

Invasion of the nervous system accounts for a high proportion of all deaths resulting from syphilis. The three principal groups of pathological change resulting from the effect of this organism upon the nervous system can be classified as meningeal, vascular and parenchymatous. Meningeal and vascular symptoms tend to appear relatively early in the course of the disease, often during or just after the secondary stage and within one to five years of the primary infection; these can generally be treated very effectively. Manifestations of parenchymatous cerebral and spinal cord disease, which usually develop in the tertiary and quaternary stages of the illness, do not appear for some ten to twenty years, or exceptionally even later; treatment of these conditions is considerably less effective, though considerable improvement can nevertheless be expected in a high proportion of cases. It is apparent that the secondary manifestations of syphilis are more acute and florid, and tertiary manifestations (gummata, skeletal involvement) are more common, in populations and communities in which syphilis is a relatively recent acquisition. When the disease has been present in a population for many hundreds of years the quaternary or parenchymatous neurosyphilitic manifestations are much more frequent. Tertiary syphilis is comparatively rare nowadays in Great Britain, but quaternary neurosyphilis is by comparison relatively common.

It should be remembered that **asymptomatic neurosyphilis** is not infrequent. This term is utilised to describe cases in which there are no clinical symptoms or signs indicating disease of the nervous system but nevertheless there are changes in the cerebrospinal fluid (pleocytosis, raised protein, abnormal gold colloidal curve, positive Wassermann reaction) indicating activity of the disease. The positive serological reaction reveals that the nervous system has been invaded, while the cell count usually parallels the degree of activity. Marked abnormality of the cerebrospinal fluid usually heralds the eventual development of clinical neurosyphilis. If the fluid is normal in every respect it can be assumed with a reasonable degree of confidence that affection of the nervous system has not occurred or that it is no longer active.

An acute **meningitic illness** (luetic meningitis) can occur during the secondary stage of the illness, within two years of the primary infection. This is characterised by fever, headache and neck stiffness and sometimes there is confusion or semicoma and even papilloedema. There are usually many hundreds of lymphocytes per cubic millimetre in the cerebrospinal fluid, the Wassermann reaction is strongly positive and the Lange curve is meningitic in type. The condition can resemble closely lymphocytic and tuberculous meningitis and usually responds well to anti-syphilitic treatment.

The term **meningovascular syphilis** is applied to a group of clinical manifestations of luetic infection which are generally manifest between two and five years after the primary infection. They result from a subacute or chronic inflammatory change in the leptomeninges (arachnoiditis) on the one hand or from a syphilitic endarteritis of cerebral and/or spinal cord arteries on the other. There may be symptoms of a subacute meningitis with intermittent headache, low fever and neck stiffness, but more often the arachnoiditis at the base of the brain results in strangulation of one or more cranial nerves to give clinical signs of a cranial nerve palsy. The third and sixth nerves are particularly vulnerable; sometimes affection of the eighth nerve will give unilateral or bilateral deafness, while an optic chiasmal arachnoiditis is known to occur giving progressive bilateral, but often asymmetrical, visual failure. Manifestations of a partial communicating hydrocephalus are also seen from time to time and convulsions are a not uncommon complication. The arterial changes, if involving cerebral, brain stem or cerebellar arteries, may result in infarction, particularly if a vessel is suddenly occluded, and the clinical effects are indistinguishable from any episode of cerebral 'thrombosis' (*see* Chap. 17). Hemiplegia, monoplegia, aphasia and vertigo can all occur. Syphilis was once the commonest cause of the syndrome of cerebral 'thrombosis' in relatively young people, but this is no longer the case. The arteries of the spinal cord may also be involved; one mode of presentation is with a relatively acute episode suggesting a transverse cord lesion or so-called luetic transverse myelitis. Sometimes the arterial changes are more insidious and the pyramidal tracts, which are supplied by the peripheral branches of the anterior spinal artery, are increasingly starved of blood so that a gradually progressive spastic paraplegia develops (Erb's syphilitic spastic paraplegia). It is not infrequent for arachnoidal and vascular lesions to be combined in the cervical region; as a result of strangulation of nerve roots produced by the arachnoiditis there is weakness and wasting of muscles in the upper limbs, while in the lower limbs there is frequently a spastic paraplegia, due to ischaemia of long tracts. This condition, which can resemble motor neurone disease (*see* Chap. 18) has been referred to as luetic amyotrophic lateral sclerosis, or, because of macroscopic changes in the cervical meninges, pachymeningitis cervicalis hypertrophica. The cerebrospinal fluid in meningovascular syphilis is always abnormal, showing a lymphocytic pleocytosis, an increase in protein, a positive Wassermann reaction and a Lange curve which is usually of luetic or meningitic type (*see* Chap. 3).

TABES DORSALIS

Tabes dorsalis (locomotor ataxia) is the name which has been given to one of the quaternary or parenchymatous varieties of neurosyphilis, in which the spirochaetes have actually invaded nervous tissue, though they cannot always be demonstrated. The principal pathological change is degeneration at the root entry zone of many of the posterior spinal roots, with secondary involvement of ascending fibres in the posterior columns of the spinal cord. Typically patients with this disease experience so-called 'lightning pains' which are probably due to constriction and fibrosis of the posterior roots. These are often described as 'like red hot needles sticking into the legs'. Generally, too, there is a severe ataxia of sensory type, and the unsteadiness in walking which the patients describe is very much worse in the dark. Paraesthesiae, particularly in the lower limbs, and subjective numbness are also common. Sometimes in this disease, transient episodes or 'crises' occur whose aetiology is not fully explained. In laryngeal crises there is spasm of the vocal cords with stridor and difficulty in breathing; in gastric crises acute upper abdominal pain and vomiting occur, and sometimes last for several days, while renal crises (like renal colic) and rectal crises (rectal pain and tenesmus) have also been described. Urinary symptoms (delayed or difficult micturition) are not infrequent and the normal sensation indicating a need to micturate may eventually be lost, while impotence is also frequent.

On physical examination, patients with tabes show a characteristically ataxic, high-stepping gait, and Romberg's sign is positive. The Argyll–Robertson pupil is for practical purposes invariable. The pupils are small, irregular and unequal, they fail to react to light but do so on accommodation–convergence; there is atrophy of the iris and loss of the ciliospinal reflex (dilatation of the homolateral pupil on pinching the skin of the neck). Bilateral optic atrophy, with pallor of the disks and concentric constriction of visual fields, is seen in about 10 per cent of patients. Some degree of ptosis is usual, contributing to the characteristic long, drooping, so-called 'tabetic facies'. There is usually some loss of superficial pain sensibility (i.e. to pinprick) over the bridge of the nose, the centre of the sternum, the perineum, and in variable degree over the lower limbs. Deep pressure over the Achilles tendons is often painless. Generally the deep tendon reflexes, and certainly those in the lower limbs, are greatly depressed or absent and there is severe impairment of position and joint sense and of vibration sense in the legs. Loss of pain sensation can lead to the development of a degenerative arthropathy (Charcot's joint) in the feet, ankles or knees.

In early cases of tabes dorsalis the Wassermann reaction is usually positive in the blood and cerebrospinal fluid and the latter shows a pleocytosis and luetic Lange curve. In 20 per cent of late or so-called 'burnt-out' cases, the Wassermann reaction is negative and the cerebrospinal fluid is normal in every respect. These investigations are nevertheless important in the distinction between tabes dorsalis and various forms of peripheral neuropathy; in so-called diabetic pseudotabes there may actually be pupillary changes as well as involvement of peripheral nerves. Tabes dorsalis is the least satisfactory of all syphilitic conditions to treat, as there is sometimes little or no improvement. Nevertheless, the attempt should certainly be made (*see* Chap. 20).

GENERAL PARESIS

General paresis (general paralysis of the insane or G.P.I.) is a form of progressive dementia, in which there are extensive inflammatory and degenerative changes throughout the cerebral cortex, and the treponema pallidum can generally be demonstrated in the brain. In the beginning the symptoms can take the form of little more than impairment of memory and concentration, and undue fatigue. Subsequently, however, judgement and personality deteriorate and there is increasing neglect of responsibility and personal hygiene. Often the patients are confused, apathetic and show a poor memory for recent events, combined with a singular lack of insight and concern. A grandiose variety of the disease is relatively uncommon, but such patients are often euphoric, hypomanic and have delusions of great personal power or ability. They may confabulate wildly, describing in great detail personal experiences which have no foundation in fact. It seems that these manifestations occur particularly in individuals of previously extraverted personality. In due course even patients of this type become simple, grossly demented and bed-ridden. There are a small number of individuals in whom the disease presents more acutely with headache, sudden confusion, convulsions and focal neurological signs (aphasia, hemiparesis, etc.) but this variety of the illness is relatively uncommon. Physical examination of patients with this condition reveals evidence of a clear-cut dementia; Argyll–Robertson pupils are usual but not invariable. There are commonly tremors of the lips, tongue and outstretched hands, the tendon reflexes are generally exaggerated, and often the plantar responses are extensor. Occasionally the lower limb reflexes are absent and there are other features reminiscent of tabes dorsalis, in which case the condition is usually referred to as **taboparesis.** **Juvenile paresis** is general paresis resulting from congenital syphilis, and developing usually in adolescence. The clinical manifestations are similar to those in the disease of late onset, except that the pupils, though unresponsive to light, are often somewhat dilated; the prognosis of juvenile paresis is poor despite treatment. General paresis must be distinguished from other causes of dementia arising in the presenium (*see* Chap. 8). This is most readily achieved by means of cerebrospinal fluid examination. The fluid is always abnormal in untreated cases; the Wassermann reaction is positive, there is a lymphocytic pleocytosis, the protein content is raised, and the Lange curve is paretic in type (*see* Chap. 3). The condition, if untreated, is fatal within a few years, but most cases improve significantly with treatment and 50 per cent or more may recover completely.

Leptospirosis

In leptospirosis icterohaemorrhagica (Weil's disease) the organism, derived usually from rat's urine, attacks principally the liver (giving hepatitis and jaundice) and the kidneys (giving nephritis) but occasionally there are also symptoms and signs of a lymphocytic meningitis. A meningitic illness, clinically indistinguishable from other varieties of lymphocytic meningitis may, however, be the predominant or sole manifestation of canicola fever, which is due to the leptospira canicola, an organism which is generally carried by dogs. Hence this diagnosis should be considered in all cases of lymphocytic meningitis, particularly if the patient has been in contact with a sick dog.

FUNGAL INFECTIONS

Fungal disorders of the central nervous system are rare. **Actinomycosis** has been known to produce a subacute purulent meningitis of invariably fatal termination in certain cases, and in others vertebral involvement has resulted in extradural abscess formation with spinal cord compression. **Torulosis,** due to the cryptococcus neoformans (*Torula histolytica*), a yeast-like organism, is the commonest fungal infection of the nervous system but is also rare. It gives rise to the clinical picture of a subacute meningitic illness with increasingly severe headaches, confusion and neck stiffness. There is usually papilloedema and sometimes cranial nerve palsies are seen. Comparatively few cases have been recognised during life, but recognition is important, since although the condition to date has been invariably fatal, it now appears that amphotericin B may be an effective treatment. The organism can be grown from cerebrospinal fluid on Sabouraud's medium.

PARASITIC DISORDERS OF THE NERVOUS SYSTEM

Malaria

Cerebral symptoms are not uncommon in infections with malignant tertian malaria (*Plasmodium falciparum*), particularly in children. The manifestations are probably due to blockage of cerebral capillaries by parasites. Commonly the onset is abrupt with high fever (up to 110° F), severe headache, neck stiffness and sometimes focal neurological signs (hemiplegia, aphasia). In some cases there is papilloedema, and differential diagnosis from cerebral tumour or abscess may be difficult. The prognosis of cerebral malaria is grave, the mortality being as great as 50 per cent.

Toxoplasmosis

This condition, due to the protozoan toxoplasma, is usually congenital, being transmitted from the mother *in utero*. Often the infection in adults is asymptomatic, though some adults experience an acute or subacute illness with fever, headache and a skin rash when they are first affected. The encephalomyelitis which is the commonest manifestation of this disease in infancy usually gives rise to fits, hydrocephalus, intracerebral calcification and chorioretinitis. In some babies the disease runs an acute and fatal course, in others it becomes arrested leaving permanent mental defect with a recurrent tendency to convulse, but some few children survive with minimal disabilities. The diagnosis may be confirmed serologically; no effective treatment is available.

Trypanosomiasis

This disease occurs in African (*Trypanosomiasis gambiense* and *rhodesiense*) and South American (*Trypanosomiasis cruzi*) forms. The African form, sleeping sickness, is transmitted by the tsetse fly. After a long incubation period, there is a febrile illness followed by meningitic symptoms, irritability, indifference, somnolence and eventually after some months by coma and death. The South American form is a more acute illness, commoner in children and less grave in outlook, but often followed by mental defect and residua like those of cerebral palsy.

Trichiniasis

This disease is contracted usually as a result of eating inadequately-cooked pork containing the larvae of the *Trichina spiralis*. The larvae are released in the intestinal tract, mature and produce further larvae which penetrate the intestinal wall and enter the blood stream. The common clinical features at this stage are fever, puffiness of the eyelids, and severe generalised muscular pain and stiffness indicating invasion of the muscles. Respiratory difficulty due to diaphragmatic involvement is common. Sometimes fits or paraplegia result from blockage of cerebral or spinal blood vessels. Though the disease is occasionally fatal the illness usually resolves within a few days and the larvae become encysted. During the acute stage there is usually a striking eosinophilia.

Cysticercosis

This disorder is contracted by eating food which has been contaminated with tapeworm ova, usually those of *Taenia solium*. The ova are converted into the larval form of the parasite which then penetrates the intestinal wall and enters the circulation to reach the brain, muscles and subcutaneous tissues. The larva becomes encysted to form a cysticercus which may then calcify and often has a characteristic oval shape which can recognised on radiographs. Cysticercosis of the brain often gives rise to epilepsy but a racemose form has also been described in the cerebral ventricles (particularly the fourth) which can result in either repeated attacks of lymphocytic meningitis or in intermittent or progressive hydrocephalus suggesting the presence of a tumour in the posterior fossa.

NEUROLOGICAL COMPLICATIONS OF SPECIFIC INFECTIONS

Disorders Due To Specific Exotoxins

The principal infecting organisms which produce exotoxins with a particular affinity for nervous tissue are diphtheria, tetanus and botulism.

DIPHTHERITIC POLYNEUROPATHY

The exotoxin of the diphtheria bacillus gives rise to a polyneuropathy which generally begins in the musculature nearest to the point at which the infecting organism is situated. Since this is usually the tonsillar fossa, larynx or nasal mucosa, the muscles most often paralysed initially are those of the pharynx, larynx and soft palate, with resulting dysphagia, dysarthria or aphonia, or nasal speech. In some cases the external ocular muscles are affected. When the diphtheria bacillus has contaminated a limb wound, then the muscular weakness may begin in the muscles of that limb. Whatever the site of infection, the weakness may remain localised, but in other instances it spreads to involve the muscles of all four limbs and those of the trunk. The physical signs of generalised muscular weakness with absence of deep reflexes and variable sensory impairment are typical of any polyneuropathy, save for the almost constant involvement of bulbar muscles. Frequently the initial manifestations of diphtheritic polyneuropathy are observed within seven to ten days of the onset of the infection, and weakness can be profound and generalised in two to four weeks. Recovery soon begins to occur spontaneously and is often remarkably complete, though variable degrees of muscular weakness and depression of deep reflexes sometimes persist. Fortunately, as a result of prophylactic inoculation, diphtheria is now a rare disease.

TETANUS

This condition is due to the exotoxin of the tetanus bacillus, which, being an anaerobic organism, flourishes only in deep penetrating wounds. The exotoxin enters the central nervous system by travelling along the sheaths of the peripheral nerves from the site of the injury. If the amount of toxin produced is large there will also be more rapid dissemination via the blood stream. This toxin interferes with the activity of the reflex arc in such a way that intense muscular spasms are produced by minimal sensory stimulation. The incubation period of the illness varies from three or four days to as long as two to three weeks after the injury. The longer the incubation period, the better the prognosis, as the development of symptoms within a few days after the injury usually implies a massive infection. Usually the first symptom is one of trismus or inability to open the jaw; this is followed by stiffness of the neck, dysphagia, spasm of the facial muscles (risus sardonicus) and eventually by rigidity of the abdominal muscles and of all the limbs. Noise or minimal sensory stimulation of any kind may then provoke intense and generalised muscular spasms, with arching of the back (opisthotonus). Between spasms the muscles remain rigid and the tendon reflexes are brisk. Hyperpyrexia often develops; death can result from heart failure, asphyxia or exhaustion. If the patient survives for a few critical days the spasms gradually reduce in frequency and severity and recovery eventually occurs, though some stiffness may persist for several weeks. The disease can occur in a less severe or localised form when the bacteria are present in fewer numbers, or when the patient has previously received prophylactic inoculations. In such cases the rigidity and spasms may remain localised to the limb or part of the body in which the original injury occurred and can persist for several weeks or months. In cephalic tetanus, following a facial wound, in addition to spasm of facial and jaw muscles, facial paralysis and ophthalmoplegia often develop on the side of the face nearest to the injury.

BOTULISM

This condition is due to the ingestion of the exotoxin of *Clostridium botulinum* and is always acquired from infected foodstuffs, particularly tinned food. The toxin appears to have a direct paralysing effect upon the neuromuscular junction. Symptoms usually develop within twenty-four to forty-eight hours after eating the tainted food. The first symptoms are usually vomiting and diarrhoea but this is followed by blurring of vision (due to pupillary dilatation), diplopia, ptosis, dysphagia, dysarthria and weakness of jaw muscles. Death may result from respiratory paralysis or bronchopneumonia. Between 20 and 60 per cent of cases are fatal; paralysis can be prevented if antitoxin is administered quickly enough. The toxin can, however, be destroyed by cooking of tinned food for a few minutes and prophylaxis is much more satisfactory than treatment.

Other Neurological Complications of Specific Infections

In certain cases of **typhus fever** and other related disorders due to rickettsial infection, nervous symptoms are prominent. Headache, sleeplessness and delirium may indicate an encephalitic element of the general infection but in addition, focal neurological signs (hemiplegia, aphasia, dysarthria, facial paralysis) occasionally develop and are most probably due to occlusion of cerebral vessels by so-called typhus nodules (foci of perivascular inflammation). In **typhoid fever,** delirium and confusion are common, but rarely meningitis or cerebral abscess can result from direct invasion of the nervous system by the typhoid bacillus. Rarely, too, the bacillus of **dysentery** or even the *Entamoeba histolytica* of amoebic dysentery is responsible for intracranial abscess formation. A form of **encephalopathy** can also complicate whooping cough; in such cases multiple small cerebral haemorrhages may be demonstrated and are possibly the result of violent bouts of coughing. The clinical manifestations include convulsions, which may be repetitive and fatal, and focal neurological signs such as aphasia and hemiplegia. While a depressive syndrome of considerable severity is a common sequel of **influenza,** cases of postinfluenzal encephalomyelitis have been described, but are probably allergic in origin and related to the forms of encephalomyelitis which may complicate childhood exanthemata (*see* Chap. 15). The principal neurological complication of **acute rheumatism** is **rheumatic chorea,** which has already been mentioned in Chapter 9. Probably this condition can be regarded as a form of rheumatic encephalitis, although the pathological changes in the brain in such cases are very indefinite and the condition is not usually a complication of acute rheumatism but rather an alternative manifestation of rheumatic disease. The condition can affect the face and all four limbs or may be hemiplegic in distribution. In severe cases there are also mental confusion, restlessness and emotional lability. The involuntary movements of characteristic type sometimes persist for some months or years but as a rule recovery is complete. One further neurological symptom which deserves mention is the **meningism** or occipital headache and neck stiffness which is an occasional complication of infective illnesses and particularly of pneumonia in childhood. Under such circumstances, lumbar puncture may be necessary to exclude meningitis, but the cerebrospinal fluid is normal and the neck stiffness is difficult to explain.

ALLERGIC DISORDERS

Within recent years it has become apparent that many disorders of the central and peripheral nervous systems which were once believed to be due to unidentified infective agents are due to an allergic or hypersensitivity response occurring within the nervous substance but affecting particularly the blood vessels and connective tissue elements. The pathological changes in such cases can be regarded as inflammatory in the broadest sense and often occur as the secondary effect of an infective agent which has not invaded the nervous system itself but to which the tissues of the nervous system prove to be in some way allergic or hypersensitive. In other instances the neurological manifestations are but one element of a clinical syndrome resulting from a disorder of blood vessels and connective tissue throughout the body. The neurological sequelae of prophylactic inoculation and the nervous complications of the common exanthemata of childhood constitute an important group of disorders falling into this category; in most such instances, however, the neurological syndrome so produced is one of encephalomyelitis. This condition is generally considered to fall into the group of so-called demyelinating diseases, and will be described fully in Chapter 15. The principal conditions which warrant consideration here are serum neuropathy, 'shoulder girdle neuritis', postinfective polyneuritis and the neurological complications of the so-called 'collagen', 'collagen-vascular' or 'connective tissue' diseases.

SERUM NEUROPATHY

Serum neuropathy or neuritis is a condition which can follow upon the injection of foreign serum (e.g. antitetanic serum, antidiphtheritic serum). It is usually but one manifestation of the syndrome of serum sickness which may follow some days or weeks after such an injection, and in which fever, nausea and joint pains are usually the most prominent clinical features. The serum neuropathy generally affects the cervical nerve roots and gives rise to weakness and wasting of a group of muscles around the shoulder girdle, sometimes with localised sensory loss. Though some cases recover, in others, particularly when a single peripheral nerve appears to be involved (e.g. the nerve to serratus anterior), the weakness is permanent. The condition of so-called **shoulder-girdle neuritis** or **neuralgic amyotrophy** is similar and must be distinguished from the clinical syndrome designated by the outmoded term **brachial neuritis;** most cases so diagnosed in the past were the result of prolapse of a cervical intervertebral disk (*see* Chap. 18). The true shoulder-girdle neuritis is a disorder of sudden onset which can follow upon an acute non-specific infection (e.g. influenza) or may complicate any febrile illness (e.g. pneumonia); occasionally it develops during pregnancy, after relatively minimal trauma or without any apparent precipitating cause. The first symptom of this type of neuritis is a severe burning pain which generally develops over the shoulder and spreads down the arm to a variable extent. It can persist for days or weeks making sleep impossible except with the aid of powerful analgesics and sedatives. Within a few days the patient becomes aware of some muscular weakness and it is apparent that certain muscles (deltoid is a typical example) are completely paralysed. Occasionally the weakness is limited to a single muscle (e.g. serratus anterior) but sometimes it is very much more extensive. Areas of sensory loss are commonly found, but are much less striking than the motor deficit. Gradually the pain improves and some return of muscular function occurs during the succeeding weeks or months; in most cases recovery is eventually complete, but some degree of permanent weakness occasionally persists. No treatment, apart from analgesics, and later remedial exercises and splinting where necessary, appears to be of any value.

POSTINFECTIVE POLYNEURITIS

Postinfective polyneuritis or polyneuropathy is the term now utilised to describe the condition which was once entitled infectious polyneuritis. It is also referred to commonly as the Guillain–Barré syndrome and is one of the commonest causes of the clinical syndrome of ascending paralysis (Landry's paralysis). The principal pathological change in such cases appears to be an inflammatory response of allergic type within multiple spinal roots, so that strictly the disorder should be regarded as a radiculopathy (polyradiculitis) rather than a peripheral neuropathy. The condition can follow a preceding infective illness or else it may develop without apparent antecedent infection. Commonly the first symptom is one of paraesthesiae in the feet, which within a few hours or days spread up the lower limbs and trunk and are accompanied by an ascending flaccid paralysis. In acute cases the sensory 'level' and the motor weakness ascend rapidly to involve the upper limbs, muscles of respiration and bulbar musculature; assisted respiration and tracheotomy may be necessary. There are subacute cases in which the paralysis and sensory loss ascend slowly over the course of several weeks or even months and in which the march of the disease process apparently becomes arrested when the weakness and sensory loss has reached the mid-dorsal or lower cervical level. Sometimes there is a spontaneous remission and the motor and sensory changes regress, until complete recovery occurs within the course of a few months, but in the more severe cases the condition constitutes a severe danger to life. Typically all the tendon reflexes in the affected limbs are lost and the paralysed limbs remain flaccid throughout; the plantar responses, when obtainable, are flexor. Usually the sensory loss affects all modalities of sensation; sphincter control is sometimes impaired, though not usually so early or as completely as in transverse myelitis (*see* Chap. 15) which may present a similar clinical picture but in which the plantar responses are extensor. In occasional cases the condition affects predominantly the cranial nerves ('cranial polyneuritis') and may then be difficult to distinguish from bulbar poliomyelitis and from neoplasms or granulomas of the basal meninges. In postinfective polyneuritis, the cerebrospinal fluid typically shows a substantial increase in protein content (100–1,000 mg/100 ml) but no pleocytosis (*dissociation albuminocytologique*). Although a substantial proportion of patients with this disease recover completely, residual weakness and sensory impairment of some degree persists in some; evidence is, however, increasing to suggest that the condition may be treated effectively with cortisone or with related steroids.

NEUROLOGICAL COMPLICATIONS OF THE 'COLLAGEN' DISEASES

Many of the 'neurological' complications of the 'collagen' diseases, using neurological in its broadest sense to imply those disorders which fall into the province of the neurologist, are found to affect the voluntary muscles. The principal conditions of this type, namely polymyositis and dermatomyositis, occurring alone or in combination with other conditions such as rheumatoid arthritis or scleroderma, will be considered in Chapter 18. Chorea, as a form of rheumatic disease, has already been mentioned. The two major disorders of the collagen group which remain are **disseminated lupus erythematosus and polyarteritis nodosa.** Each of these disorders can give rise to symptoms and signs of nervous disease by producing pathological changes in relation to small blood vessels in the central or peripheral nervous system. Thus in disseminated lupus erythematosus focal lesions in the brain or brain stem may result in epilepsy, paresis of the limbs, vertigo or cranial nerve palsies, while paraplegia due to spinal cord disease has been described. In occasional cases, too, a symmetrical polyneuropathy develops. Polyneuropathy (*see* Chapter 18) is even more common in cases of polyarteritis nodosa, but can be asymmetrical or may give a clinical picture suggesting multiple peripheral nerve lesions (mononeuritis multiplex). More rarely, there are symptoms and signs indicating multiple lesions within the brain, brain stem or spinal cord. Whether disseminated lupus or polyarteritis is the underlying cause, there will usually be associated clinical features in such cases (including fever, multiple arthropathy, albuminuria, raised E.S.R.) to indicate the nature of the underlying disease, but these features are sometimes unobtrusive and 'collagen' disease should always be considered as a possible diagnosis in patients with obscure neurological syndromes which run a subacute or remittent clinical course.

REFERENCES

BRAIN, W. R., *Diseases of the Nervous System*, 6th ed., Chapters 6-10 (London, Oxford University Press, 1962).

FORD, F. R., *Diseases of the Nervous System in Infancy, Childhood and Adolescence*, 4th ed. (Springfield, Ill., Thomas, 1959).

GAYLOR, J. B., 'Meningitis', in *Modern Trends in Neurology*, Ed. Feiling, A., 1st series (London, Butterworth, 1951).

HEYMAN, A., 'Syphilis', in *Principles of Internal Medicine*, Ed. Harrison, T. R., 4th ed., Chapter 163 (New York, McGraw-Hill, 1962).

MILLER, H. G., 'Clinical manifestations of tissue reaction in the nervous system', in *Modern Trends in Neurology*, Ed. Williams, D., 2nd series, Chapter 12 (London, Butterworth, 1957).

PENNYBACKER, J. B., 'Abscess of the brain', in *Modern Trends in Neurology*, Ed. Feiling, A., 1st series, Chapter 10 (London Butterworth, 1951).

RUSSELL, W. R., *Poliomyelitis*, 2nd ed. (London, Arnold, 1956).

WALTON, J. N., 'Pyogenic infections of the nervous system', in *Principles of Internal Medicine*, Ed. Harrison, T. R., 4th ed., Chapter 152 (New York, McGraw-Hill, 1962).

WORSTER-DROUGHT, C., 'Syphilis of the nervous system', in *Modern Trends in Neurology*, Ed. Feiling, A., 1st series, Chapter 9 (London, Butterworth, 1951).

CHAPTER 15

DEMYELINATING DISEASES

THE demyelinating diseases are a group of disorders of the nervous system which are characterised pathologically by a destructive process which affects the myelin sheaths of nerve fibres within the brain and spinal cord. Although the grey matter can be secondarily involved, these are primarily diseases of the white matter. The principal conditions which fall into this group are acute disseminated encephalomyelitis, acute haemorrhagic leucoencephalitis, neuromyelitis optica, disseminated sclerosis and diffuse cerebral sclerosis. Whereas it now seems probable that an allergic or hypersensitivity response within the nervous system may underlie most cases of acute encephalomyelitis, and similar factors are possibly of importance in disseminated sclerosis, the exact aetiology and pathogenesis of this group of disorders remains obscure, so that classification and identification of the separate disease entities within the group on an aetiological basis is still impossible. Clinical differentiation is also at times a matter of considerable difficulty; although the natural history of the illness in a chronic relapsing case of disseminated sclerosis is totally different from that in a case of encephalomyelitis following measles, in other instances there may be no means of distinguishing between an acute episode of disseminated sclerosis on the one hand and an encephalomyelitic illness on the other. Pathologically, too, there is a considerable similarity between the changes discovered in the nervous system in each of these diseases. Between the acute perivascular inflammatory lesions with demyelination around blood vessels, which occur in encephalomyelitis, and the massive confluent areas of demyelination of diffuse cerebral sclerosis, there exists a spectrum of pathological change which can occur in varying permutations and combinations in each of these conditions. In some cases the axis cylinders within the areas of demyelination are destroyed early, in others they survive for some time, but the overall pattern of pathological reaction is broadly similar; this does not of course imply identity of aetiology, as the nervous system has only a limited repertoire of pathological responses and myelin destruction may be the result of a variety of noxious agents. Hence it must be appreciated that no absolutely clear-cut definition of the demyelinating diseases is at present possible, and some at least of the clinical syndromes which are customarily identified (of which neuromyelitis optica is an outstanding example) may be artificially defined, and may eventually prove, when aetiology is more fully understood, to belong in one of the other groups.

ACUTE DISSEMINATED ENCEPHALOMYELITIS

Acute disseminated encephalomyelitis can be defined as an acute inflammatory disorder of the brain and/or spinal cord of variable clinical course and severity, in which the principal pathological changes take the form of perivascular cellular infiltration and perivenous demyelination in the white matter of the brain or spinal cord. The syndrome can follow vaccination against smallpox, inoculation against rabies or other protective inoculations, or a non-specific 'influenzal' infective illness; alternatively it may develop during the course of one of the childhood exanthemata, while on occasion an illness of this type occurs without there being any clinical evidence of a preceding or concurrent infection. Probably the condition is an allergic response of the nervous system to some unidentified antigenic agent; certainly the disorder resembles closely the experimental allergic encephalomyelitis which can be produced in animals.

The clinical picture of the illness is extremely variable; sometimes it is primarily encephalitic with headache, drowsiness, confusion and possibly convulsions, but in other instances the disease process can apparently be confined to the spinal cord and a clinical picture indicative of a transverse or ascending myelitis results. Indeed at the present time, when syphilis is becoming a comparatively rare disease, post-infective encephalomyelitis and disseminated sclerosis are the most common causes of the syndrome of transverse myelitis. Less commonly the clinical features indicate that the disease process is involving brain-stem structures or cerebellar connexions, to give ataxia, nystagmus, vertigo and cranial nerve palsies. Under such circumstances, differential diagnosis from an acute episode of disseminated sclerosis can be an extremely difficult matter. In yet other cases there may be evidence of involvement of motor and sensory roots as well as the spinal cord and the condition will resemble the closely-related acute post-infective polyradiculopathy (the Guillain–Barré syndrome). Often in such a case the question as to whether or not the spinal cord is involved must depend upon the plantar responses. In any event, the appropriate treatment (steroid therapy) is the same in the two conditions. It will now be convenient to consider the clinical features of the different varieties of encephalomyelitis.

Post-vaccinal encephalomyelitis and the disorder which may follow **rabies inoculation** are broadly similar. The post-vaccinal condition is most common after primary vaccination, in children of school age, and has been known in epidemics to affect as many as 1 in 2,500 vaccinated individuals though its incidence at the present day is very much less. A considerable proportion of cases suffer a relatively mild encephalitic illness which begins with headaches, neck stiffness, drowsiness, fever and vomiting and lasts only for a few days. In others convulsions occur and there is stupor and later deepening coma. The condition must be distinguished from the so-called post-vaccinial encephalopathy which, particularly in infants and young children, gives rise to transient drowsiness and convulsions, often lasting for no more than twenty-four to forty-eight hours. Often symptoms and signs of spinal cord involvement are seen; hemiplegia is comparatively rare but often there is an ascending flaccid weakness of the limbs with loss of tendon reflexes and paralysis of the bladder and bowels. Indeed, in very occasional cases, a myelitic picture of this nature can occur without headache, neck stiffness or clouding of consciousness. The disease may be fatal in as many as 30 per cent of cases, although the prognosis is probably influenced favourably nowadays by steroid therapy. In the remaining cases eventual recovery is often complete, although occasionally neurological signs, intellectual deterioration and personality change persist for some years after the illness.

The commonest variety of **post-exanthematous encephalomyelitis** is that which complicates *measles*, though a similar disorder may also occur following *chicken pox* (varicella) or *German measles* (rubella), and very rarely in *scarlet fever* (scarlatina). The neurological complications of mumps are probably due to direct invasion of the nervous system by the causal virus, giving a lymphocytic meningitis, and those of whooping cough (pertussis encephalopathy) are likely to be due to repeated episodes of cerebral anoxia developing during bouts of coughing. The encephalomyelitis of measles usually develops some two to four days after the appearance of the rash but can even antedate it; it has been known rarely to develop in contacts who do not develop a rash. The usual pattern of the illness is one of encephalitis which, if mild, gives rise to headache, neck stiffness, drowsiness and confusion for a few days, but if severe there are convulsions and deepening coma. Less commonly an acute hemiplegia develops, or a cerebellar ataxia of acute onset, while some few cases give the clinical picture of a transverse myelitis or polyradiculitis. About 10 per cent of cases end fatally; many recover completely but some few remain disabled by hemiplegia, paraplegia, fits or mental deterioration. In *chicken pox* the clinical picture is broadly similar, but most cases of encephalitis occurring in cases of this illness are mild and recover completely, while cerebellar ataxia occurs in an unusually large proportion. An explosive encephalomyelitic illness

K

can occasionally complicate rubella, but more often in this disease the encephalitic or myelitic illness, if it occurs, is mild and transient.

The form of **postinfective encephalomyelitis** which can follow non-specific infective illnesses or which may occur without clinical evidence of preceding infection, is even more protean in its manifestations. Sometimes there is a clinical picture indicating severe disseminated encephalomyelitis with deepening coma, convulsions and flaccid paraplegia, or the illness may be mild with headache, drowsiness, fever and transient limb or bulbar pareses. Alternatively, a transverse myelitis may be the presenting feature, while in a considerable proportion of cases the disease process affects the brain stem, giving nystagmus, impairment of conjugate ocular movement, dysphagia, facial weakness and variable long-tract signs. Under such circumstances it may be almost impossible to distinguish the clinical features of this condition from those produced by an initial episode of disseminated sclerosis. In early childhood the condition which has been referred to as 'acute cerebellar ataxia of infancy' is probably a variant of encephalomyelitis and can also occur in a subacute form.

The changes in the cerebrospinal fluid in all varieties of encephalomyelitis are similar, though by no means diagnostic. There is a variable pleocytosis, usually lymphocytic, but in acute cases polymorphonuclear leucocytes are present for a few days; the protein content of the fluid is invariably raised.

ACUTE HAEMORRHAGIC LEUCOENCEPHALITIS

This condition, which in the United States is generally entitled acute necrotising haemorrhagic leucoencephalopathy, is very probably a fulminating form of acute encephalomyelitis. A closely related condition is brain purpura which can be fatal within a few hours and is probably the result of an acute hypersensitivity reaction affecting cerebral blood vessels. In haemorrhagic leucoencephalitis the pathological changes are those of widespread vascular necrosis in the white matter of one or both cerebral hemispheres, with large areas of demyelination which may be confluent. The onset of the illness is often catastrophic and apoplectiform, with headache, convulsions and coma which deepens rapidly. Remarkably the physical signs are often in the first instance unilateral so that an onset with hemiplegia is not infrequent. Death often occurs within twenty-four to forty-eight hours; comparatively few cases are recognised during life, but a considerable polymorphonuclear reaction in the cerebrospinal fluid with a moderate rise in protein can be a valuable guide to the diagnosis, even though the clinical features may mimic those of massive cerebral infarction or cerebral abscess. It is possible that in certain cases of myelitis of exceptionally acute onset, the pathological process in the spinal cord is similar.

NEUROMYELITIS OPTICA

It is doubtful whether neuromyelitis optica (Devic's disease) can reasonably be considered to be a separate disease entity, as the clinical features which are regarded as typical of this syndrome can occur as one episode in the course of the illness in a patient with disseminated sclerosis. Rarely, too, cases of postinfective encephalomyelitis present in this way. The symptoms of the condition are, however, sufficiently distinctive for it to be regarded as a separate syndrome even though its pathogenesis and nosological status remain uncertain. The condition may develop at any age and in either sex. Typically it begins with pain in the eyes and visual loss which is generally unilateral at first but involves the other eye within hours or days. Blindness may rapidly become complete with subsequent slow regression but in other cases some useful vision is retained throughout. Usually the optic disks are swollen and the visual fields show bilateral central scotomas, though one eye is sometimes much more severely affected than the other. Soon afterwards the typical picture of a transverse myelitis appears with flaccid paralysis of the limbs, loss of sphincter control, absence of tendon reflexes, extensor plantar responses, and an ascending sensory 'level' below which all forms of sensation are impaired. Sometimes the spinal cord symptoms precede the visual loss, and it is also possible that some cases of bilateral retrobulbar neuritis without other neurological signs are in fact abortive examples of this syndrome. The cerebrospinal fluid shows simply a non-specific rise in protein and mononuclear cells. The disorder is fatal within the course of a few weeks in as many as one-third of affected individuals. Some make a slow but complete recovery; in this instance one may assume in retrospect that the pathological process was probably one of acute encephalomyelitis. However, a significant number of patients have residual visual loss and optic atrophy with paraplegia, and some of these eventually turn out to be suffering from disseminated sclerosis. Probably all cases of this syndrome should be treated initially with steroids (cortisone or one of its derivatives).

DISSEMINATED SCLEROSIS

Disseminated or multiple sclerosis is a disease of obscure aetiology characterised clinically by symptoms which indicate the presence of multiple lesions in the white matter of the brain and spinal cord. In most cases the disease process extends in an episodic manner, with remissions of variable duration separating the relapses, but in other individuals the condition presents as an intermittently progressive disease with spastic paraparesis and added signs indicating cerebellar or brain-stem disease. Although there is a considerable proportion of relatively mild cases in which relapses occur at intervals of several years and even then are comparatively transient and incapacitating, it is equally true that in some individuals the disease is inexorably progressive, giving rise to almost total disability and rarely death within one to two years of the onset. Eventually the great majority of cases become disabled with progressive paraplegia and/or ataxia. Pathologically there are multiple plaques of demyelination and gliosis of varying age throughout the nervous system; these principally involve the white matter of the brain and cord and are often perivenous or periventricular in distribution, but the grey matter is sometimes involved as well.

The **aetiology** of the disease remains obscure. It is commonest in temperate climates, being rare in the tropics, and although it is principally a disease of the white races it does appear sometimes in Negroes living in Europe or North America. It occurs equally in the two sexes and usually begins between the ages of twenty and forty, although it rarely develops in the first and second decades or in the fifth and sixth. It certainly occurs more often in several members of a family than could be accounted for by chance, but rarely afflicts more than one of a pair of identical twins, so that the genetic factor cannot be very powerful. Probably there is an inherited susceptibility in some cases to the agent or agents which are responsible for the demyelinating process. The rarity of conjugal cases is against an infective theory of aetiology, and there is no concrete evidence to indicate that the disease is due to infection by a virus or spirochaete, as has been suggested by several workers. Other theories implicating excessive fat in the diet, heavy-metal poisoning, vasospasm or venous thrombosis also have a few adherents. Current opinion favours the view that the disease is due to a recurrent allergic response of the nervous system to one or several unknown allergens. Although evidence in favour of the allergic hypothesis is much less convincing in this disease than in acute encephalomyelitis, it receives modest support from the fact that the Y-globulin in the cerebrospinal fluid is often raised, while the changes in the fluid which follow the injection of intrathecal tuberculin in a Mantoux-positive patient with the disease appear to be modified, as in the cortisone-treated animal. It is also apparent that relapses can repeatedly follow infective illnesses in certain individuals, and have also been described following prophylactic inoculation. The fact that onset or relapse may also follow trauma and/or emotional stress is much less easy to explain.

The **clinical manifestations** of the disease can be very variable, depending upon the situation and intensity of the pathological changes. A single discrete lesion occurring at the outset may be responsible for a wide variety of symptoms and signs depending upon its site, but if multiple lesions occur simultaneously in eloquent areas of the nervous system a much more specific clinical picture will result. This variation in spatial distribution of the areas of demyelination is responsible for the remarkable clinical pleomorphism of the disease. Symptoms due to a single localised lesion almost always remit within a few days or weeks as do those attributable to multiple lesions which have developed acutely. In such cases, numerous relapses may occur, each followed by a partial remission, but each leaving in its wake further evidence of permanent neurological deficit upon which every succeeding manifestation is superimposed. In the end the clinical picture is often indistinguishable from that observed in cases which from the beginning can be recognised as harbouring multiple and widespread lesions, all progressing inexorably at much the same rate. The relapsing type with multiple acute or subacute episodes is commoner in young patients, whereas in cases with an onset in middle life the course of the disease is more often slowly progressive and the brunt of the disease process falls upon the spinal cord. Although it is possible that in a small proportion of cases the disease becomes arrested, and that in fewer still a remission may be complete and permanent, most cases eventually follow a final common path of increasing ataxia and/or spasticity, immobility, respiratory or urinary infection and death.

Although it is true that almost any symptom of neurological disease can at some time be observed in cases of disseminated sclerosis, there are a number of symptom-complexes which occur particularly often, usually as the presenting features of the disease.

One of the most frequent initial symptoms is *visual failure*, which is generally unilateral but occasionally bilateral, and is the result of *retrobulbar neuritis*. There is often pain in the eye with progressive blurring or dimming of vision over a period of several hours or days. Often vision is totally lost but spontaneous improvement generally occurs and recovery may be complete within a few weeks or months, although a central scotoma not infrequently persists. In the acute stage the optic disk is usually swollen, but subsequently waxy pallor of the temporal half of the disk or optic atrophy is seen. An alternative presenting symptom, which can also precede the development of other neurological manifestations by several years, is *diplopia*, lasting for several hours or days. Occasionally this is due to involvement of the nucleus of one of the oculomotor nerves, but more often it is of central or internuclear type, occurring without an objective ocular palsy. An almost pathognomonic sign of this disease is Harris's sign, or ataxic nystagmus, in which, on attempted lateral gaze, there is a gross nystagmus in the abducting eye and a failure of medial movement of the abducting eye.

An alternative mode of onset is with *transient weakness or loss of control of the limbs*. The weakness can take the form of a monoparesis or hemiparesis, but paraparesis, involving both lower limbs, is more common. There is weakness and clumsiness of the affected limb or limbs with difficulty in walking. Physical examination during the episode reveals either spasticity with increased reflexes and extensor plantar responses, or cerebellar ataxia. These initial manifestations may resolve over the course of a few days or weeks to be succeeded by other manifestations in the subsequent months or years.

Sensory symptoms are also common as the initial manifestations of the disease. Paraesthesiae in a limb lasting for a few days can easily be overlooked; often these spread in a typical manner, indicating centrifugal spread of a plaque of demyelination in the posterior columns of the cord. In such a case the tingling and numbness may spread up one leg and down the other or from an arm to the trunk and then to the face and leg on the same side of the body. The so-called 'useless hand' syndrome is often due to such a lesion which so impairs proprioceptive sensation in one hand that the patient is virtually unable to use it even though motor power remains intact. In such a case there will be impairment of position and joint sense, of vibration sense and two-point discrimination in the affected limb or limbs, while if the legs are involved, Romberg's sign will be positive. Less frequently the patient will observe, particularly on entering a hot bath, that pain and temperature sensation is diminished in one leg, and examination will reveal the clinical features of a partial Brown–Séquard syndrome, indicating the presence of a plaque of demyelination in one lateral column of the spinal cord. Sensory symptoms of this nature almost invariably remit over the course of a few weeks or months.

Symptoms indicating primary *involvement of brain-stem structures* are also common. One mode of presentation is with an acute episode of vertigo and vomiting due to involvement of vestibular centres; evidence of sensory or motor long-tract lesions are occasionally seen in such cases. Alternatively, there is sometimes an ataxia of relatively acute onset with signs of cerebellar disease affecting the co-ordination of all four limbs; this is generally associated with severe nystagmus on lateral gaze and with dysarthria (Charcot's triad). A similar constellation of signs may also develop at a later stage in established cases. Combined lesions involving cranial-nerve nuclei and long tracts are also seen occasionally in bewildering variety. Some patients develop a unilateral facial anaesthesia which is followed months later by tic douloureux on the same side of the face and later still by evidence of spinal cord disease. Tic douloureux can also develop in patients who have suffered from the disease for some years.

As already mentioned, a significant group of cases demonstrates a *slowly-progressive weakness and clumsiness of the limbs*. When this is the case in the younger patients there is usually clinical evidence of widespread lesions. Thus it is common to find in such individuals temporal pallor of the optic disks (even without a previous history of retrobulbar neuritis), nystagmus, cerebellar ataxia, and spastic weakness of the limbs with absent vibration sense at the ankles. In the common intermittently-progressive form of disseminated sclerosis which begins in middle life the main brunt of the disease falls upon the pyramidal tracts in the spinal cord, and the signs are those of a spastic paraparesis or quadriparesis with impaired or absent perception of vibration in the lower limbs, but without any evidence of cranial nerve involvement.

Acute episodes of disseminated sclerosis can involve almost any area of the central nervous system. Thus in some cases the onset is explosive with headache, vomiting, vertigo and facial pain and with a succession of symptoms indicating severe involvement of the brain stem, optic nerves or spinal cord. Indeed an episode indistinguishable from other forms of transverse myelitis may occur. Rarely a cerebral illness with mental changes, convulsions, aphasia, hemiplegia or hemianopia develops at the onset. Under such circumstances, differentiation from acute encephalomyelitis is difficult or impossible.

Mental symptoms are not infrequent in patients with this disease. Often hysterical features are present at the outset and may mask the organic nature of the illness. Euphoria is the prevailing mood of many patients, but some are depressed; in the late stages a progressive dementia sometimes develops.

Sphincter involvement is common; precipitancy of micturition is a constant feature in most established cases, but as the paraplegia advances, urinary retention with overflow and faecal incontinence commonly ensue.

The **prognosis** of the disease is variable. Many patients live for as long as thirty or forty years from the onset, while some die within one to two years. The prognosis can certainly be regarded as being much more favourable in patients who are not significantly disabled within five years of the onset. The average duration of the disease is from twenty to twenty-five years; the final state of the bedridden incontinent patient, racked by painful flexor spasms of the lower limbs and shaken by febrile episodes of intercurrent infection, is one of the most distressing in medicine.

The **cerebrospinal fluid** may be entirely normal, particularly in chronic or advanced cases. During an acute episode there is often a moderate mononuclear pleocytosis of up to fifty cells/mm^3 and the protein content of the fluid (particularly the γ-globulin) is often raised to more than 25 per cent of the total protein. A raised proportion of γ-globulin in a fluid with a normal total protein is very suggestive of this disease. In about 25 per cent of cases the colloidal gold (Lange) curve is paretic in type.

The **diagnosis** in a typical case in which there has been a remittent course and the clinical features indicate the presence of lesions widely disseminated throughout the central nervous system, is not a difficult matter. It is indeed a useful axiom that this disease should not be diagnosed when all the symptoms and signs could be accounted for by a single lesion. Whereas this rule must sometimes be ignored in the presence of one of the typical symptom-complexes described above, it is nevertheless a useful guide. Acute episodes may mimic epidemic vertigo, meningovascular syphilis and even encephalitis; the first of these can only be recognised by the course of the illness and then not with certainty, but the other two conditions will generally be identified by means of cerebrospinal fluid examination. Distinction from acute encephalomyelitis may also be particularly difficult but the latter is usually a monophasic self-limiting disease. In the more chronic cases, diagnosis from the familial ataxias is made by virtue of the consistent pattern of inheritance and stereotyped clinical pattern of the latter group of diseases, while motor neurone disease is identified by the presence of muscular wasting and fasciculation, features which are very rare in disseminated sclerosis. Subacute combined degeneration can occasionally be mimicked and when 'posterior column' and 'pyramidal' symptoms and signs predominate, examination of the blood and of the gastric juice for the presence of hydrochloric acid is obligatory. In patients who present with a progressive spastic paraplegia it is sometimes impossible to exclude spinal tumour and cervical spondylosis with certainty except by myelography, and in such individuals the diagnosis of disseminated sclerosis may have to be made by exclusion, although a raised γ-globulin or abnormal Lange curve in the cerebrospinal fluid will give valuable confirmatory evidence.

The **treatment** of this and other conditions will be considered in Chapter 20, but it may be said that no single form of therapy is uniformly successful, though there is some evidence that steroid therapy may favourably influence the course of the disease in a few cases and that others may obtain temporary benefit from physiotherapy. In advanced cases with painful and disabling extensor spasticity or flexor spasms, intrathecal phenol injections may be of great value. It is usually wise not to reveal the nature of the illness to patients who have had one or two transient episodes of disability, and to use terms such as 'neuritis' in explaining the nature of their symptoms, but when the disease process is established and progressive, there is usually little advantage in withholding the true facts of the situation; in appropriate cases it is useful to stress how benign the disorder can be in some cases.

DIFFUSE CEREBRAL SCLEROSIS (LEUCODYSTROPHY)

This group of disorders, of which the commonest variety was first described by Schilder in 1912, is characterised pathologically by a progressive massive demyelination, usually beginning posteriorly, and spreading more or less symmetrically throughout the white matter of the two cerebral hemispheres. A variety of clinical and pathological forms of diffuse sclerosis have been described. Clinically, the form which begins in early childhood is usually entitled **Schilder's disease** or **encephalitis periaxalis diffusa,** and the pathological changes are characteristic macroscopically in that the white matter is replaced by greyish, rubbery translucent material; the arcuate fibres of the occipital lobe are typically spared. Schilder's disease may rarely occur in later life, but the familial form which usually begins in late childhood has been entitled the Pelizaeus–Merzbacher disease. In these conditions phagocytes within the demyelinated area are generally filled with sudanophilic lipid. Other less-common pathological varieties are seen in which curious globoid bodies are found between nerve fibre bundles, and in one variety much of the degenerate material is found to stain metachromatically. In the latter condition, which may be familial, and which has been called late-infantile metachromatic leukoencephalopathy, there is also widespread degeneration of oligodendrocytes.

The **clinical features** of all forms of diffuse sclerosis are similar. The disease is commonest in childhood, and occurs in either sex. It often begins with progressive visual failure, which is succeeded by focal or generalised fits, aphasia, mental deterioration and variable degrees of paresis of the limbs, leading eventually to total blindness, dementia and spastic quadriplegia. Rarely the onset is sudden with headache, stupor and convulsions. The disease is progressive, uninfluenced by treatment, and usually leads to death in one to three years from the onset. Generally the cerebrospinal fluid is normal but occasionally there is a slight rise in its protein content. Most commonly in childhood the condition can be confused with other disorders which give rise to fits, progressive dementia and paralysis, of which cerebral lipidosis and subacute encephalitis are the most prominent. In adult life the condition must be distinguished from other forms of progressive cerebral degeneration and particularly from general paresis and presenile dementia.

REFERENCES

BRAIN, W. R., *Diseases of the Nervous System*, 6th ed., Chapter 11 (London, Oxford University Press, 1962).

MCALPINE, D., COMPSTON, N. D. and LUMSDEN, C. E., *Multiple Sclerosis* (Edinburgh, Livingstone, 1955).

MCALPINE, D., LUMSDEN, C. E. and ACHESON, E. D., *Multiple Sclerosis. A Reappraisal* (Edinburgh, Livingstone, 1965).

MILLER, H. G., 'Clinical manifestations of tissue reaction in the nervous system', in *Modern Trends in Neurology*, Ed. Williams, D., 2nd series (London, Butterworth, 1957).

WALTON, J. N., 'Demyelinating diseases', in *Principles of Internal Medicine*, Ed. Harrison, T. R., 4th ed., Chapter 287 (New York, McGraw-Hill, 1962).

CHAPTER 16

NEOPLASMS AND THE NERVOUS SYSTEM

ABOUT 1 per cent of all deaths are due to intracranial tumours. These occur in great variety; the majority are locally malignant, and constitute about 15 per cent of all malignant tumours occurring in man. Of these, most arise primarily within the cranial cavity and, being invasive, can rarely be removed surgically, but a considerable proportion are metastatic from a malignant neoplasm which is growing elsewhere in the body, and which has given secondary deposits within the brain or in the bones of the cranial cavity. There exist, however, a significant number of benign neoplasms which may grow within the skull, and it is particularly important that these should be recognised as they can generally be extirpated in whole or in part at operation, with excellent results. The proportion of intraspinal tumours which compress the spinal cord and are benign is much higher, and diagnosis of these removable growths is even more imperative. The symptomatology of intracranial neoplasia is extremely variable, as it depends not only upon the character of the neoplasm but also upon its situation and rate of growth. There are limitless permutations and combinations of these three factors which may influence the clinical picture. It can, however, be said that intracranial tumours in general tend to produce a series of general symptoms, upon which the specific features produced by different varieties of tumour arising in individual situations are superimposed. Before considering these general symptoms and some of the more common and important tumour syndromes, it will first be necessary to formulate a working classification of tumours of the nervous system, in order to provide an understanding of the basic pathological features of intracranial and intraspinal new growths, and to give an approximate outline of their relative incidence.

CLASSIFICATION OF NEOPLASMS IN THE NERVOUS SYSTEM

In the absence of any convincing information concerning the aetiology of intracranial or intraspinal tumours, they must at present be classified according to their cells or tissues of origin. Of the **primary neoplasms,** those arising from the nerve cells and fibres themselves or from their cells of embryonic origin (neuroblastomas and neurocytomas) are extremely rare. Commonest are the gliomas, of which

279

the most malignant is the glioblastoma multiforme, the least invasive the astrocytoma. According to one modern classification all gliomas are called astrocytomas and are graded in Groups I to IV according to the characteristics of the predominant cells in the tumour; Group I is the least, and Group IV the most anaplastic and malignant. Accurate grading can be a matter of considerable difficulty, since in a single tumour it may be possible to find certain cells which are characteristic of glioblastoma and others which are those of a typical slowly-growing astrocytoma. The rapidly-growing medulloblastoma, a common malignant tumour of the posterior fossa in infancy and childhood, which tends to metastasise throughout the subarachnoid space, is probably best classified with the gliomas, although its predominant cell is very different from the astrocyte and its precursors. Other tumours of the nervous supporting tissues are first, the relatively slow-growing and benign oligodendroglioma, which has a particular tendency to calcify, and the ependymoma, which, because of the cells from which it originates, tends to grow in relation to the cerebral ventricles or to the central canal of the spinal cord.

Of the primary neoplasms which arise in the meninges, the benign meningioma is the most common, but occasionally a fibrosarcoma, a reticulum cell sarcoma, or a melanoma may arise in this situation. Turning to the commoner growths which arise from organs which are attached to or lie in close relationship to the brain, though not strictly a part of it, one must consider the adenomas of the pituitary · gland (the hypophysis), pinealomas, and papillomas of the choroid plexus. Neoplasms of developmental origin ('rest cell' tumours) include: the craniopharyngioma which arises from remnants of Rathke's pouch; haemangioblastomas which are usually found in the cerebellum; arteriovenous angiomas or hamartomas (which are more properly regarded as vascular malformations rather than tumours); chordomas, which are generally found either in relation to the brain stem or in the sacral region and grow from primitive remnants of the notochord; epidermoid (cholesteatoma) and dermoid cysts, some of which are teratomas; and an uncommon tumour called a colloid cyst which is generally found in the third ventricle and is believed to arise from vestiges of the primitive paraphysis. Primary neoplasms of the cranial or vertebral bones which secondarily involve the brain or spinal cord are relatively uncommon but deserve mention. These include osteomas, osteogenic sarcomas and haemangiomas of vertebral bodies. Lastly, in considering primary tumours, one must remember those which grow from or in relation to nerve trunks, as these may form upon cranial nerves or spinal nerve roots to give symptoms and signs indicating the presence of an intracranial or intraspinal tumour. By far the commonest is the neu-roma, neurolemmoma, neurinoma, or neurofibroma (as it is variously called), which grows from the sheath of Schwann; usually a neoplasm of this nature takes the form of an encapsulated swelling upon a nerve, but occasionally it infiltrates between nerve fibres, with which it becomes inextricably intermingled to give a so-called plexiform neuroma. This latter type of growth is seen particularly on peripheral nerves. It should be remembered that neurofibromas sometimes grow in relation to nerve plexuses or single peripheral nerves outside the nervous system, when they give a clinical picture indicating a peripheral nerve or plexus lesion (*see* Chap. 13) and there is usually a palpable swelling over the nerve trunk. Fibrosarcomas also occur occasionally on or in peripheral nerves.

When one comes to consider **secondary tumours,** those which are most common are secondary carcinomas, arising as blood-borne metastases from tumours in other sites, of which the lung, breast, kidney, ovary and colon are the most frequent. Sarcomas of bone and other tissues and malignant melanomas also sometimes metasta-sise to the brain. Another common group of cases are those in which malignant tumours involve the cranial bones, vertebral bodies or extradural tissues and subsequently involve the brain or spinal cord. Of these the most prominent are carcinoma of the nasopharynx or paranasal sinuses, metastatic carcinoma involving the bone (lung, prostate, breast, thyroid) and multiple myelomatosis. Deposits of lymphadenoma (Hodgkin's disease) and of the other reticuloses are rarely found in the brain but not uncommonly involve the cranial and spinal meninges.

Last of all it is important to remember that certain conditions which are not strictly neoplastic can give a clinical picture suggesting the presence of a space-occupying lesion within the skull or spinal column. That this is true of certain cases of cerebral abscess has already been mentioned (*see* Chap. 14) but in such individuals there is usually clinical evidence of infection. In certain individuals, however, an intracranial or intraspinal mass of inflammatory origin develops in an indolent manner without clear clinical evidence of infection. This is true of certain granulomas (gumma, tuberculoma, sarcoidosis) and parasitic cysts (e.g. cysticercosis).

There is much evidence to suggest that the relative incidence of these tumours has changed considerably in recent years. Thus the once common granulomas (gumma, tuberculoma) are now rare and the incidence of metastatic tumours is probably increasing. The most common intracranial tumours are gliomas, metastases and menin-giomas in that order. In adult life, most gliomas are supratentorial, and over half are glioblastomas; more males than females are affected. In childhood, most gliomas occur in the posterior fossa and are generally either medulloblastomas or cerebellar astrocytomas. Gliomas developing in adult life are most common in middle-age; but in women, with increasing age there is an increasing probability that a supratentorial neoplasm will be a meningioma. In the spinal canal, gliomas are comparatively rare, and neurofibromas, which occur at any spinal level and equally in the two sexes, are much more common. Spinal meningiomas usually occur in the dorsal region, and nearly always in women. For ease of reference, an outline of this classification and approximate figures of incidence are shown in the accompanying table.

INTRACRANIAL TUMOURS

It is important first to consider the means by which intracranial tumours alter the physiology of the brain and so give rise to symptoms and signs indicating their presence. It should be remembered that the brain and its membranes are contained within a rigid bony box, the skull; any increase in volume of the intracranial contents means that cerebrospinal fluid is displaced from the cranial cavity, so that the pressure of this fluid within the spinal theca, which can usually be regarded as giving a reasonably faithful indication of the intracranial pressure, rises. As would be expected from the principles elucidated in Chapter 4, headache is an almost invariable accompaniment. In extreme cases the pressure is raised to such a degree that there is a greatly increased resistance to the entry of blood into cerebral arteries, so that the cerebral blood flow is reduced. This increased arterial resistance leads in turn to a reflex raising of arterial blood pressure in an attempt to overcome it, so that temporary hypertension develops. Rarely the blood flow may nevertheless be reduced sufficiently for infarction to occur. The local cerebral oedema which is almost invariable in the immediate vicinity of an intracranial tumour contributes to the increasing intracranial tension. Not only is the pressure of the cerebrospinal fluid increased in the spinal theca but in all extracranial extensions of the subarachnoid space. Thus the pressure in the meningeal sheaths around the optic nerves also rises; this in turn leads to a diminished venous return from the retinae, with engorgement of retinal veins, swelling of the optic nerve heads or disks (papilloedema) and in severe cases, retinal haemorrhages and even exudates around their edges. Another effect of increased intracranial pressure is that there is compression of the respiratory and cardiac centres in the brain stem so that both respiration and the heart rate become much slower; a full, slow pulse is characteristic. In severe cases which are showing progressive deterio-

	Incidence in cranium
I. *Primary tumours*	
1. Neuroblastomas and neurocytomas.	Rare
2. Gliomas and other supporting cell tumours.	
(a) Glioblastoma.	
(b) Astrocytoma.	
(c) Medulloblastoma.	40 per cent
(d) Oligodendroglioma.	
(e) Ependymoma.	
3. Meningeal tumours.	
(a) Meningioma.	15 per cent
(b) Fibrosarcoma and reticulum cell sarcoma.	
(c) Melanoma.	Rare
4. Tumours of secretory or glandular tissues.	
(a) Pituitary adenomas (acidophil, chromophobe).	
(b) Pinealoma.	8 per cent
(c) Papilloma of choroid plexus.	
(d) Glomus tumours.	
5. Tumours of developmental origin.	
(a) Craniopharyngioma.	
(b) Haemangioblastoma.	
(c) Arteriovenous angioma.	10 per cent
(d) Chordoma.	
(e) Epidermoid and dermoid cysts.	
(f) Colloid cyst of third ventricle.	
6. Primary tumours of cranial vertebral bones.	
(a) Osteoma.	
(b) Osteogenic sarcoma.	Rare
(c) Haemangioma of vertebral body	
7. Tumours of nerves and nerve roots.	
(a) Neurinoma (neurofibroma) and plexiform neuroma.	10 per cent
II. *Secondary tumours*	
1. Intracranial and intraspinal metastases.	
(a) Carcinoma (lung, breast, kidney, thyroid, ovary, colon).	15 per cent
(b) Sarcoma.	
(c) Melanoma.	
2. Tumours involving cranial bones, vertebral bodies and meninges.	
(a) Carcinoma of nasopharynx and paranasal sinuses.	
(b) Metastic carcinoma of bone (lung, prostate, breast, thyroid).	
(c) Multiple myelomatosis.	
III. *Granuloma* (gumma, tuberculoma, sarcoid, parasitic invasion).	2 per cent

ration, brain-stem centres (the reticular substance) can be compressed to an extent sufficient to lead to unconsciousness. In these later stages, respiration becomes irregular or of Cheyne–Stokes type and eventually ceases altogether, while a terminal tachycardia, rather than bradycardia, is common.

The severity of the symptoms attributable to a rise in the intracranial pressure depends not only upon the size and rapidity of growth of the tumour but also upon its situation. Thus a slowly-growing meningioma in one or other frontal region will produce few symptoms due to this cause, at least initially, when manifestations of focal brain damage are predominant. Growths in the posterior fossa, however, which interfere with the free circulation of cerebrospinal fluid at an early stage, either through aqueductal pressure, or through blockage of foramina in the fourth ventricle, give 'pressure symptoms' from the beginning. Additional complications may arise as a result of herniation of brain tissue under the free edge of the falx cerebri, through the tentorial notch, or the foramen magnum. The falx is the longitudinal and vertical fold of dura mater which separates the medial surfaces of the two cerebral hemispheres, while the tentorium is the horizontal fold whose curved free edge encircles the upper brain stem, and which separates cerebrum from cerebellum. A mass in either cerebral hemisphere can give rise to the gradual extrusion of a part of the hemisphere across the free edge of one of these folds. Pushing downwards of the medial aspect of the temporal lobe through the tentorial notch is particularly important. As the third (oculomotor) cranial nerve crosses this notch, it is often compressed, and the first sign of tentorial herniation may be a fixed dilated pupil, ptosis or later a complete third-nerve palsy on the side of the lesion. Subsequently there is compression of the upper brain stem with stupor or coma and occasionally homolateral pyramidal signs develop due to compression of the contralateral crus cerebri against the opposite free edge of the tentorium. Reduction of the pressure below the tentorium, say by lumbar puncture, will greatly increase the tentorial herniation, giving a rapidly fatal termination to the illness owing to brain-stem compression. The risks of lumbar puncture are equally as great when a tumour lies in the posterior fossa, but in this instance it is herniation of the cerebellar tonsils through the foramen magnum (a pressure cone), with compression of the medulla oblongata, which is responsible for the condition.

General Symptoms

Since all cerebral tumours, whatever their character and situation, can be expected to give rise to an increase in the intracranial pressure, the characteristic symptoms and signs so produced appear eventually in virtually every case. These symptoms and signs are headache, vomiting and papilloedema.

The **headache** of cerebral tumour has little localising value, although it is sometimes unilateral and then generally affects the side of the head upon which the tumour is situated. More often it is frontal or occipital or both. It may be more severe posteriorly in patients harbouring posterior fossa tumours, but this is not invariable. The headache is often paroxysmal and generally 'throbbing' or 'bursting' in character. It is generally most severe on waking and tends to improve as the day wears on; typically it is made worse by coughing, stooping or straining at stool. But these features are not invariable and in some cases the pain is vague and indefinite.

The **vomiting** experienced by patients with intracranial neoplasms often has no specific characteristics, though it tends to be worse in the mornings, like the headache, and is sometimes precipitate and projectile, occuring without preceding nausea.

Papilloedema, though a characteristic physical sign, does not as a rule produce symptoms in the early stages. Typically the retinal veins are blurred, the optic disk is pinker than normal, the physiological cup is obliterated, and the edges of the disk (including its temporal edge) are blurred. It should be remembered that there is some blurring of the nasal edge of the disk in most normal persons. As papilloedema increases, haemorrhages may be seen in 'flare' formations around the disk and the patient will often complain of some blurring of vision, or of the fact that he sees haloes around lights. The latter is an ominous symptom, since although very gross degrees of papilloedema can exist without apparent impairment of visual acuity, visual failure, when it comes, is often rapid, complete and irreversible.

The increased intracranial pressure produced by a tumour in any site sometimes gives rise to mental symptoms and false localising signs. **Mental symptoms** may take the form of a progressive apathy leading in the end to stupor and coma, but at an earlier stage there is often evidence of a mild dementia with impairment of memory, intellect and social adaptation. Frequently there is incontinence of urine and faeces. Confusion and disorientation in time and place are common and in occasional cases there is a fully-developed Korsakoff syndrome (*see* Chap. 7). The commonest **false localising signs** are a unilateral or bilateral sixth-nerve palsy (due to pressure upon the nerve trunks in their long intracranial course), a partial third-nerve paralysis (due usually to tentorial herniation) or an extensor plantar response on one or both sides due to brain-stem compression.

Having considered the general symptoms attributable to intracranial tumour, it will next be convenient to describe the various **modes of clinical presentation** of these lesions. As in the majority of nervous diseases it can be said that the physical signs are generally of most assistance in localisation of a lesion, whereas one will be dependent upon the clinical history in attempting to identify the nature of the growth. As a general rule the onset is relatively rapid when the tumour is a glioblastoma, a medulloblastoma or a metastasis, but when it is an astrocytoma, an oligodendroglioma, a meningioma, an acoustic neuroma or pituitary adenoma, the development of symptoms usually proceeds in an insidious manner. In a considerable proportion of cases, and particularly when the tumour is a supratentorial glioma or meningioma, the clinical picture is one of progressive focal symptoms and signs indicating cerebral compression or destruction, combined with symptoms and signs of increased intracranial pressure. In other instances, particularly when the tumour is slowly-growing, the focal symptoms progress insidiously but there are no clinical features indicative of raised pressure when the patient attends for examination. Another common history is one of focal or generalised epileptiform seizures. When the fit has focal or Jacksonian features the suspicion that it may be the result of a focal lesion such as a tumour is immediately raised, but if the seizures are generalised from the start, they may have occurred intermittently for months or exceptionally for several years before symptoms (headache, vomiting) or physical signs (papilloedema, monoparesis or hemiparesis) arise to indicate that they are not idiopathic in origin. Another common group of cases is that in which there are symptoms and signs clearly indicating that the intracranial pressure is raised, but there is no clinical evidence whatever to indicate the situation of the neoplasm. While this may be the case in a patient harbouring a glioblastoma, even in one cerebral hemisphere, it is particularly common in children with medulloblastomas and in adults with tumours in the posterior fossa or in the upper brain stem or third or fourth ventricle. A final but most important group of cases is that in which the symptoms of indefinite headache, intermittent giddiness, vague memory loss and lack of concentration are ill-defined but nevertheless progressive. These are the most difficult cases of all, as the clinical picture is indefinite and easily confused with disorders of emotional origin. Under these circumstances it is often a matter of the greatest difficulty to decide how far investigations ought to be pursued in an attempt to demonstrate an intracranial neoplasm. Cases of this type are unfortunately common and it is in just such an individual that diagnostic errors are particularly easy to make. Hence before discussing specific tumour syndromes it will be appropriate to consider a number of cardinal points which are of value in the management of cases in which the diagnosis of intracranial tumour is suspected.

Management of the Tumour Suspect

When the patient's clinical history suggests that an intracranial tumour is a possible cause of his symptoms, a careful physical examination is of course imperative. If papilloedema is observed as well as evidence of a hemiparesis in a patient with a few weeks' history of increasing headache and drowsiness, it is not difficult to decide that a glioblastoma in one cerebral hemisphere is the most probable diagnosis, while, alternatively, unilateral ataxia will point to one lateral lobe of cerebellum as the most probable site. Jacksonian epilepsy, too, indicating in all probability the presence of a hemisphere lesion near to the motor or sensory cortex, is of great localising value. It is when the physical signs are minimal and indefinite that difficulties arise. In such a case the importance of palpation, percussion and auscultation of the skull should not be overlooked. A localised area of bony tenderness or hyperostosis is sometimes present in the skull overlying a meningioma, while in young children with tumours in the posterior fossa, there may be separation of the cranial sutures and a typical 'cracked-pot' note on percussion, as in hydrocephalus from any cause. Similarly, the presence of a cranial bruit or of enlarged arteries in the scalp is a valuable guide to the presence of an intracranial arteriovenous angioma.

If clinical examination is uninformative, the next investigations which should be performed are radiography of the skull and chest. The plain films of the skull may reveal a shift of the pineal gland from the midline, intracranial calcification, or erosion of the internal auditory meatus on one side (in a patient with an acoustic neuroma). In the chest film a shadow indicating the presence of a silent bronchogenic neoplasm will indicate that the intracranial lesion is probably a metastasis. Echo-encephalography may then be useful in confirming that mid-line structures are displaced. An electroencephalogram should next be performed, and may localise the lesion to one cerebral hemisphere. The advisability of lumbar puncture is a matter of debate. This investigation is certainly contraindicated in the presence of papilloedema or other evidence of greatly raised intracranial pressure. Indeed it is probably best avoided whenever there is a strong clinical presumption that an intracranial tumour is present. In doubtful cases, however, it can be a valuable test, as the pressure of the fluid can be recorded and its protein content measured. The pressure is usually raised in a patient with an intracranial neoplasm, unless it is very slow-growing or infiltrating in character, and in most cases there is also an increased quantity of protein in the fluid. The protein level is often exceptionally high (up to several hundred milligrams per 100 ml) if the tumour is an acoustic neuroma, while the protein tends in general to be higher in patients with extracerebral lesions such as meningiomas than in those with gliomas. If the pressure of the fluid is normal, and suspicion of an intracranial neoplasm persists, it is then usual to carry out air encephalography (*see* Chap. 3) using the fractional technique if a posterior fossa lesion is suspected. When the pressure is raised, however, and certainly in the presence of papilloedema, the next investigation must depend upon the presence or absence of clinical or electroencephalographic localising signs. If there is clinical evidence that a tumour is likely in one cerebral hemisphere, the appropriate investigation is carotid arteriography, as this technique will not only localise the tumour but the vascular pattern may indicate its nature. Gamma-encephalography is also useful in localisation. When there are no localising features, however, and particularly if a neoplasm in the posterior fossa is suspected, air ventriculography should be carried out, and in occasional cases it will be necessary to inject myodil into the cerebral ventricles for accurate localisation of the neoplasm. Although it is difficult to generalise, it can be said that surgical exploration should be considered in all cases in which a tumour appears to be at all accessible, and particularly if there is any possibility, however remote, that it may be benign. On the other hand, if the presence of a glioma is confirmed and unless the pressure is greatly raised indicating that decompression is necessary as a life-saving procedure, exploration and biopsy may be better avoided as many patients deteriorate rapidly after this procedure.

Tumour Syndromes

Having considered the general symptomatology and the management of cases of suspected intracranial tumour, it will now be appropriate to describe briefly a number of the syndromes which may result from specific tumours in different parts of the cranial cavity.

GLIOMA

Between the rapidly-growing glioblastoma on the one hand, and the insidiously invasive astrocytoma on the other, a great variety of gliomatous tumours are seen, each with its own pathological characteristics and rate of growth. As the clinical history of the illness produced by such a lesion depends upon the rapidity of its development, it is impossible to describe fully all the possible variations in clinical presentation and course which can be observed in such cases. Typically, however, the patient with a glioblastoma gives a history of increasingly severe headache, drowsiness, nausea and vomiting, with or without focal or generalised epileptiform attacks and often with recent disorders of memory, of speech or of movement of the limbs; usually in such a case the duration of the illness can be measured in days or weeks. By contrast, in the patient with a slowly-growing astrocytoma, it is common to obtain a history of occasional major seizures and of vague headache or failure of concentration, beginning some years previously and not giving rise to undue alarm until some new symptom (aphasia, monoparesis, vomiting) made its appearance. Much depends, of course, upon the situation of the tumour. Those in the **frontal lobe** often produce a progressive dementia without other localising features until the motor cortex or speech area is irritated or invaded, when Jacksonian epilepsy, or hemiparesis or aphasia will result. Rarely there are attacks of turning of the head or eyes away from the side of the lesion (adversive attacks). Occasionally a contralateral grasp reflex can be elicited. Lesions in the anterior part of the **temporal lobe** may produce initially any of the features regarded as characteristic of temporal lobe epilepsy (attacks of fear, *déjà vu*, unreality, hallucinations of smell or taste, and lip-smacking or chewing) while the proximity of the arm area of the motor cortex means that Jacksonian seizures affecting the contralateral hand or else weakness of the hand and arm are commonly seen. Should the lesion extend more posteriorly, it is usual to find an upper quadrantic defect in the visual field, or sensory aphasia if the dominant hemisphere is involved. Lesions of the **parietal lobe** will generally result in impairment of the appreciation of the finer and discriminative aspects of sensibility in the opposite limbs, while disorders of the body image (*see* Chap. 10) or apraxia and agnosia, if the lesion involves the dominant hemisphere, may occur. Formed auditory or visual hallucinations may be experienced if a tumour is present in the auditory or visual association areas of the cortex, but when, as rarely happens, the tumour involves the **occipital lobe**, visual hallucinations are generally crude (e.g. unformed flashes of light) and a contralateral homonymous hemianopia, either partial or complete, is invariable. Involvement of the **thalamus and basal ganglia** usually leads to contralateral patchy impairment of all forms of sensation, somnolence and a dense hemiplegia due to damage to the internal capsule, while tumours of the **corpus callosum** are characterised particularly by progressive apathy, drowsiness and disorders of memory, followed usually by generalised convulsions, unilateral and then bilateral pyramidal signs. When a glioma develops in the **mid-brain**, symptoms and signs of increased intracranial pressure develop early owing to aqueductal compression but in addition there is generally impairment of conjugate ocular deviation upwards or laterally or both, with bilateral ptosis and/or ophthalmoplegia and variable long-tract signs. Gliomas of the **pons or medulla** tend to be particularly slow-growing ('benign hypertrophy of the pons'); diplopia is usually the first symptom and is followed by additional cranial nerve palsies, often combined at first with contralateral sensory or pyramidal signs ('crossed paralysis') but subsequently the 'long-tract' signs are bilateral. Gliomas rarely develop in one **optic nerve or chiasm,** usually in children, or in adults with neurofibromatosis, and produce progressive unilateral visual failure with optic atrophy and visual field defects which tend to be unusual in outline and unlike those seen in other diseases. Astrocytomas of one **cerebellar hemisphere** are particularly common in childhood but do occur in adult life. In such cases the intracranial pressure is increased early, but there is usually evidence of cerebellar ataxia in the limbs on the side of the tumour with nystagmus on lateral gaze to the same side. When the growth involves central cerebellar structures (the vermis and roof nuclei) the patient's gait is grossly ataxic ('truncal ataxia') but there may be no nystagmus and no clear evidence of ataxia in the limbs when these are tested individually.

Occasionally multiple areas of gliomatous infiltration can develop, apparently simultaneously, throughout the brain and brain stem **(gliomatosis cerebri).** In such a case the clinical picture, indicating the presence of multiple lesions, may suggest a diagnosis of multiple metastases.

MEDULLOBLASTOMA

This common tumour of infancy and early childhood grows almost invariably in midline cerebellar structures and has the property of seeding throughout the meningeal space so that tumour cells may be discovered in the cerebrospinal fluid. The characteristic clinical picture is one of progressive ataxia, with frequent falls, followed by drowsiness and vomiting in a young child. Papilloedema is almost invariable and the cranial sutures are separated at an early stage.

OLIGODENDROGLIOMA

These uncommon tumours, which almost invariably grow in one cerebral hemisphere, and particularly in the temporal lobe, are remarkably benign, and most patients have experienced intermittent focal or generalised seizures for several years before additional symptoms are experienced. These neoplasms commonly calcify and a characteristic punctate area of calcification seen on a skull radiograph can be virtually diagnostic.

EPENDYMOMA

This rare tumour is most commonly found in the fourth ventricle; it rapidly produces symptoms and signs of raised intracranial pressure and other signs are rare, although there may be evidence of cerebellar dysfunction or of compression of long tracts in the brain stem. Positional vertigo and morning vomiting are common in the early stages, and may indeed be the only symptoms, while nystagmus with variable neck stiffness or vertigo provoked by attempted neck flexion are often the only physical signs.

MENINGIOMA

A meningioma compressing one cerebral hemisphere often produces a clinical picture indistinguishable from that resulting from an astrocytoma arising in a similar situation, although Jacksonian epilepsy seems to be particularly common with these benign neoplasms. There are, however, a number of specific syndromes which have been recognised as being due to meningiomas arising in particular situations. The **olfactory groove meningioma** which lies beneath one frontal lobe typically gives unilateral anosmia and dementia, often with inappropriate jocularity (*Witzelsucht*) due to frontal-lobe compression. As it extends posteriorly it can compress the homolateral optic nerve to give unilateral optic atrophy, and when this is combined with contralateral papilloedema, this combination of signs is known as the Foster Kennedy syndrome. A **parasagittal meningioma,** growing between the two cerebral hemispheres, typically compresses the foot and leg areas of the motor or sensory cortex in both cerebral hemispheres, giving rise to Jacksonian seizures in both legs and/or a spastic paraplegia. Urinary retention or incontinence sometimes occur. A meningioma in the **cerebellopontine angle** can be responsible for a clinical picture indistinguishable from that resulting from an acoustic neuroma (*vide infra*), while a similar tumour growing above the sella turcica (**parasellar meningioma**) typically produces progressive unilateral and later bilateral visual failure with a visual field defect indicating chiasmal compression. The meningiomas which arise from the **sphenoidal ridge,** on the lesser wing of the sphenoid, protrude into the orbit to produce unilateral proptosis, optic atrophy (due to compression of the optic nerve), ptosis and diplopia (due to involvement of the oculomotor nerve). Rarely a growth arising from the basal meninges may gradually involve multiple cranial nerves as they approach the exit foramina by which they leave the skull (**meningioma en plaque**).

PITUITARY ADENOMAS

There are two principal varieties of pituitary adenoma which

produce similar neurological signs but have different endocrino-
logical effects. The adenoma of the acidophil cells gives rise to gigan-
tism if it develops before puberty and to acromegaly afterwards,
while the non-secreting chromophobe adenoma eventually produces
signs of hypopituitarism. Basophil adenomas are extremely rare and
do not usually grow sufficiently large to give symptoms or signs of an
intracranial space-occupying lesion. They produce the endocrine
features of Cushing's syndrome which is, however, more often
produced by over-activity of the adrenal cortex. Both the acidophil
and chromophobe tumours are generally large enough to cause
expansion of the sella turcica (which can be recognised radiologically)
and also tend to extrude above the sella to compress the medial
aspect of both optic nerves and the chiasm. A bitemporal hemianopia
is the typical field defect but many variations may be observed.
Occasionally a chromophobe adenoma expands rapidly and compresses one third nerve and the optic nerve to give sudden severe
headache, unilateral hlindness, a third-nerve palsy and sometimes
subarachnoid haemorrhage (the syndrome of 'pituitary apoplexy').

PINEALOMA, PAPILLOMA AND GLOMUS TUMOUR

The *pinealoma* is a comparatively uncommon tumour which generally develops in children or young adults and usually presents solely
with symptoms of increased intracranial pressure; however, compression of the corpora quadrigemina and upper mid-brain can
give a characteristic impairment of upward conjugate gaze. *Papillomas* of the choroid plexus, too, are usually responsible for recurrent subarachnoid haemorrhage or for a hydrocephalus without
other specific features. The characteristic manifestations of the rare
tumour of the glomus jugulare are multiple lower cranial nerve palsies
(deafness, facial palsy, dysphagia, hemiatrophy of the tongue) combined sometimes with a vascular polyp in the inner ear or a palpable
mass anterior to the mastoid bone.

CRANIOPHARYNGIOMA

This relatively common tumour, arising from developmental
remnants of Rathke's pouch, may be solid, but more often takes the
form of a cholesterol-containing cyst which is suprasellar in situation. It compresses the optic chiasm to give unilateral or bilateral
optic atrophy and progressive visual-field defects, and also extends
upwards into the hypothalamus. In childhood it can give rise to
delayed physical and sexual development (pituitary infantilism), or
diabetes insipidus; in some cases symptoms indicating the presence of
the tumour do not develop until early adult or even middle life, when
diminished libido, mental dullness and signs of hypopituitarism are

often apparent. The sella turcica is generally enlarged but shallow, unlike the typical ballooning produced by a pituitary adenoma, and there is calcification in the tumour, visible radiologically in up to 50 per cent of cases.

HAEMANGIOBLASTOMA

This tumour occurs almost invariably in one cerebellar hemisphere in children or young adults and gives symptoms indistinguishable from a cerebellar astrocytoma. It may be familial and is often associated with angiomatosis of the retina or abdominal organs (Lindau-von Hippel disease). Polycythaemia is often present.

ARTERIOVENOUS ANGIOMA

The characteristic clinical features produced by these vascular malformations, which will be given further consideration in Chapter 17, are epilepsy, subarachnoid haemorrhage, focal neurological signs, depending upon their situation, and a cranial bruit.

CHORDOMA

This soft jelly-like tumour usually grows either between the basisphenoid and the anterior aspect of the brain stem, or in the sacral canal. When it develops intracranially there are typically multiple cranial-nerve palsies; in the sacrum it produces signs of involvement of multiple roots of the lower cauda equina.

EPIDERMOID OR DERMOID CYSTS

These rare pearly tumours or cholesteatomas are most commonly found in the posterior fossa, and are usually indistinguishable clinically from other posterior fossa tumours. Diagnosis is generally made at operation.

COLLOID CYST OF THE THIRD VENTRICLE

This uncommon tumour arises within the third ventricle from vestigial remnants of the primitive paraphysis. Usually it produces clinical features indicating merely a progressive increase in the intracranial pressure, but the presence of such a lesion may be suspected when the patient experiences repeated attacks of hydrocephalus with intervals of freedom; in such cases it seems that the pedunculated cyst may act as a ball-valve, giving intermittent blockage of the foramina of Monro.

NEUROFIBROMA (NEURINOMA)

This relatively common intracranial neoplasm is sometimes single, sometimes multiple; if the latter is the case the patient is usually suffering from neurofibromatosis, and other stigmata of the disease will generally be apparent on careful enquiry. Thus there may be a family history of the disease and careful examination will reveal cutaneous neurofibromas and pigmentation. Whereas in the cranial cavity these neoplasms can grow upon the fifth or seventh nerves, the commonest site by far is the eighth or acoustic nerve (the acoustic neuroma). This tumour is commonest in middle-aged and elderly patients (except in individuals with neurofibromatosis). Unilateral nerve deafness is an almost invariable physical sign and may be associated with some indefinite vertigo. Next in frequency is unilateral facial sensory loss (absence of the corneal reflex is sometimes the initial sign), and later as a rule comes homolateral facial paresis or twitching due to compression of the facial nerve. Minimal cerebellar ataxia on the side of the lesion is frequently observed and there may be pyramidal signs which are usually contralateral but occasionally ipsilateral. The protein content of the cerebrospinal fluid is generally greatly raised and radiographs commonly demonstrate erosion of the internal auditory meatus. Neuro-otological studies (audiometry and caloric tests—*see* Chap. 3) are valuable aids to early diagnosis in such cases.

'PSEUDOTUMOUR CEREBRI' (BENIGN INTRACRANIAL HYPERTENSION)

The clinical picture of this condition, which has also been entitled toxic hydrocephalus or serous meningitis, can closely resemble that of cerebral tumour, as the predominant symptom is headache and bilateral papilloedema is discovered. Ventriculography, however, which is necessary for diagnosis, reveals that the cerebral ventricles are either normal in size and situation or more often they are unusually small. The condition can complicate otitis media, pregnancy, or cachexia, or may follow head injury. It is due either to thrombosis of one or more intracranial venous sinuses or to diffuse brain swelling of unknown aetiology. It is a self-limiting condition which recovers completely in a few weeks or months, but during the acute stage the papilloedema constitutes a danger to vision and urgent decompression is occasionally required. Most such patients are surprisingly well considering the severity of the papilloedema; bilateral sixth-nerve palsies are sometimes present as false localising signs.

INTRACRANIAL METASTASES

Intracranial deposits secondary to extracranial malignant disease are generally carcinomatous, and the most common sites of primary growths which spread to the cranial cavity are the lung, breast, kidney, ovary and colon, although occasionally the primary tumour may be in some other organ. Sarcomas too may metastasise to the brain, as may malignant melanomas, while rarely a reticulum cell sarcoma appears to arise primarily within the cranial cavity, either in the meninges or within the substance of the brain itself. The clinical picture produced by one or more intracranial metastases can be very variable, but does not appear to be dependent in any sense upon the nature or situation of the primary growth. Subarachnoid haemorrhage is a rare complication of intracranial metastases except that it frequently occurs in cases of malignant melanoma when the metastatic deposits are very numerous and very vascular. In many cases the manifestations of intracranial disease precede those attributable to the primary tumour and the symptoms and physical signs usually resemble closely those produced by a glioblastoma in one or other cerebral hemisphere, or by a rapidly-growing tumour in the posterior fossa. The discovery of an opacity in a chest radiograph may be the first indication that the tumour is metastatic. Although cerebral metastases are frequently multiple it is comparatively uncommon though not unknown for the symptoms or physical signs to indicate the presence of more than one lesion. On occasion the clinical picture is even more indefinite, with vague headache, forgetfulness, lack of concentration, depression and intermittent confusion, and a diagnosis of presenile dementia may be seriously considered. Rarely there are widespread carcinomatous deposits in the leptomeninges and the clinical picture is then one of headache, neck stiffness, confusion and usually paresis of one or more cranial nerves (*carcinomatosis of the meninges*). In such a case there is generally a moderate pleocytosis and rise in protein in the cerebrospinal fluid, the sugar content of the fluid is greatly diminished and carcinoma cells can be recognised by means of cytological techniques.

Carcinomatous deposits in the bones of the skull may produce headache and tenderness of the scalp, but only rarely do neurological signs result from involvement of the underlying brain. It is not uncommon, however, for a *nasopharyngeal carcinoma* to erode the base of the skull and to destroy multiple cranial nerves in succession, at first unilaterally and later bilaterally. Hence in any case in which there is progressive paralysis of the third, fourth, sixth or seventh nerves and later perhaps of those arising from the lower part of the brain stem, this diagnosis should be strongly suspected. A somewhat similar picture, in which deafness and involvement of multiple lower cranial nerves on one side occurs, may be the result of invasion of the cranial cavity by a *glomus tumour* arising from the glomus jugulare. A carcinoma in the maxillary sinus can also involve multiple cranial nerves, while a malignant neoplasm in the ethmoid sinus more often gives an asymmetrical proptosis with lateral displacement of the eye

Proptosis is also occasionally seen as a result of a *myeloma* of the orbit, although in general, multiple myelomatosis involving the skull does not give rise to neurological symptoms and signs.

INTRACRANIAL GRANULOMAS AND PARASITIC CYSTS

A *gumma* is now an uncommon lesion, although this diagnosis should always be suspected when a patient with proven syphilis develops clinical features suggesting the presence of an intracranial space-occupying lesion. *Tuberculomas* are equally rare, and while the rupture of such a lesion into the subarachnoid space can be the cause of tuberculous meningitis, they are rarely of sufficient size to give rise to symptoms of focal brain disease. Cysticerci within the brain are an occasional cause of epilepsy, particularly in those who have served in the Forces in India, and typical calcified 'oval' lesions may be recognised radiologically. Occasionally cysticerci of racemose type form in the cerebral ventricles and are then responsible for repeated attacks suggesting lymphocytic meningitis, followed by a progressive or intermittent hydrocephalus of the type which occurs in any patient with an intraventricular tumour.

SPINAL TUMOURS

The tumours which arise within or encroach upon the spinal cord can be divided into three groups. These are: first, those which arise in the bones of the spinal column or in the extradural space (extradural tumours); secondly, those which lie within the dura mater but outside the spinal cord (intradural–extramedullary); and thirdly, those which grow within the substance of the spinal cord itself (intramedullary). In a general hospital, about 40 per cent of all spinal space-occupying lesions are extradural, and of these the majority are **metastases,** although deposits of a reticulosis, extradural granuloma (due often to tuberculous caries of the spine), chordoma (in the sacral region) or a haemangioma of a vertebral body can produce similar effects. Intradural–extramedullary tumours constitute about 50 per cent of all spinal growths and intramedullary neoplasms about 5 per cent. The common intradural–extramedullary tumours are first, the **neurofibroma,** and secondly the **meningioma.** A neurofibroma may occur at any level of the spine and in either sex. It tends to grow from a spinal root to give a mass which lies partly inside and partly outside the spinal canal, eroding generally the intervertebral foramen and adjacent vertebral pedicles (a 'dumbbell' tumour). Meningiomas are nearly always found in the dorsal region and usually in women. The commonest intramedullary tumours are the **glioma** and the **ependymoma,** though arteriovenous angiomas, or other small and discrete vascular malformations of small blood vessels (telangiectases) occur from time to time.

Although the clinical presentation of a spinal tumour will clearly depend upon its character and situation, it can be said that the initial symptoms are usually those of compression of one or more spinal roots, of the spinal cord, or more often of both. If the tumour is intramedullary there is progressive destruction or distortion of long tracts resulting in motor and sensory change in the limbs and trunk below the level of the lesion, depending upon which pathways are principally involved. Extradural growths are particularly liable to give pain of a persistent aching character in the back at the level where the tumour is situated; sometimes, if spinal roots are compressed, the pain will radiate along the dermatomes innervated by the roots concerned. These symptoms are often present for some time before symptoms and signs of spinal cord compression appear, but this is not invariable and if a carcinomatous deposit causes collapse of a vertebral body, a sudden paraplegia may result. Pain in root distribution is also a characteristic symptom of an intradural–extramedullary tumour, particularly the neurofibroma, but is not invariable, and the clinical picture may be predominantly that of progressive spinal cord compression, as described in Chapter 13. If the tumour is situated in the cervical region there will often be muscular wasting, weakness and sensory loss in one or both arms, indicating a lesion of one or more spinal roots or nerves, in addition to the evidence of spinal cord disease, but if it is dorsal in situation these signs are unobtrusive and it may be impossible clinically to determine whether the lesion is intramedullary or extramedullary. A Brown–Séquard syndrome can be an early result of an extramedullary tumour, but a clinical picture suggestive of syringomyelia of unusually rapid progression generally implies that the lesion is intramedullary, and very probably an ependymoma. When the neoplasm lies below the termination of the spinal cord, the characteristic clinical features of involvement of one or more roots of the cauda equina are seen and there is commonly some pain over the lumbar and sacral regions. Urinary retention and impotence usually develop and if the lower sacral roots are involved there is generally perianal or 'saddle' anaesthesia. A tumour at the eleventh and twelfth dorsal or first lumbar level can compress not only the roots of the cauda equina but also the termination of the spinal cord to give a combination of upper and lower motor neurone signs. The commonest tumours involving the cauda equina are a neurofibroma, an ependymoma of the filum terminale, or a chordoma which may produce massive erosion of the sacrum, clearly visible radiologically. Rarely a solitary myeloma of the sacrum will produce similar effects.

The accurate diagnosis of spinal tumours is a matter of the greatest importance, as so many are benign and can be successfully removed; if irreversible damage due to restriction of blood supply to the cord has not occurred, most patients recover completely. On suspicion that a tumour may be present, the obligatory investigations are radiography of the spine, which may reveal excessive separation of the pedicles or bony erosion, and lumbar puncture. A spinal block on Queckenstedt's test is almost diagnostic, but even if there is a free rise and fall of the fluid in the manometer following compression and the subsequent release of pressure on the jugular veins, a moderate rise in the protein content of the fluid will be a suggestive finding. For accurate localisation of the neoplasm it is essential to carry out opaque myelography, and indeed this investigation is the only means of excluding an extramedullary neoplasm with certainty if suspicion persists despite negative findings on straight X-ray and lumbar puncture. Unfortunately the diagnosis of an intramedullary neoplasm cannot always be substantiated by myelography, even though in some cases the spinal cord is seen to be expanded. It is, however, the extramedullary lesions which are particularly important to recognise, as these are so eminently treatable, and in this myelography rarely fails.

NEUROLOGICAL COMPLICATIONS OF MALIGNANT DISEASE

It has become apparent within recent years that a number of specific neurological manifestations may develop in patients with malignant disease and that these are not dependent upon the development of metastases within the brain or spinal cord. The symptoms of nervous disease can indeed antedate those attributable to the primary growth. The aetiology of these disorders is obscure; nutritional, toxic and allergic theories have been proposed to explain these reactions of the nervous system to the presence of the neoplasm elsewhere in the body, but up to the moment none of these theories has been substantiated. The primary neoplasm is most often a bronchogenic carcinoma but neurological complications of this type have now been described in occasional cases of malignant disease in many different sites and even in some patients suffering from a reticulosis. The two principal syndromes have been entitled **carcinomatous neuropathy** and **carcinomatous myopathy**. In patients suffering from a neuropathy the most common features are those of a progressive peripheral neuropathy (*see* Chapter 18) affecting principally the lower limbs and sometimes involving motor function predominantly, sometimes sensory function. Unilateral and subsequently bilateral footdrop may be the initial manifestation, or alternatively the patient complains of aching pain in the legs on exertion; gradually then over a period of weeks or months the tendon reflexes become depressed and are eventually lost. Peripheral sensory impairment often develops subsequently but occasionally a severe sensory neuropathy is present from the beginning. In some cases there is also a symmetrical **cerebellar ataxia,** affecting all four limbs, and a typical spinocerebellar degeneration has been demonstrated pathologically in such individuals. Sometimes this cerebellar syndrome can occur alone. Occasionally, too, the neuropathy is associated with a severe depressive psychosis or else this emotional disturbance may be the sole manifestation. **Carcinomatous myopathy** gives rise to a progressive weakness and atrophy of proximal limb and girdle muscles without sensory loss. In some such cases the clinical and pathological features resemble those of polymyositis (*see* Chap. 18) but in others the muscular changes are mild and indolent, myasthenic features with some improvement following an edrophonium injection may be seen and the pathological changes in the muscle are scanty; the pathogenesis of this condition remains obscure.

REFERENCES

BAKER, G. S. and MULDER, D. W., 'Spinal cord tumours', in *Clinical Neurology*, Ed. Baker, A. B., 2nd ed., Chapter 33 (New York, Hoeber, 1962).

BRAIN, W. R., *Diseases of the Nervous System*, 6th ed., Chapters 3 and 17 (London, Oxford University Press, 1962).

ELSBERG, C. A., *Tumours of the Spinal Cord* (New York, Hoeber, 1925).

NORTHFIELD, D. W. C. and RUSSELL, D. S., 'Intracranial tumours,' in *Modern Trends in Neurology*, Ed. Feiling, A., 1st series, Chapter 11 (London, Butterworth, 1951).

PEYTON, W. T., FRENCH, L. A. and BAKER, A. B., 'Intracranial neoplasms', in *Clinical Neurology*, Ed. Baker, A. B., 2nd ed., Chapter 9 (New York, Hoeber, 1962).

RUSSELL, D. S. and RUBINSTEIN, L. J., *Pathology of Tumours of the Nervous System* (London, Arnold, 1959).

WEBSTER, H. DE F. and ADAMS, R. D., 'Tumours of the brain and spinal cord', in *Principles of Internal Medicine*, Ed. Harrison, T. R., 4th ed., Chapter 286 (New York, McGraw-Hill, 1962.)

CHAPTER 17

VASCULAR DISORDERS OF THE NERVOUS SYSTEM

THE effects of disease in the cranial and/or spinal blood vessels upon the functioning of the nervous system may be profound. Indeed the clinical syndromes or 'strokes' produced by disorders of the cerebral circulation are the most common of nervous diseases. In 1952, 170,000 people in the United States died of cerebral vascular accidents, and many more were left hopelessly crippled in body or in mind by a stroke or series of strokes which were not sufficiently severe to end their lives. While it is true that many of the patients afflicted in this way are elderly, the effects of cerebral vascular disease are nowadays seen with increasing frequency in patients under the age of sixty and even in relatively young adults. It should be remembered that although cerebral vascular disease is usually manifest through symptoms and signs indicating a disorder of brain function, 'stroke syndromes' cannot be regarded as specific diseases, but rather as stereotyped combinations of clinical features which can be produced by many different diseases of the cerebral arteries and veins and which only secondarily affect the behaviour of the nervous system. Most of these disorders are in fact complications of hypertension and atherosclerosis, while other cardiovascular factors, including disease of the heart and great vessels, and variations in the systemic blood pressure, may be of the greatest importance in their genesis. Hence it is important always to bear in mind the possibility in any patient showing evidence of a cerebral vascular syndrome, that the primary abnormality may lie in the heart or kidneys. In this chapter, the common vascular disorders of the brain will first be considered and then brief reference will be made to the much less common vascular syndromes of the spinal cord.

CEREBRAL VASCULAR DISEASE

The commonly-occurring cerebral vascular accidents fall into two principal categories, namely spontaneous intracranial haemorrhage on the one hand and cerebral infarction or ischaemia on the other. The word spontaneous is taken to exclude intracranial haemorrhage resulting from an obvious traumatic cause, which is usually evident in cases of extradural haemorrhage and in subdural haematoma (*see*

300

Chapter 13), though the latter condition masquerades in a variety of guises and is a common pitfall for the unwary. Probably about 70 per cent of cerebral vascular accidents are the result of infarction or ischaemia (50 per cent 'thrombotic', 20 per cent 'embolic') while primary cerebral haemorrhage accounts for approximately 20 per cent and subarachnoid haemorrhage for about 8 per cent of all cases.

Spontaneous Intracranial Haemorrhage

The two principal varieties of intracranial haemorrhage are first, primary intracerebral haemorrhage, which is usually of hypertensive origin, and secondly, subarachnoid haemorrhage, which generally results from the rupture of an intracranial aneurysm or angioma. The term 'subarachnoid haemorrhage' is in many cases a misnomer, since in 50 per cent of cases at least the haemorrhage involves brain tissue and is not purely subarachnoid in situation; furthermore, in many cases of primary cerebral haemorrhage the bleeding extends into the cerebral ventricles or subarachnoid space. As will be seen, these facts can give rise to considerable diagnostic difficulty in certain cases.

PRIMARY INTRACEREBRAL HAEMORRHAGE

This condition is responsible for the classical stroke or apoplexy which was recognised by the earliest physicians. It usually arises as a result of rupture of small perforating arteries, either in the putamen and internal capsule (the territory of the lenticulostriate artery), in one cerebellar hemisphere, or in the pons. Hypertension is clearly the most important cause and the condition commonly develops during exertion or emotion when the blood pressure is at its height. Little is known of the pathological changes in the blood vessels which are finally responsible for the arterial rupture, though recent work confirms the 'classical' view that microaneurysms on small arteries are frequently present within the brain in hypertensive patients and it seems likely that rupture of such a microaneurysm frequently initiates the haemorrhage. The condition is commonest in the elderly (sixty–eighty age group) but can occur in severely hypertensive individuals at any age. There is a rapid outpouring of arterial blood and, after ploughing up the brain tissue surrounding the site of origin of the haemorrhage, this frequently enters the ventricular system; if the bleeding is massive, the patient may die within a few hours. More often the patient, who has had no prodromal symptoms, complains of a sudden ill-defined sensation that something is wrong within the head. Within a few moments the face becomes twisted, weakness of one arm and leg develops and consciousness is soon lost.

L

The period of evolution of the stroke is rarely as brief as that observed in cases of cerebral embolism and the onset is less abrupt than that of subarachnoid haemorrhage; the full clinical picture can take up to half or one hour to develop. By this time the patient is usually deeply comatose, with stertorous respiration, neck stiffness, a slow, bounding pulse, deviation of the head and eyes away from the side of the lesion, and a dense, flaccid hemiplegia. Vomiting is usual and the patient is generally incontinent of urine and faeces. Occasionally 'decerebrate attacks', or generalised or focal convulsions occur at the onset. When the site of the haemorrhage is the cerebellum, the clinical picture is sometimes indistinguishable from that produced by a severe cerebral haemorrhage, but if the bleeding is less quick to develop or if it is not too extensive, the early clinical features are vertigo, repeated vomiting and ataxia, often of truncal or central type; sometimes, however, unilateral ataxia confirms that the bleeding has occurred in one cerebellar hemisphere. When the primary site of bleeding is the pons, the patient is as a rule comatose from the beginning, but in addition there are often inequality of the pupils, of which one may be pin-point in size, hyperpyrexia and a quadri-plegia rather than a hemiplegia.

About 80 per cent of patients die, some within the first twenty-four hours, the remainder during the course of the next few days. A fluctuant clinical course, and clinical features indicative of recurrent bleeding, are not usually observed; deterioration is generally remorseless in the severe cases. Of the patients who survive, about half remain helpless neurological cripples, but there are some in whom the haemorrhage is relatively small, loss of consciousness brief, and residual disability comparatively slight. These cases are, however, difficult to recognise clinically, and are easily confused with examples of cerebral infarction.

Unfortunately, cerebral haemorrhage presents a distinctly gloomy picture from the therapeutic standpoint. Save in exceptional cases little, apart from nursing care, can be done. In selected cases it now appears that surgical evacuation of the intracerebral clot, after localisation by angiography or ventriculography, can occasionally be of benefit, but this procedure is only justifiable in certain of the less severe cases occurring in the younger age group. Lumbar punc-ture is of no therapeutic value and carries considerable risks of tentorial or cerebellar herniation. The administration of powerful hypotensive agents after the haemorrhage has occurred is not indi-cated, as lowering the blood pressure may, in the presence of wide-spread vascular spasm (which is an almost invariable concomitant of intracranial haemorrhage) give rise to the further complication of infarction. Clearly, prevention of cerebral haemorrhage (perhaps by the treatment of severe hypertension), rather than treatment, must be the aim.

SUBARACHNOID HAEMORRHAGE

This is the second major category of spontaneous intracranial bleeding and therapeutically it is much more hopeful. In about 85 per cent of cases the condition results from rupture of an intracranial aneurysm on one of the major arteries which form the circle of Willis, while in about 10 per cent a developmental anomaly of cerebral blood vessels, an arteriovenous angioma, may be present. The remaining 5 per cent of cases include patients with intracranial neoplasms, cerebral venous sinus thrombosis, blood diseases, and other conditions of which the subarachnoid bleeding is symptomatic. The so-called berry aneurysms, which are the commonest cause, are probably due to the coexistence of a congenital defect in the media of a cerebral artery with an early atheromatous lesion in the intima which breaches the internal elastic lamina. Mycotic aneurysms are now rare and syphilitic arterial dilatations are virtually non-existent. Aneurysms are particularly common at arterial bifurcations and are multiple in as many as 16 per cent of cases. Their commonest sites are upon the internal carotid artery, below or near its bifurcation, the region of the anterior communicating artery, and the middle cerebral artery, although they can arise upon any major cerebral vessel.

The patient, who may be a young adult or even a child, but who is usually between forty and sixty years of age, is suddenly struck down by an intense and catastrophic headache. Consciousness is often lost at the outset, and convulsions are common, but quite often the senses are retained, though the patient is drowsy and confused and complains bitterly of headache. The headache, which is usually frontal or occipital in situation to begin with, then mounts in severity and becomes generalised, severe neck stiffness and other symptoms and signs of meningeal irritation become apparent and vomiting is usual. Papilloedema is sometimes seen immediately or within the course of a few days or weeks, but a more characteristic sign observed on ophthalmoscopy is an extensive brick-red subhyaloid haemorrhage, spreading outwards from the edge of one or both optic disks. In many cases there is evidence of damage to the cranial nerves or to the brain itself. Unilateral or bilateral sixth-nerve palsies are common, or alternatively one third cranial nerve may be paralysed. Depending upon the situation and severity of the intracerebral extension of the haemorrhage, aphasia, a monoparesis, hemiparesis or hemiplegia may be found. Similar signs are sometimes the result of a coexistent cerebral infarction which is a common complication of subarachnoid haemorrhage and which probably results, at least in part, from arterial spasm. The compression or distortion of vessels produced by local collections of blood in the subarachnoid space either between the frontal lobes or within the Sylvian fissure may be another factor responsible for this complication. When the patient is comatose with a dense hemiplegia, diagnosis from primary intracerebral haemorrhage with rupture into the subarachnoid space can be a matter of considerable difficulty and must depend usually upon the patient's age and upon the presence or absence of evidence of severe hypertension and atherosclerosis. It should, however, be remembered that in the initial stages of the illness, transient arterial hypertension is common, resulting probably from hypothalamic compression, and temporary albuminuria and glycosuria can also result from this cause.

Although in many cases the diagnosis is self-evident, a lumbar puncture is generally necessary for confirmation, and also in order to distinguish the condition from such disorders as meningitis or cerebral abscess, with which it may occasionally be confused, particularly if the onset is less abrupt than usual. This investigation should be performed with great care, particularly if there are signs indicating intracerebral haemorrhage, in view of the risks of tentorial herniation. The cerebrospinal fluid is found to be deeply and uniformly bloodstained, unlike the early tingeing with blood, disappearing as the fluid flows, which can result from damage to vertebral veins produced by the exploring needle. Furthermore, on centrifuging, the supernatant fluid is found to have a faint orange tinge (due to oxyhaemoglobin) within four to six hours of the onset, and becomes deeply yellow or xanthochromic (due to bilirubin) within thirty-six to forty-eight hours.

With conservative treatment, including such measures as complete bed rest and sedation and relief of headache by pethidine or similar drugs, along with prophylactic antibiotics given to avoid respiratory and urinary infection, between 40 and 50 per cent of patients die within eight weeks of the ictus. Of these, some two-thirds die from the effects of the first bleed, often within twenty-four hours, but the remaining one-third succumb to a second, more catastrophic haemorrhage, which is particularly liable to occur within the second week after the first attack. About 10 per cent of those patients who are still alive eight weeks after the onset will die of recurrent bleeding before six months have elapsed and another 10 per cent in the subsequent months or years. Of the long-term survivors, only one-third are symptom-free, while another third have severe and disabling sequelae, including hemiparesis, headache, epilepsy and psychoneurosis, and the remainder have less severe residual symptoms.

Although the indications are not yet absolutely clear, it is now apparent that the prognosis of the condition can be radically improved by the judicious application of surgical methods of treatment. Nothing can at present be done to save those patients who die within the first two or three days, as surgical procedures carried out on the unconscious patient during this period carry almost a 100 per cent mortality. And there are also a proportion of patients who for reasons of age and general condition are unsuitable candidates for surgical treatment. But most patients who survive beyond the first few days should be considered with the possibility of operative procedures in mind. First, however, the surgeon must have full information concerning the situation and nature of the lesion responsible for the haemorrhage. Unfortunately clinical examination is of little help in this regard; for although it is reasonable to conclude in a patient with a hemiplegia that the bleeding point is on the opposite side of the head, it is virtually impossible to localise a bleeding aneurysm or angioma by clinical means with any degree of accuracy. While the electroencephalogram may help, it too is insufficiently precise, and all must depend upon the results of cerebral angiography, which should ideally be performed within four or five days after the first bleed. Both carotid arteries should be injected because of the possibility that multiple aneurysms may be present and also in an attempt to study the collateral circulation. If carotid arteriography gives negative results, as it does in 20-25 per cent of cases, this may mean that the causal aneurysm has clotted or that it lies on the vertebral system of vessels. However, vertebral arteriography should not be undertaken lightly, first because this investigation carries more risks than carotid injection, and secondly because aneurysms on the vertebral system of vessels are difficult to treat surgically. Nevertheless, in the conscious patient in good condition in whom bilateral carotid arteriography is negative, it should generally be performed. There is some evidence that in cases with negative arteriograms the prognosis is considerably better than the average. If, however, an aneurysm or angioma, or some other causal lesion is demonstrated, the surgeon can decide whether the lesion is surgically accessible and will then choose his time to operate depending upon the size and situation of the lesion and the age and condition of the patient. The most appropriate time is often at about seven days after the haemorrhage, when there is a chance of preventing those fatal recurrent haemorrhages which are particularly common in the second week and when arterial spasm, which greatly increases the risks of surgical treatment because of the danger of infarction, has usually passed off. The angiograms may also demonstrate complications of aneurysmal rupture such as intracerebral or subdural haematoma which require surgical treatment in their own right. The use of hypothermia as an aid to anaesthesia has been a valuable aid in such cases as it reduces cerebral metabolism. With further improvements in surgical and anaesthetic techniques it is reasonable to predict an increasing reduction in the mortality of this condition.

Cerebral Infarction

A cerebral infarct can be caused by the sudden embolic occlusion of a cerebral artery, by the gradual thrombosis of an artery, or by a combination of arterial narrowing with other factors which cause the blood supply of a part of the brain to be reduced below a critical level. An increased coagulability of the blood (as in pregnancy), haemoconcentration (due to dehydration) and an increase in circulating red cells (as in polycythaemia vera) are occasional factors of importance.

CEREBRAL EMBOLISM

In cerebral embolism the onset is usually abrupt and if the artery blocked is a major one, loss of consciousness or even sudden death may occur. In less severe cases, consciousness is retained but the patient develops a hemiplegia or other evidence of a rapidly developing focal cerebral lesion. Headache is not usually a feature. When a minor artery is blocked there may simply be transient confusion, speech disturbance or monoparesis, a 'little stroke', which clears up rapidly owing to establishment of the collateral circulation. Indeed in many cases of cerebral embolism, even those with a complete hemiplegia, there is rapid improvement, leading sometimes to complete recovery within a few days or weeks, though some patients do remain seriously disabled. For every embolus there must be a source, generally in the heart or great vessels. Cerebral embolism in subacute bacterial endocarditis and in mitral stenosis is a well-recognised complication, but the frequency of its occurrence following mural thrombosis in the chambers of the heart after cardiac infarction, as well as embolism from thrombi forming on atheromatous plaques in the aorta and carotid arteries, are less well appreciated. Hence in any patient with a sudden onset of a hemiplegia or of less striking focal signs, a careful search should be made for a source of emboli, and particularly for evidence of antecedent cardiac disease. This is of considerable importance, as cerebral embolic episodes are for obvious reasons likely to be multiple and there is now some evidence to indicate that this danger can sometimes be averted by long-term anticoagulant therapy.

CEREBRAL THROMBOSIS

The remaining conditions which give rise to cerebral infarction have for long been grouped together under the broad general heading of 'cerebral thrombosis'. This title is often a misnomer, as there are a great many cases in which no actual arterial occlusion can be demonstrated. The condition is commonest in patients over sixty years of age but is nowadays occurring with increasing frequency in patients who are aged between forty and sixty or even younger. Characteristically, the patient retires to bed perfectly well and wakes up next morning to find that one arm and leg are paralysed and perhaps that he cannot speak; or he may not discover the weakness until he attempts to stand and the leg gives way. Often there is no headache and no serious impairment of consciousness, though mild or moderate confusion is common. A great deal depends, of course, upon the size of the infarct and its situation. If it is large, the patient may be comatose, owing to swelling of the affected hemisphere, while if the brain stem is affected, rather than the cerebral hemisphere, vertigo, vomiting and diplopia are often prominent features. A mild attack of confusion, and transient weakness or numbness of one arm may be the only evidence of a small infarct. The differential diagnosis between a large infarct and a small intracerebral haemorrhage is often difficult; often one may be helped by examination of the cerebrospinal fluid, which usually contains frank blood or a good many red cells, in a patient with a cerebral haemorrhage. But even in cerebral infarction, red cells may be present and a slight to moderate rise in white cells and in protein content of the fluid is not uncommon.

The size and anatomical delimitation of the infarct and hence the neurological signs depend upon a great many factors. In some typical cases it is true that autopsy reveals a large thrombus in, say, the internal carotid artery or in the middle cerebral, giving an infarct in the expected distribution. In many others, however, no arterial thrombosis can be demonstrated, although arterial narrowing produced by atheroma is widespread, affecting some arteries more than others, and the infarct lies in the territory supplied by the narrowest of these vessels. There is some evidence that in many such cases a fall in blood pressure may have been the final precipitating factor which produced infarction without arterial occlusion, due to a selective fall in blood flow through a particularly narrow vessel. Sometimes a cardiac infarct can present with cerebral symptoms in this way, or else the reduction in blood pressure which occurs during sleep may be sufficient to tip the scales. Another important determining factor is the efficiency of the collateral circulation through the circle of Willis and through arterial anastomoses in the meninges. Furthermore, the importance of narrowing of the main trunks of the carotid, vertebral and basilar ateries is being increasingly recognised. Atheroma is the all-important aetiological factor, but contrary to the position which obtains in cases of cerebral haemorrhage it is a temporary fall in blood pressure, rather than hypertension, which is sometimes an important subsidiary factor. This is a good argument against the over-enthusiastic use of drugs designed to reduce blood pressure in patients who are probably atherosclerotic as well as hypertensive. On the other hand, severe hypertension may itself precipitate spasm of small arteries and arterioles and this may cause infarction so that in such cases a moderate reduction in the blood pressure should be achieved.

RECURRENT CEREBRAL ISCHAEMIA

It has been suggested that transient falls in blood pressure or other haemodynamic factors may account for many so-called recurrent cerebral ischaemic attacks. While this may be true of some, the majority seem to be due to recurrent micro-embolism. The emboli consist either of platelets or of cholesterol and seem to arise from mural thrombi or from atheromatous plaques in the large vessels in most cases. The consistency of the clinical pattern of these attacks can probably be accounted for by laminar flow in the cerebral arteries which determines that a particle becoming free in the lumen at the same point will generally reach the same peripheral branch of the vessel. These attacks are particularly common in patients with carotid or vertebro-basilar insufficiency and were previously attributed, erroneously as it now proves, to hypertensive encephalopathy or to vascular spasm. Patients with severe narrowing or even occlusion of one internal carotid artery often experience at frequent intervals over several days, weeks or months, recurrent brief attacks of weakness or paraesthesiae in the contralateral limbs, and particularly in the hand and arm. Often there are episodes of transient blindness in the homolateral eye, owing to reduction in blood flow through the ophthalmic artery, a branch of the internal carotid. Micro-emboli in the retinal arteries in such cases have often been observed with the ophthalmoscope. Pulsation in the affected internal carotid artery may be reduced on palpation, and the arterial pressure in the retinal arteries on the same side is also often reduced, a finding which can be confirmed by ophthalmodynamometry. The presence of a systolic bruit over one common or internal carotid artery is a valuable sign, often indicating carotid stenosis. Patients suffering from basilar insufficiency experience similar transient attacks involving a variety of brain-stem structures, now on one side of the body and now on the other, and including such features as vertigo, diplopia, transient hemianopia or bilateral blindness due to posterior cerebral artery insufficiency, paraesthesiae and weakness of one limb, of one arm and leg, or of all four limbs. It is important to recognise the significance of these symptoms as early as possible, since total occlusion of the artery can produce a complete hemiplegia (in carotid occlusion) or quadriplegia and death (in basilar occlusion). Carotid stenosis or thrombosis can be confirmed by arteriography, but vertebrobasilar insufficiency must generally be diagnosed on clinical grounds, as vertebral arteriography in such a case carries considerable risks. Arteriography after catheterisation of the aortic arch is a safer procedure and the origins of all the major vessels may be visualised. The practical value of early diagnosis in such a case is that occasionally the attacks can be terminated, and catastrophic complete occlusion prevented, by the institution of long-term anticoagulant therapy. Sometimes when carotid stenosis is present, it is possible to remove the blood clot and the atheromatous plaque or to insert an arterial graft; in some cases the attacks cease spontaneously, despite complete occlusion of the artery, owing to the opening up of collateral arterial channels.

THE SYNDROMES OF THE CEREBRAL ARTERIES

A great many eponymous clinical syndromes have been attributed to the occlusion of individual cerebral arteries. Of these, some occur consistently, and in a stereotyped manner, while others are rare. The fact that many cases of unquestionable cerebral infarction do not fulfil the diagnostic criteria of any of these classical syndromes is good evidence of the variability in distribution of some of the cerebral arteries and of the anastomotic channels which exist in the meninges. Broadly speaking, however, perforating arteries are true end-arteries and occlusion of these vessels can often be recognised clinically. A diagrammatic representation of the cortical distribution of blood from the major cerebral arteries is given in Fig. 12.

INTERNAL CAROTID ARTERY THROMBOSIS. The syndrome of recurrent cerebral ischaemic attacks resulting from narrowing of this vessel has already been described. When a complete occlusion occurs, however, there is often a complete contralateral hemiplegia, with aphasia if the dominant hemisphere is involved. Alternatively, if the collateral circulation is satisfactory, the clinical features may resemble those of middle cerebral artery occlusion, while on occasion, symptoms are transient, and disability trivial. Occlusion of this artery has nowadays replaced meningovascular syphilis as the commonest cause of hemiplegia in adults in the third and fourth decades. It may complicate pregnancy and can follow trauma to the neck. A carotid arteritis with occlusion, sometimes due to a spread of inflammation from cervical lymph nodes, probably accounts for many cases of acute infantile hemiplegia.

L.*

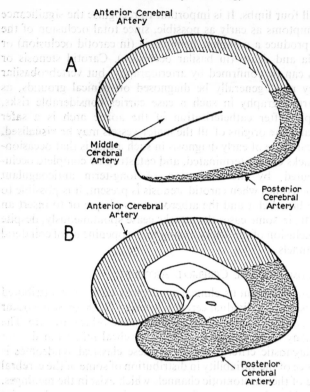

FIG. 12. A diagrammatic representation of the distribution of blood from the three major cerebral arteries to the cerebral hemispheres.

THE MIDDLE CEREBRAL ARTERY. Occlusion of the main trunk of the middle cerebral artery gives a contralateral hemiplegia and sensory loss of cortical type. When the obstruction is situated more distally the weakness involves mainly the face, arm and hand. Motor aphasia is common, sensory aphasia less so, but the latter does occur from time to time, and a hemianopia occasionally results owing to infarction of the optic radiation in the temporal lobe.

THE ANTERIOR CEREBRAL ARTERY. When the main trunk of this artery is occluded, this results in a contralateral hemiplegia with crural dominance (i.e. greater weakness of the leg than of the arm). Cortical sensory loss and aphasia are often present. When Heubner's artery, a penetrating branch which supplies the anterior limb of the internal capsule, is occluded, there is paralysis of the contralateral face and upper limb and often some sensory loss of spinothalamic type in the contralateral limbs.

THE POSTERIOR CEREBRAL ARTERY. The principal effect of thrombosis of this artery is a contralateral homonymous hemianopia. When perforating branches to the thalamus are involved, a contralateral thalamic syndrome may develop, while lesions of the visual association area in the dominant hemisphere occasionally result in visual agnosia.

THE BASILAR ARTERY. The type of recurrent ischaemic attacks attributable to basilar artery insufficiency have been mentioned above. Total occlusion of the artery is generally soon fatal, with loss of consciousness, a decerebrate state, or quadriplegia, but a myriad of clinical syndromes can occur as a result of occlusion of individual perforating branches of the artery. Thus Weber's syndrome consists of a unilateral third cranial nerve palsy and a contralateral hemiplegia. The Benedikt syndrome is a third nerve palsy with ipsilateral cerebellar ataxia. A paralysis of the sixth and seventh cranial nerves on one side with a contralateral hemiplegia constitutes the Millard–Gubler syndrome, while the Foville syndrome consists of a sixth nerve palsy, paralysis of conjugate ocular deviation to the side of the lesion, and again, as a rule, a contralateral hemiparesis. Occlusion of the internal auditory artery may give sudden unilateral deafness and severe vertigo. Apart from these classical syndromes, a great many other clinical phenomena may be attributable to basilar artery insufficiency, including such features as cranial nerve palsies in various combinations, ipsilateral cerebellar signs, and contralateral hemiplegia or hemianalgesia.

THE SUPERIOR CEREBELLAR ARTERY. The characteristic features of superior cerebellar artery occlusion are first, ipsilateral cerebellar ataxia and often choreiform movements; and secondly, contralateral hemianaesthesia of 'spinothalamic' type.

THE POSTERIOR INFERIOR CEREBELLAR ARTERY. Occlusion of this branch of the vertebral artery gives a typical clinical picture which is probably the commonest of the brain-stem vascular syndromes (Wallenberg's syndrome). The onset is usually abrupt with vertigo and vomiting, and sometimes with pain in one side of the face. There is often dysphagia at the outset and the palate is paralysed on the side of the lesion, while there are also clear-cut 'cerebellar' signs in the limbs on this side. An ipsilateral Horner's syndrome is often present, while there is usually dissociated anaesthesia to pain and temperature on the same side of the face and over the opposite half of the body below the neck. This sensory loss is, however, variable and a complete contralateral hemianalgesia is not uncommon.

Although a great many other syndromes of the cerebral arteries have been described, these are the commonest. It is particularly important to recognise the nature of recurrent cerebral ischaemic attacks as it is possible that these can be treated effectively.

PROGNOSIS

Cerebral infarction is fatal in about 20 per cent of cases. When the infarct has been small or the causal ischaemia relatively transient, complete recovery can take place within a few days and this is also true in about 20 per cent of patients. In the remaining 60 per cent some degree of disability persists. For instance, up to 20 per cent of patients are liable to develop focal or generalised seizures as a sequel of the illness. Even after a complete hemiplegia has developed, remarkable degrees of recovery may be expected and the great majority of patients are eventually able to walk after some weeks or months, although in cases of middle cerebral or carotid insufficiency little recovery of function in the affected hand may be expected. Aphasia, too, can recover to a surprising extent, either spontaneously or with appropriate speech training which may have to be continued in selected cases for many months. Recovery from brain-stem vascular syndromes is also surprisingly complete in a definite though small proportion of cases. Recurrent infarction seems to occur after a greater or lesser period in about half the survivors, but the remaining half appear to remain remarkably free from such episodes, often for several years.

Hypertensive Encephalopathy

This term should be reserved for a disorder of acute onset in which severe arterial hypertension is associated with headache, nausea, vomiting, confusion, convulsions and stupor or coma. Usually the condition occurs only in patients with malignant hypertension or in the terminal stages of chronic nephritis; papilloedema and advanced retinopathy are invariably present. Focal neurological symptoms and signs are not a part of this syndrome as a rule but imply the presence of complicating factors such as 'thrombosis', embolism, or haemorrhage.

Cerebral Atherosclerosis

This term is utilised to describe the progressive degenerative disorder which results from widespread atheroma of the cerebral vasculature with consequent intermittently-progressive ischaemia of the brain. The condition gives rise to an irreversible dementia, but the progress of the disorder is invariably step-like, and it is not possible to accept this diagnosis as a cause of dementia arising in the presenium or in the elderly unless there have been transient episodes

of confusion, paraesthesiae, aphasia or paresis, to indicate that one
or more 'little stroke' has occurred. In the late stages dementia is
severe, the patient is doubly incontinent, but often has an enormous
appetite, and may have remarkably few signs of neurological
abnormality.

A clinical picture which develops in some such cases is that of so-
called **pseudobulbar palsy.** This syndrome is characterised by over-
emotionalism with sometimes pathological laughing and crying and
gross lability of the affect, along with spasticity of the muscles of
speech and swallowing, due to bilateral pyramidal tract lesions in
the upper mid-brain or cerebral hemispheres. Some degree of
dysarthria and dysphagia and of pathological overemotionalism is
often seen in cases of **atherosclerotic Parkinsonism** in which hypertensive and atherosclerotic patients show facial masking, a shuffling
gait and progressive rigidity of the limbs with increased reflexes and
usually extensor plantar responses. This condition is closely related
clinically and pathologically to pseudobulbar palsy.

Cerebral Venous Sinus Thrombosis

The effects of suppurative thrombosis of intracranial venous sinuses
have already been described in Chapter 14. Aseptic thrombosis of
the cavernous sinus is rare but this pathological process can occur,
apparently spontaneously, in the lateral or sagittal sinuses, giving
rise to the syndrome of so-called benign intracranial hypertension,
or pseudotumour cerebri. The characteristic features are headache
and high papilloedema in a patient whose consciousness is unimpaired, who looks well, shows no localising neurological signs,
and is found to have normal cerebral ventricles on ventriculography.
The condition can complicate otitis media or malignant disease, it
may develop during pregnancy or after head injury, and sometimes
it appears spontaneously, particularly in young and rather obese
women. Cortical thrombophlebitis in childhood or in pregnancy is
sometimes different in its presentation and may give rise to focal
fits and to neurological signs (e.g. hemiplegia) which may resolve
unusually rapidly. Occasionally, when the thrombosis of the sagittal
sinus is extensive, the patient is semicomatose and has fits and focal
neurological signs (hemiparesis or paraplegia) due to venous infarction of the superior aspect of the cerebral cortex; subarachnoid
haemorrhage sometimes occurs as a result of this pathological
change.

Temporal or Cranial Arteritis

This condition, which is commonest in patients over sixty-five years
of age, is related to the other diseases of the 'collagen' or connective

tissue group. Characteristically the patient has a period of general malaise with vague aches and pains in the limbs and joints, fever and loss of appetite. There is also temporal headache and tenderness of the neck and scalp. The temporal and occipital arteries are found to be thrombosed, nodular and tender. The most important complication is occlusion of the central retinal artery, and this condition is the commonest cause of sudden unilateral blindness in the elderly. If the disease is not treated the second eye can be involved soon afterwards. Rarely, the carotid, cerebral and coronary arteries are affected to give a clinical picture of cerebral or cardiac infarction. The erythrocyte sedimentation rate is invariably raised and the condition responds readily to steroid therapy.

Buerger's Disease

Rarely, thromboangiitis obliterans may involve the cerebral vasculature to give a clinical picture which is generally dominated by fits, progressive dementia and variable palsies of the limbs.

Pulseless Disease (*Takayasu's Disease*)

This is the name which has been given to a condition in which non-specific arteritis of the aortic arch occurs in young people and results in slow progressive occlusion of medium-sized arteries. No limb pulses may be palpable. As the carotid and vertebral arteries are involved, a variety of symptoms and signs of progressive or repeated cerebral infarction commonly appear in such cases. True pulseless disease is rare in Great Britain and the United States, but a similar syndrome may occur in middle-aged or elderly patients due to atherosclerosis.

Unruptured Saccular Aneurysms

Unruptured aneurysms of the cerebral vessels often give no symptoms, but they can simulate basally-situated space-occupying lesions if they become large enough to compress cranial-nerve trunks or other important structures. The supraclinoid aneurysm of the internal carotid artery is a common cause of an isolated third nerve palsy, while a suprasellar aneurysm can be responsible for chiasmal compression and hence for appropriate visual-field defects. An aneurysm within the cavernous sinus may give a paralysis of the third, fourth and sixth cranial nerves on the affected side, along with sensory loss in the distribution of the first and second divisions of the ipsilateral fifth nerve. If an aneurysm in this situation ruptures, a pulsating exophthalmos develops and a loud bruit can be heard over the affected eye.

Arteriovenous Angioma

Small angiomas in the substance of the cerebrum may give rise to no symptoms until they bleed, resulting in subarachnoid haemorrhage. Others are associated with headaches closely resembling migraine, which are often strictly limited to the side of the head upon which the angioma lies, while yet others give rise to focal fits and neurological signs (aphasia, hemiparesis), as they expand in size. Large angiomas are occasionally big enough to starve the surrounding brain of blood, resulting in dementia. A cranial bruit is often heard on the scalp overlying the intracranial lesion or over the appropriate internal carotid artery in the neck. Similar angiomas of the brain stem and posterior fossa are comparatively rare, but they can be responsible for repeated episodes of brain-stem dysfunction occurring over a period of several years, resembling in some respects attacks of basilar artery insufficiency and in others, repeated brain-stem episodes of disseminated sclerosis.

Sturge–Weber Syndrome

This is a congenital malformation of precapillaries in the cerebral cortex, involving usually one parietal and occipital lobe and giving rise to a characteristic radiological pattern of subcortical calcification outlining the cerebral gyri. Usually such patients have frequent fits and a contralateral hemiplegia. An invariable feature of the syndrome is a 'port-wine' naevus of the face on the affected side, with which is often associated a unilateral congenital ox-eye (buphthalmos).

VASCULAR DISORDERS OF THE SPINAL CORD

By comparison with cerebral vascular disease, disorders of the spinal vasculature are uncommon.

Spinal Subarachnoid Haemorrhage

This rare variety of subarachnoid haemorrhage gives rise to sudden pain in the back of considerable severity. This spreads into the arms and legs, depending upon which spinal roots are principally affected through being in close proximity to the bleeding point. Headache and neck stiffness often develop subsequently if the haemorrhage is sufficiently extensive and extends to the cranial subarachnoid space. There may be neurological signs of variable extent in the limbs, depending upon the aetiology of the bleeding and the amount of damage to the spinal cord and/or nerve roots which has taken place. The commonest cause of this syndrome is an arteriovenous angioma of the spinal cord but it can also be symptomatic of a cauda equina tumour, such as an ependymoma of the filum terminale and occasionally a neurofibroma.

Intramedullary spinal haemorrhage is an extremely rare event; this spontaneous variety of haematomyelia gives a clinical picture resembling that of the traumatic condition (*see* Chapter 13). It is usually the result of bleeding from small vascular anomalies (angiomas, telangiectases) within the cord.

Anterior Spinal Artery Thrombosis

The anterior spinal artery, formed by the fusion of branches from each vertebral artery at the level of the foramen magnum, descends in the anterior median fissure of the spinal cord and supplies, by means of its perforating branches, the greater part of the spinal cord apart from the posterior columns. The latter area receives its blood supply from two posterior spinal arteries which are also branches of the vertebral arteries and descend on the posterolateral aspect of the cord but which are smaller and less constant. Throughout the dorsal region the anterior spinal artery receives contributions from radicular arteries which are derived from the intercostals, and indeed in the mid-dorsal region (at about the level of the D10 cord segment) the major blood flow in the anterior spinal artery is received from the intercostals. Thrombosis of the anterior spinal artery gives massive infarction of the spinal cord with a complete flaccid paraplegia, retention of urine and sensory loss to pain and temperature below the level of the lesion. Only some light touch and position and joint sense may be retained. The condition is generally due to atherosclerosis and hence occurs in the elderly. When it develops in the upper cervical region there is a complete quadriplegia with respiratory paralysis, and death follows rapidly. More commonly the upper level of the paralysis and sensory loss is at about the D10 dermatome and in such a case occlusion of the intercostal arteries may be responsible. The latter syndrome is an important immediate complication of a dissecting aneurysm of the aorta which occludes the mouths of its intercostal branches. The paraplegia is irreversible and most patients so afflicted soon die from urinary or respiratory infection. It is, however, increasingly clear that a syndrome of incomplete infarction due to occlusion of radicals of the anterior spinal artery is not uncommon, and in such a case there is paresis rather than paralysis and partial recovery often occurs. Some patients even prove to have episodes of transient spinal cord dysfunction comparable to recurrent cerebral ischaemic attacks, often following exertion ('intermittent claudication of the spinal cord'). Occasionally, in such cases, the cord is found to be compressed, say by a central disk protrusion, and surgical decompression may abolish the attacks.

Spinal Venous Thrombosis

A form of subacute necrotising myelitis, giving a slowly ascending paraplegia, has been attributed to widespread thrombosis of vertebral veins, but is rare. It is particularly liable to occur in patients with chronic cor pulmonale and myelography may demonstrate dilated veins on the surface of the cord.

REFERENCES

CARTER, A. B., *Cerebral Infarction* (Oxford, Pergamon Press, 1964).

FISHER, C. M., DALAL, P.M. and ADAMS, R.D., 'Cerebrovascular diseases and the stroke Syndrome', in *Principles of Internal Medicine*, Ed. Harrison, T. R., 4th ed., Chapter 284 (New York, McGraw-Hill, 1962).

MILLIKAN, C. H., SIEKERT, R. G. and WHISNANT, J. P., *Cerebral Vascular Diseases* (New York, Grune and Stratton, 1961).

SYMONDS, C. P., 'Occlusion of the internal carotid arteries', in *Modern Trends in Neurology*, Ed. Williams, D., 2nd series, Chapter 7 (London, Butterworth, 1957).

WALTON, J. N., *Subarachnoid Haemorrhage* (Edinburgh, Livingstone, 1956).

WRIGHT, I. S. and MILLIKAN, C. H., *Cerebral Vascular Diseases* (New York, Grune & Stratton, 1958).

CHAPTER 18

DISORDERS OF THE LOWER MOTOR NEURONE AND VOLUNTARY MUSCLES

THERE exists a large and important group of diseases and symptom-complexes, often referred to as the neuromuscular disorders, which are characterised by weakness and/or wasting of the voluntary muscles, due to disordered function of the lower motor neurones or of the muscles themselves. A considerable number of these conditions are chronic, progressive, and uninfluenced by any form of treatment which is at present available, but others, which are superficially similar, can be treated effectively. Hence differential diagnosis of the disease entities falling into this group is a matter of considerable importance, and apart from the clinical criteria which are of value in this connexion, and which will be outlined below, certain special investigations, including techniques of electro-diagnosis and muscle biopsy (*see* Chapter 3) have an important place. The first step in diagnosis must be to identify the site of the pathological change; the lesion may lie in the motor nuclei of the cranial nerves, in the anterior horn cells of the spinal cord, in the spinal roots, in the peripheral nerves, in the neuromuscular junction, or in the skeletal muscles themselves. The coexistence of abnormalities of sensation in some cases can be of considerable assistance in this process of identification. Next it will be necessary to determine if possible the nature and aetiology of the pathological process. Unfortunately there are still a great many diseases in this group whose causation and pathogenesis remains obscure. Several of those of known cause have been considered in previous chapters. Thus muscular weakness and/or atrophy is a striking feature of many cases of acute anterior poliomyelitis, of postinfective polyradiculitis, and of 'collagen' disease affecting the peripheral nerves (*see* Chap. 14). Involvement of the anterior horn cells of the spinal cord, with resulting muscular atrophy, is often a feature of degenerative disorders of the spinal cord such as syringomyelia, and amyotrophy due to lesions in the cord or peripheral nerves is seen in certain conditions of the hereditary ataxia group (*see* Chap. 12). Furthermore, intra- or extra-medullary spinal neoplasms (*see* Chap. 16) or traumatic disorders of the spinal cord, of roots, of plexuses and of peripheral nerves (*see* Chap. 13) may have a similar effect. This chapter will be devoted to a consideration of those conditions to which reference has not previously been made.

SPINAL MUSCULAR ATROPHY

Three conditions can provisionally be classified in this group. The first is an infantile variety of progressive degeneration of the anterior horn cells, the second is adult motor neurone (or motor system) disease, and the third is peroneal muscular atrophy (it is not yet certain whether the principal lesion in the latter disease lies in the anterior horn cells, motor roots, or peripheral nerves).

Infantile Progressive Spinal Muscular Atrophy

This condition (Werdnig–Hoffman disease), which typically begins in the second six months of life, but can also develop shortly before, or shortly after birth, affects babies of either sex. It appears to be genetically determined and is inherited as an autosomal recessive factor, so that it commonly affects more than one member of a sibship. Indeed the number of affected children in any one family often exceeds the expected one in four incidence. Usually the parents observe that the child is not moving his limbs normally, that he is unable to hold up his head or to sit, that he is generally limp and 'floppy' and when picked up he tends to slip through the hands. Gradually muscular weakness and generalised hypotonia increase, affecting first the muscles around the shoulder girdle and pelvis and later those of the chest wall, so that there is a characteristic indrawing of the lower ribs at the diaphragmatic attachment on inspiration. The infant, which is at first sight healthy and well-nourished, is seen to lie in a typical posture with the arms abducted on either side of the head, and with the legs abducted and externally rotated at the hips. Later there is weakness of the muscles of deglutition, and fasciculation in the tongue is clearly apparent. Most of the affected children die from respiratory infection before the end of the first year of life but in a few cases the disease process appears to become arrested before paralysis is complete and the affected child survives, though often helplessly crippled by muscular weakness, contractures and consequent skeletal deformity, for several years. Unfortunately the disease is uninfluenced by any form of treatment. In recent years it has become apparent that the condition is sometimes much more benign than the classical descriptions would suggest; for instance, weakness may first appear in the proximal limb muscles later in the first decade or even in the second, when the picture is easily mistaken for that of muscular dystrophy (these are cases of 'pseudomyopathic' spinal muscular atrophy, the so-called Kugelberg–Welander syndrome).

Motor Neurone Disease

This is a disease of adult life which usually begins after the age of forty, though appearing occasionally in younger individuals. In Britain and in the United States the condition generally occurs sporadically, but in isolated instances it may occur in typical form in several members of a family, often following the genetic pattern attributable to an autosomal dominant gene. There is some evidence that in certain affected families the inherited variety of the disease follows an atypical and unusually benign course, but in the Chamorros, a people who inhabit the island of Guam in the Pacific, the disease occurs very frequently in a clinically typical but clearly inherited form. The pathogenesis of the condition is obscure; some few cases have been described as developing many years after an attack of paralytic poliomyelitis and occasionally after encephalitis lethargica, while trauma has been implicated as a contributory factor in isolated instances, but the significance of these observations remains dubious. There is certainly no evidence available to identify the nature of the progressive degenerative changes which occur in the motor nuclei of the cranial nerves, in the anterior horn cells of the spinal cord, and in the pyramidal tracts. Even though pathological changes have been discovered in sensory pathways in certain cases of this disease it is a diagnostic axiom that clinically-recognisable sensory disturbances are absent. Although they merge with one another, three distinctive clinical syndromes, namely progressive bulbar palsy, amyotrophic lateral sclerosis and progressive muscular atrophy, have been described as typifying the variable clinical presentation of the disease. In progressive bulbar palsy the motor cranial nerve nuclei are predominantly affected, in amyotrophic lateral sclerosis the pyramidal tracts, and in progressive muscular atrophy the anterior horn cells of the cord, but in practically all cases there is eventually evidence of lesions in all three sites.

Progressive Bulbar Palsy

The first symptom of this condition is usually dysphagia, and dysarthria soon follows. Food, particularly solid particles, sticks in the back of the throat, choking is frequent and later there is often regurgitation of fluid down the nose owing to palatal paralysis; the voice, in addition to being slurred, acquires a nasal quality. On examination there is paralysis of palatal, pharyngeal and tongue muscles; profuse fasciculation of the tongue is evident, and the jaw jerk is exaggerated. Fasciculation is also observed as a rule in the muscles around the shoulder girdle and there are usually signs of pyramidal tract dysfunction in the limbs. The disease is progressive, leading to complete bulbar palsy with the serious nursing problems which this state entails, along with weakness and spasticity of the limbs. Most patients die from respiratory infection within a year or eighteen months of the onset.

AMYOTROPHIC LATERAL SCLEROSIS

The usual presenting symptom in this variety of motor neurone disease is difficulty in walking due to stiffness of the legs, or else dragging of one leg with subsequent involvement of the other. Physical examination reveals a spastic quadriparesis with a striking increase of the tendon reflexes in all four limbs and extensor plantar responses. There is no abnormality of sensation and the abdominal reflexes are often retained despite the severity of the 'pyramidal' signs. In the early stages there are comparatively few indications of lower motor neurone dysfunction but there is generally some fasciculation in the muscles of the shoulder girdles and thighs and subsequently muscular atrophy makes its appearance. However, in some cases the clinical picture is one of bilateral pyramidal tract disease for some years before signs of lower motor neurone lesions develop. Symptoms and signs of bulbar paralysis appear late; in cases of this type it is spasticity and weakness due to the upper motor neurone lesions which are the principal cause of disability. Nevertheless it is weakness of the bulbar muscles which in the end leads to death in most cases, usually in two to five years from the time of appearance of the first symptom.

PROGRESSIVE MUSCULAR ATROPHY

In this, the most benign variety of motor neurone disease, the first symptom is usually weakness of the muscles in one hand or forearm; less commonly leg muscles are first affected, when a progressive foot drop is the most common manifestation. The weakness progresses insidiously; in the first instance the only symptom may be a clumsiness of fine movements of the fingers (inability to fasten buttons, to sew or to write) but subsequently the grip is affected or a complete wrist drop develops, and the weakness spreads up the arm. In the early stages, fasciculation is often scanty, though later it is usually a prominent feature. There may be considerable difficulty in distinguishing the early manifestations of this disease from those due to cervical spondylosis or to peripheral nerve or plexus lesions, but subsequently it becomes apparent that the distribution of muscular weakness and wasting is more extensive than could possibly be accounted for by involvement of a single peripheral nerve or of one or two motor roots. Eventually there is extensive involvement of the muscles of the limbs and trunk, but the signs are usually asymmetrical at first. Because of the extensive muscular atrophy, the tendon reflexes subserved by the affected muscles are commonly lost, and evidence of pyramidal tract involvement is often lacking for some time, but in the end the plantar responses usually become extensor and some degree of bulbar palsy develops. The absence of sensory loss generally serves to distinguish this condition from the many varieties of peripheral neuropathy, but when fasciculation is scanty, diagnosis from a predominantly motor polyneuropathy can be extremely difficult if not impossible, though motor nerve conduction velocity measurements, usually normal in motor neurone disease and reduced in polyneuropathy, may be helpful. The natural history of this condition is extremely variable; the average duration of the illness before it ends fatally, again as a rule from respiratory infection, is between eighteen months and five years, but in some proven cases the total duration has been as long as ten or fifteen years.

Peroneal Muscular Atrophy

This condition, to which reference has already been made in Chapter 12, is related to the other conditions of the hereditary ataxia group, and is in many respects the most benign of all the chronic progressive neurological diseases. It is inherited as either an autosomal dominant character or as an autosomal recessive, affects either sex, and begins usually in adolescence or early adult life. The first symptoms are usually those of unilateral or bilateral foot drop. Subsequently the calf muscles are involved so that there is severe weakness of dorsiflexion, plantar-flexion, inversion and eversion of the feet and there is a striking atrophy of all muscles below the knee. The picture of an 'inverted champagne bottle' limb, in which the thin legs contrast strikingly with the normal thighs, is characteristic. In most cases the intrinsic muscles of the hands are also affected to give a bilateral 'claw hand', but the muscular involvement does not spread to involve the upper arms. Usually there is loss of vibration sense in the lower limbs, but impairment of cutaneous sensibility is rare. Despite their disability, most patients remain remarkably active and survive to a normal age.

LESIONS OF MOTOR CRANIAL NERVES, OF SPINAL ROOTS AND OF PERIPHERAL NERVES

Many of the disorders which could reasonably be considered under this heading have already been described. Thus dysfunction of the nerves supplying the extrinsic ocular muscles was discussed in

Chapter 8. Infective and allergic conditions involving spinal roots were described in Chapter 14, while trauma to roots, plexuses and peripheral nerves was considered in Chapter 13. There remain to be considered certain abnormalities of the facial nerve and of other motor cranial nerves, the clinical effects of intervertebral disk prolapse, of cervical spondylosis, and the differential diagnosis of disorders which cause pain in the arm or wasting of the small muscles of the hands.

Facial Paralysis

A lower motor neurone lesion of the facial nerve can be distinguished from the type of facial paralysis which results from a lesion of the upper motor neurone by the fact that in the former all the facial muscles on one side are equally affected, while in the latter the weakness involves principally the muscles of the lower face, and movement of those around the eye is comparatively unimpaired. A complete unilateral facial palsy can be the result of a nuclear lesion, as in cases of poliomyelitis, disseminated sclerosis, pontine infarction or tumour, or motor neurone disease. It can also result from lesions of the nerve trunk in its intracranial course, when it is involved in a cranial polyneuropathy, constricted by inflammatory exudation in the subarachnoid space (meningitis, meningovascular syphilis) or compressed by a tumour (e.g. an acoustic neuroma). The commonest conditions giving facial palsy due to involvement of the nerve in its course through the temporal bone are otitis media and herpes zoster of the geniculate ganglion (the Ramsay Hunt syndrome). In its extracranial course the nerve may be damaged by disease of the parotid glands; bilateral facial palsy is rarely a presenting feature of acute leukaemia or sarcoidosis.

The commonest variety of unilateral facial palsy is, however, the so-called **Bell's paralysis** which can occur at any age and in either sex and is of unknown aetiology, although a swelling of the nerve in the narrow bony canal above the stylomastoid foramen has been postulated as its cause. It may follow exposure to cold or a draught but often arises without any apparent precipitating cause. Often the patient awakens to find that one side of his face is paralysed, that he is unable to close the eye on the affected side, that the furrows on this side of the forehead are lost, and that the mouth is drawn over to the sound side. Occasionally there is hyperacusis in the ipsilateral ear due to involvement of the nerve to the stapedius. In some cases the paralysis is incomplete; when this is the case, if there is no progression over the course of the first two or three days, complete recovery generally occurs within one to two weeks. More often the paralysis remains complete for two or three weeks and then begins to recover;

and recovery then is complete as a rule within two or three months. In a comparatively small proportion of cases there is an actual dissolution in continuity of certain of the nerve fibres (neuronotmesis) and regeneration is necessary. In such a case recovery may take several months and even then it is generally incomplete, as some of the regenerating nerve fibres go astray. Commonly under these circumstances some degree of permanent facial contracture develops, a factor which improves the appearance of the face while at rest, though paralysis is still evident on movement (e.g. smiling). Occasionally, too, clonic facial spasm (*vide infra*) is a sequel. Another rare complication is involuntary lacrimation when the patient eats (the syndrome of 'crocodile tears') due to the fact that regenerating autonomic fibres intended for the salivary glands reach the lacrimal glands instead. During the acute stage, it may be necessary to protect the cornea of the eye which cannot be closed. The cosmetic appearance can be improved by the use of strips of transparent adhesive tape (e.g. 'Sellotape'). Cortisone therapy has been advocated but has no real value, and surgical decompression of the facial canal is usually performed too late to help, as it is only done when it is apparent that spontaneous recovery is not taking place. Unfortunately, electromyography can give little information of prognostic value until about three weeks after the onset. Galvanic stimulation of the paralysed muscles is often given but is of dubious value and may increase contracture. In long-standing facial paralysis, cosmetic plastic surgery has a limited but definite place. Some patients suffer repeated attacks of Bell's palsy, now on one side of the face and now on the other, but such attacks are comparatively uncommon.

Hemifacial Spasm

This condition, which is also known as clonic facial spasm, is commonest in middle-aged or elderly women. It is believed to be due to a benign irritative lesion of unknown aetiology which involves the nerve in its bony canal. It gives rise to intermittent fine twitching in the orbicularis oculi and later spreads to involve the remainder of the facial muscles on one side. The spasms can eventually be quite powerful, and rapidly though irregularly repetitive. In the early stages it may resemble a tic and is certainly accentuated by emotional stress, but tics are almost always bilateral so that the strictly unilateral movements of hemifacial spasm are diagnostic. The EMG is often helpful in demonstrating 'grouped' motor unit discharges (each consisting of two or three motor unit action potentials) which repeat rhythmically. Eventually in many cases a progressive facial paralysis develops on the affected side and the movements cease. The condition is embarrassing and inconvenient and is unfortunately uninfluenced by drugs. Decompression of the facial canal has been advocated but is only occasionally successful, and sometimes alcohol injection or operative division of certain fibres of the nerve are necessary in order to relieve the patient's distress, although the spasm is then usually exchanged for a facial paralysis.

Lesions of other Motor Cranial Nerves

Isolated lesions of the other motor cranial nerves are rare, but the nuclei of these nerves can be damaged by lesions of the brain stem, while the nerves themselves may be compressed by space-occupying lesions or involved in inflammatory exudate either intracranially or extracranially. A lesion of the motor root of one **trigeminal nerve** gives rise to atrophy and weakness of the masseter, temporalis and pterygoids on the affected side with consequent asymmetrical jaw movement. The **glossopharyngeal** nerve supplies only the stylo-pharyngeus muscle, so that its motor function cannot be tested. The **vagus** nerve, however, supplies the muscles of the soft palate, pharynx and larynx, so that a unilateral lesion of this nerve will paralyse these structures on the affected side. When such a lesion is present, the soft palate and uvula deviate to the side away from the lesion, and there is a 'curtain' movement of the posterior pharyngeal wall, again to the opposite side, which can often be seen when the patient says 'ah'. Unilateral paralysis of laryngeal muscles, which can also be the result of a lesion of the recurrent laryngeal branch of the vagus (due to secondary neoplasm or reticulosis in mediastinal lymph nodes, to an aortic aneurysm, or thyroid carcinoma) gives hoarseness of the voice and a paralysis of the ipsilateral vocal cord which can be seen on laryngoscopy. When there is a lesion of the eleventh or **spinal accessory** nerve there is atrophy and weakness of the trapezius and sternomastoid on the affected side, while a unilateral **hypoglossal** palsy results in atrophy and fasciculation of one half of the tongue, which, when protruded, deviates to the affected side.

Prolapsed Intervertebral Disk

The intervertebral disks consist of an outer fibrocartilaginous ring, the annulus fibrosus, and a central semifluid portion, the nucleus pulposus. As a result of a degenerative process of unknown aetiology, the annulus fibrosus may be breached, allowing the nucleus pulposus to herniate through the gap so formed. If this gap lies posteriorly in the annulus, as usually occurs, the prolapsed portion of the disk may encroach either upon the spinal canal (a central protrusion) or upon an intervertebral foramen (a lateral protrusion). An acute lateral prolapse of a cervical disk will usually compress a spinal root, giving rise to the clinical syndrome of brachial neuralgia, while a similar lateral protrusion of a lumbar disk is the commonest cause of sciatica. An acute central protrusion developing in the cervical region produces sudden compression of the cervical cord, with symptoms and signs of partial, or even complete, paraplegia or quadriplegia depending upon the size of the protrusion and the level of the lesion, while in the lumbar region a similar acute prolapse may give a cauda equina syndrome of acute onset. Disk protrusions in the dorsal region are comparatively rare, but when they do occur, the spinal canal is so narrow in this situation that there is generally clear evidence of spinal cord compression.

The clinical syndromes resulting from disk prolapse can occur in either sex, but are considerably more common in men; they are more frequently observed in middle and late life, as increasing age clearly contributes to disk degeneration, but may occur in early adult life. It is apparent that trauma plays an important role, as symptoms often develop first after sudden exertion (a twisting movement, hyperextension of the neck, straining to lift a heavy object). The first symptom is generally pain in the neck or back, with tenderness over the spinous processes of the affected vertebrae and also with pain and tenderness in the spinal muscles (possibly owing to protective spasm). This is why the first symptoms of an acute intervertebral disk prolapse are commonly attributed to 'stiff neck', 'fibrositis' or 'lumbago'. Movements of the affected area of the spine may be intensely painful. When the protrusion has occurred centrally, weakness and paraesthesiae in the lower limbs and retention of urine are often seen immediately. If the lesion is cervical there will be clinical evidence of a symmetrical paraparesis, while if it is lumbar, there are usually lower motor neurone and sensory signs in the lower limbs indicating involvement of multiple roots of the cauda equina. In the case of a laterally-situated prolapse in the cervical region, pain of an intense burning character spreads over the shoulder and down the arm, along the dermatome innervated by the affected root. In the lumbar region the pain travels down the back of the thigh and leg and often into the foot, although occasionally in a case of high lumbar disk protrusion the pain may radiate down the front of the thigh. Typically the pain is made worse by movement, and by coughing or by straining, which temporarily increase the pressure in the spinal canal. Peripheral nerves (e.g. the sciatic) which receive contributions from the affected root, are tender and painful when stretched. When the lesion is cervical, lateral movement of the head towards the side of the prolapse is painful (Spurling's sign) while in a case of sciatica, straight-leg raising on the affected side is restricted and painful (Lasègue's sign).

Compression of a motor root by the prolapsed disk is often

responsible in due course for muscular weakness, fasciculation, atrophy and reflex changes, depending upon which root is involved; affection of the sensory root is responsible for subjective numbness and paraesthesiae and objective sensory loss in the appropriate dermatome. In the cervical region, the commonest levels of disk prolapse are at C5-6 in which case the fifth cervical root is principally involved and at C6-7, giving compression of the C6 root. In either case, the deltoid, biceps and brachioradialis muscles may be weak or atrophic and the biceps and radial jerks are commonly depressed. In the lumbar region the sites of election are L4-5 (L5 root) and L5-S1 (S1 root). In either event a partial foot drop may result, but when the disk is at the higher of these two levels the pain usually radiates down into the dorsum of the foot and the reflexes are intact, while compression of the S1 root gives pain along the outer border and sole of the foot and absence of the ankle jerk. In a case of acute disk prolapse, radiographs of the spine are often normal, but in some instances the affected disk space is seen to be narrowed. A moderate rise in the cerebrospinal fluid protein (up to 100 mg/100 ml, or more if there is a complete block) is not uncommon.

Commonly with rest alone the symptoms of an acute disk prolapse resolve within a few days or weeks, but exertion may be responsible for the recurrence of symptoms, often after an interval of months or years. Under such circumstances, immobilisation in plaster or else in a plastic cervical collar or lumbar support is necessary; alternatively spinal traction may be tried. Manipulation has many advocates, and is occasionally very successful, though in the cervical region particularly, it carries considerable risks of damage to the spinal cord. Surgical decompression is usually indicated when there is evidence of severe muscular weakness, extensive sensory loss or impairment of sphincter control, or in occasional cases without extensive neurological signs but in which all other measures have failed.

Cervical Spondylosis

This term is utilised to describe the chronic changes which occur in the cervical spine as a result of long-standing multiple or single intervertebral disk lesions, and which can be responsible for a variety of symptoms and physical signs which are attributable to compression of cervical nerve roots and of the spinal cord (cervical myelopathy). This name should not be used to describe the syndrome of acute cervical disk prolapse, either central or lateral. When a portion of an intervertebral disk has been prolapsed for some time the protruding portion becomes at first fibrotic but later it is calcified and bony-hard. A firm bar of tissue is thus created along the posterior aspect of the intervertebral disk (and often on its anterior aspect as well); this is commonly associated with overgrowth of the margins of the contiguous vertebrae to give bony spurs or osteophytes (so-called lipping). Commonly these bars and lips also encroach upon the intervertebral foramina, and this encroachment may be apparent in oblique radiographs of the spine. These changes are usually observed at the level of several intervertebral disks and are responsible for a clinical syndrome attributable to progressive compression of multiple roots and of the spinal cord. The changes are clearly seen on radiographs of the spine and are often referred to as indicating 'osteoarthritis'. Appearances of this type are observed in a considerable proportion of manual workers and in a fewer number of sedentary workers after middle-age; some such individuals have no neurological symptoms and signs whatever. Hence, it is apparent that these radiological changes will sometimes be observed coincidentally in patients with other neurological diseases, including disseminated sclerosis, syringomyelia and even spinal tumour; therefore it is unwise to assume that such changes are necessarily responsible for the patient's symptoms though this may well be the case.

The syndrome of **cervical myelopathy** resulting from spondylosis is a disorder of middle- and late-life and is much commoner in men than in women. There may have been symptoms in the past (episodes of stiff neck, or 'neuritis' in the arms) to indicate previous acute incidents of disk prolapse, while even in the chronic stage the patient sometimes complains of intermittent pain or stiffness in the neck, or of pain down the arm. Variable degrees of wasting and weakness of upper limb muscles, sometimes with fasciculation, may be observed on one or both sides, but these changes are as a rule unobtrusive and most symptoms are referable to the lower limbs. The muscles usually involved in the arms are the spinati, deltoid, biceps and triceps, as the roots which are most often compressed are those of the C5, 6 and 7 segments; involvement of intrinsic hand muscles is rare. A common and valuable sign is inversion of the biceps or radial reflex. The biceps jerk is said to be inverted if tapping the biceps tendon produces contraction of the triceps; while the radial jerk is inverted if a tap on the brachioradialis tendon produces no contraction of this muscle, but finger flexion. These signs, if present, imply that there is a lesion of the C5 or C6 segment of the cord, breaking the reflex arc for reflexes which utilise these segments of the cord, but at the same time compressing the pyramidal tract to give exaggeration of reflexes whose pathways pass through lower cord segments. The usual symptoms and signs in the lower limbs are those of a progressive spastic paraplegia, often beginning in one leg, and later involving the other. Indeed, this syndrome is probably the commonest cause of a spastic paraparesis developing in late middle-life. Commonly the patient describes a gradual onset with dragging and stiffness of one leg or with some aching pain in the limb after walking any distance. Paraesthesiae are relatively uncommon, but occasionally 'electric shocks' in the trunk and legs on flexion of the neck (Lhermitte's sign) are experienced. On examination there are signs of a spastic paraparesis with exaggerated tendon reflexes and extensor plantar responses. Absence of vibration sense in the lower limbs is common, due to posterior column involvement, but sensory loss of spino-thalamic type is seen less often. In other words, the syndrome can mimic cervical cord compression due to a tumour or a focal cord lesion resulting from any cause. The symptoms are on the whole slowly progressive, less rapidly than in a case of cord tumour, while the absence of remissions is helpful in distinguishing the condition from disseminated sclerosis. However, diagnosis may in the end depend upon myelography, which reveals in such cases multiple indentations of the column of myodil opposite the disk spaces. An ever-present danger in cases of this type is complete quadriplegia due to cervical cord contusion, which, as a result of narrowing of the cervical canal, may follow a relatively mild hyperextension injury of the neck. In the average case, although disability slowly increases, patients are not totally disabled and in a proportion, the symptoms of cord compression seem after a time to become no worse. Although used extensively, a cervical collar is often of little value in these cases except to relieve pain; surgical decompression of the cervical canal may be indicated when deterioration is comparatively rapid and when there is myelographic evidence of a large central disk protrusion at one or at the most two levels, but the results of this measure are often disappointing.

The Causes of Pain in the Arm

It will be convenient at this point to mention briefly some of the important causes of the syndrome of brachial neuralgia or pain in the arm. The anatomical situation of the cause of the pain must first be considered; the conditions mentioned have all been discussed previously in this volume. Among the spinal disorders which may cause pain of root distribution in the upper limb are poliomyelitis, syringomyelia, disseminated sclerosis and intramedullary tumour (intramedullary lesions); shoulder girdle neuritis (neuralgic amyo-trophy), arachnoiditis and extramedullary tumours (extramedullary lesions); acute cervical disk prolapse, cervical spondylosis, and neoplasia in a vertebral body (lesions of the spinal column). Outside the spinal column, the commonest causes are cervical rib (pain down the inner side of the arm), the ill-defined costoclavicular outlet syndrome, tumours (i.e. neurofibroma or metastases in the root of the neck) of the brachial plexus or peripheral nerves, and, at the wrist, compression of the median nerve in the carpal tunnel. A bronchogenic carcinoma at the apex of the lung (Pancoast's superior pulmonary sulcus tumour) is a not infrequent cause of pain in the arm associated with an ipsilateral Horner's syndrome from involvement of the cervical sympathetic. A pericapsulitis of the shoulder joint, giving an immobile painful joint with a tender capsule, is often associated with pain at the insertion of the deltoid and occasionally with painful brawny swelling of the hand (the shoulder-hand syndrome); the latter, if long-standing, may lead to atrophy and decalcification of bones (Sudeck's atrophy). Commonly, too, patients referred to neurological clinics with pain in the forearm, spreading down the dorsum into the fingers, prove to be suffering from a 'tennis-elbow' syndrome with local tenderness over the neck of the radius.

The Causes of Wasting of Small Hand Muscles

The pathological conditions which may be responsible for wasting of the small muscles of the hands can be similarly classified. The commonest lesions of the spinal cord to have this effect are haematomyelia, poliomyelitis, motor neurone disease, syringomyelia and peroneal muscular atrophy. A similar effect may result from an extramedullary tumour at the D1 level, or from arachnoiditis, but is rare in cervical spondylosis or acute disk lesions as the appropriate root is not commonly compressed. Wasting of all the small hand muscles can be the result of any lesion of the inner cord of the brachial plexus; common lesions at this site include birth injury (Klumpke's paralysis) or a hyperabduction injury during anaesthesia, compression by the neck of the humerus following shoulder dislocation, tumours of the brachial plexus, and compression by a cervical rib or in the thoracic outlet. All the small hand muscles become atrophic as a rule in cases of severe polyneuropathy, but when there is a lesion of the ulnar nerve, those of the lateral half of the thenar eminence are spared, while the latter muscles are selectively involved when there is a lesion of the median nerve (as in the carpal tunnel). Hence atrophy of all the small hand muscles usually indicates disease of the D1 segment of the cord, of the D1 root, of the inner cord of the brachial plexus, or a generalised disorder of all peripheral nerves; atrophy of the lateral half of the thenar eminence generally indicates a median nerve lesion, while sparing of these muscles but atrophy of the others, giving a 'claw hand', indicates an ulnar nerve lesion. The presence or absence of associated sensory signs, and their distribution, are of additional value in differential diagnosis. Wasting and weakness of these muscles is rare in myopathic disorders but may occur late in muscular dystrophy of the limb-girdle type; it is, however, an early sign of the rare distal variety of this disease.

Peripheral Neuropathy

This condition, which has long been entitled peripheral neuritis or polyneuritis, is more properly called peripheral neuropathy or polyneuropathy as inflammatory changes are rarely discovered in the affected nerves. It is a clinical syndrome of multiple aetiology in which there are features indicating simultaneous involvement of many peripheral nerves. The clinical picture therefore is one of weakness or paralysis of lower motor neurone type with eventual atrophy, in the peripheral muscles of the limbs; there is usually symmetrical sensory impairment in 'glove and stocking' distribution, and the tendon reflexes are absent. In contradistinction to 'glove and stocking' sensory loss of hysterical origin, that due to polyneuropathy does not show a sharp margin between the area of sensory impairment and that of normal sensation, but the change is gradual. Furthermore, a 'flare' response following a scratch is absent in polyneuropathy if sensory fibres are severely involved, but is present in hysteria. Sometimes motor activity is predominantly affected (motor neuropathy) and sometimes sensation (sensory neuropathy), but it is comparatively uncommon for one or the other to be involved exclusively. Often the affected skeletal muscles, and particularly those of the calves, are tender. Considerable variations in the clinical picture occur from case to case and depend in part upon the aetiology of the illness. It is therefore essential initially to classify and define the known causes of this syndrome according to present knowledge. A provisional classification, which is not intended to embrace all causes of the syndrome but simply those which are the most important, is given below.

CLASSIFICATION

1. INFECTIVE: leprosy.
2. POSTINFECTIVE: (*a*) due to specific exotoxins — diphtheria; (*b*) postinfective (probably allergic) — the Guillain–Barré syndrome, serum neuropathy; (*c*) complicating specific infections — typhoid fever, dysentery, etc.
3. METABOLIC: (*a*) nutritional — vitamin B$_1$ deficiency, alcoholism, pregnancy, etc.; (*b*) heavy metal poisoning — arsenic, mercury, gold, copper, etc.; (*c*) other poisons — triorthocresyl phosphate, isoniazid, organic poisons; (*d*) diabetes mellitus; (*e*) hyperinsulinism; (*f*) primary amyloidosis; (*g*) acute porphyria.
4. VASCULAR: polyarteritis nodosa; disseminated lupus erythematosus.

5. GENETICALLY-DETERMINED: familial intestitial hypertrophic polyneuropathy (Dejerine–Sottas); hereditary sensory neuropathy; heredopathia atactica polyneuritiformis (Refsum's syndrome).

6. UNKNOWN AETIOLOGY: carcinomatous neuropathy; chronic progressive polyneuropathy.

The infective and postinfective varieties of polyneuropathy have been described elsewhere (*see* Chap. 13). In **leprosy** the clinical picture is one of progressive involvement of individual peripheral nerves with thickening of the nerve trunks themselves and patchy cutaneous anaesthesia. The polyneuropathy due to the exotoxin of **diphtheria** usually begins within ten days of the acute infection and first involves the muscles near to the infected area, so that dysphagia and palatal palsy are often the first manifestation; in the more severe cases, there is a symmetrical polyneuropathy of all four limbs which may not appear for four to six weeks. The **Guillain–Barré syndrome** is the commonest cause of acute ascending paralysis, but more often gives rise to a subacute symmetrical peripheral neuropathy of the limbs, associated with a raised protein in the cerebrospinal fluid. Indeed, a rise in the protein content of the fluid is a feature common to cases of nearly every variety of polyneuropathy, but the values recorded in the postinfective group of cases are generally the highest of all. It is also true that a polyneuropathy of non-specific type can occasionally complicate a wide variety of specific infective disorders. In many of these it is probable that the neuropathy should strictly be regarded as postinfective in character, and may well result from allergy.

Turning to the metabolic group of cases, the polyneuropathy resulting from a **deficiency of vitamin B^I** (thiamine) has been well-recognised for many years. Sensory symptoms are generally predominant, and the condition begins with paraesthesiae in the hands and feet; these symptoms are followed by pain and tenderness of calf muscles and by the development of bilateral foot drop, weakness of the grip and later wrist drop. There is peripheral blunting of all forms of sensation. This syndrome can be the result of a primary dietary deficiency of vitamin B$_1$; in such a case there is commonly associated tachycardia, enlargement of the heart and peripheral oedema, giving the fully-developed syndrome of beri-beri. In less severe cases the polyneuropathy develops alone. The condition sometimes begins during pregnancy, following hyperemesis gravidarum, or may result from the anorexia which is an occasional feature of psychiatric disorders such as depression or chronic anxiety and is the predominant symptom of anorexia nervosa. The polyneuropathy which is a frequent complication of **chronic alcoholism** is due to thiamine deficiency and not to the alcohol itself; it only develops as a rule when the consumption of alcohol has increased to such an extent that

it interferes with the intake of food. Pain and cutaneous hyperaesthesia are particularly severe in alcoholic neuropathy. Wernicke's
encephalopathy (*see* Chap. 19) and the Korsakoff syndrome (*see*
Chap. 7) are sometimes present in addition. The polyneuropathies
resulting from **heavy-metal poisoning** are similar. Thiamine, as co-
enzyme A, is important in the metabolism of pyruvate; heavy metals,
by competing with thiamine for certain essential SH groups, interfere
with this activity and hence they produce polyneuropathy through
conditioned thiamine deficiency. A pyruvate tolerance test (*see* Chap.
3) will often aid in identifying this form of polyneuropathy; if the
result is at first abnormal but returns to normal following treatment
with thiamine, then a primary deficiency of the vitamin is indicated,
whereas if it remains abnormal after this treatment, occult heavy
metal poisoning may be suspected. Lead poisoning in adults (*see*
Chap. 19) commonly gives a neuropathy which begins with localised
weakness of one muscle group (e.g. wrist drop) but polyneuropathy
due to other heavy metals is more often generalised. One variety of
polyneuropathy which is usually due to mercury poisoning (from the
use of teething powders) and which is now becoming rare as fewer
of these powders are used, is pink disease (acrodynia). This condition
produces in infants a profound state of irritability with hypotonia of
the limbs, weight loss and a reddened, scaly condition of the hands
and feet. **Triorthocresylphosphate,** a cholinesterase poison, which
was a common contaminant of alcoholic liquors in America in the
1930s, produced many cases of severe polyneuropathy, in which
paralysis and sensory impairment were often permanent (Jamaica
ginger paralysis). It was the cause of a recent 'epidemic' of polyneuropathy in Morocco and was there due to the use of lubricating
oil for cooking purposes. A similar syndrome may follow the use
of **apiol,** taken to procure abortion. In recent years, a number of
cases of polyneuropathy have been described following the use of
various drugs, of which **isoniazid** is a good example. Usually in such
cases the neuropathy recovers in a few weeks or months after the
offending drug has been withdrawn. Isoniazid probably produces its
effect through pyridoxine deficiency, but the exact mechanism by
which other drugs and certain **industrial organic poisons** produce
polyneuropathy is unknown. The neuropathy following **sulphonamide
therapy** is very probably due to hypersensitivity and is in many cases
related to that which may complicate polyarteritis nodosa or disseminated lupus (*vide infra*).

Peripheral neuropathy is a common and important complication
of **diabetes mellitus.** Two principal clinical varieties exist. One, which
is particularly common in the elderly, produces pain and cramp in
the calves, symptoms which are particularly troublesome at night.

M

The ankle and/or knee jerks are absent and there is some impairment of the appreciation of vibration at the ankles. The second form, which usually occurs in younger patients, is often a more severe and generalised form of polyneuropathy, affecting motor power and sensation in all four limbs. It has been suggested that the first type is due to atherosclerosis of the vasa nervorum, the second to some as yet unidentified metabolic disorder associated with diabetes. Whether this is the case remains to be proved; however, most cases of both clinical types improve when the diabetic condition is properly controlled. The syndrome of so-called **diabetic amyotrophy** is one in which wasting and weakness develops in one or both quadriceps muscles and there may also be pain in the affected muscles. It may well be due to a localised femoral neuropathy and this condition too tends to improve when the diabetes is controlled. Another rare variety of polyneuropathy, which is, however, predominantly motor in type and may therefore mimic motor neurone disease, is an occasional complication of **hyperinsulinism** due to an adenoma of the islets of Langerhans.

Primary amyloidosis is yet another uncommon cause of poly-neuropathy, but is seen more often in certain parts of the world (e.g. Portugal) where it produces progressive weakness and sensory loss in the limbs, and is often associated with trophic ulceration of the feet; in these areas it is probably genetically-determined. Occasionally amyloid deposits in the peripheral nerves, giving rise to this clinical picture, are found in association with **multiple myelomatosis.** An asso-ciation between peripheral neuropathy and episodes of abdominal pain and mental confusion, during which port-wine coloured urine is passed, favours a diagnosis of another rare condition, **acute porphyria,** which will be considered further in Chapter 14.

The varieties of peripheral neuropathy which complicate cases of so-called **'collagen' disease,** probably depend upon pathological changes in the vasa nervorum of peripheral nerves. Whatever the aetiology, an asymmetrical involvement of multiple peripheral nerves (mononeuritis multiplex) is a common feature of **polyarteritis nodosa,** while a symmetrical polyneuropathy develops in a propor-tion of cases of **disseminated lupus erythematosus** (*see* Chap. 14). In such cases, steroid therapy may not only control the primary illness but also the neuropathic syndrome. And, as previously mentioned (*see* Chap. 12) a progressive peripheral neuropathy can be an in-herited phenomenon, either in a form which clinically resembles peroneal muscular atrophy, but in which the peripheral nerves are greatly thickened (**Dejerine–Sottas disease**), or else in a form associ-ated with nerve deafness and cerebellar ataxia (**Refsum's syndrome**). In **hereditary sensory neuropathy** a progressive degeneration of posterior root ganglia gives rise to progressive peripheral sensory loss, often accompanied by perforating ulcers of the feet and necrosis of phalanges.

Finally we come to certain varieties of peripheral neuropathy of unknown aetiology. It has become increasingly apparent in recent years that a progressive peripheral neuropathy is a common complication of **bronchogenic carcinoma** and less commonly of malignant disease in other sites. Sometimes the symptoms and signs of the peripheral nerve disorder precede those of the primary neoplasm by months or even years. Although the earliest cases to be described showed signs of an almost pure sensory neuropathy, it is now clear that in the majority of cases the affection is predominantly motor, though minor degrees of peripheral sensory loss are often found. Numerous variations in clinical history occur, but a common story is one of vague pain in the legs on exertion, followed by gradual diminution and finally loss of the lower limb reflexes and then by foot drop and sensory changes. A negative chest X-ray is never sufficient to exclude the diagnosis of bronchogenic carcinoma in such a case, and the primary neoplasm may appear in subsequent radiographs. In occasional cases, the neuropathy has remitted after successful removal of the primary growth, but the exact nature of the relationship between the malignant disease and the neuropathy remains unexplained. The final category included in the above provisional classification is **chronic progressive polyneuritis.** It is unfortunately true that a significant number of cases exist in which a progressive polyneuropathy develops without obvious cause. The number of cases classified in this group nowadays is steadily diminishing and there is substantial evidence to suggest that many of these, and particularly certain cases of recurrent polyneuropathy, are due to an allergic or hypersensitivity reaction involving peripheral nerves and that steroid therapy may be beneficial.

MYASTHENIA GRAVIS

The phenomenon of myasthenia consists of an abnormal degree of fatigability of skeletal muscle. If repeated contractions of an affected muscle are induced, either voluntarily or electrically, the power of these contractions becomes progressively less powerful. Hence in patients suffering from myasthenia, it is a common experience to observe that they become weaker as the day wears on, or after exceptional effort, and improve after rest. The exact mechanism of myasthenic fatigability is unknown; the nature of the phenomenon, and the fact that it can be corrected by the use of neostigmine (prostigmine) or edrophonium (tensilon), suggest that the principal site of the abnormality is at the myoneural junction, where acetyl-choline is destroyed unusually rapidly, perhaps because an excessive quantity of cholinesterase is present. However, it is now apparent that this simple explanation is not adequate to explain all the characteristics of myasthenia, and there may be an abnormality in the behaviour of the muscle-fibre membrane as well as in the myo-neural junction. On the other hand, there is some evidence to suggest that the amount of acetylcholine produced by individual nerve terminals is defective, while even more recently it has been suggested on the basis of clinical and immunological evidence that this disease may be one of the so-called auto-immune disorders, resulting from an antigen-antibody reaction involving end-plate protein.

A myasthenic syndrome has been described in certain patients suffering from bronchogenic carcinoma, and myasthenic fatigability is occasionally observed in others with polymyositis or muscular dystrophy, but it is much more common for myasthenia to occur alone without other evidence of disease in the skeletal muscles or elsewhere; this syndrome is referred to as myasthenia gravis, though the benign course of many cases belies the name. The condition occurs in association with thyrotoxicosis much more often than could be accounted for by chance. It is seen in either sex but is much more common in females than in males. It can begin at any age, in child-hood, in adolescence or early adult life, or in late life. An infant born of a myasthenic mother may suffer from neonatal myasthenia for the first few days of life, but then recovers completely; this fact suggests that some unidentified humoral factor is conveyed across the placenta from mother to child.

The disease usually affects first the external ocular, pharyngeal or jaw muscles. In a considerable proportion of cases the condition remains limited to the extraocular muscles indefinitely and in such individuals the condition is extremely benign. A common first symptom is ptosis, either unilateral or bilateral, and/or diplopia, which become worse towards the end of the day. Difficulty in swallowing or in chewing are common in more severe cases, and sometimes the jaw may become so fatigued after a brief meal, that it hangs open. In other severe cases, there is a similar severe fatigability of the limb and trunk muscles, and respiratory paralysis is an impor-tant and sometimes fatal complication. After some months or years permanent muscular weakness and wasting, uninfluenced by treat-ment, develop in a proportion of cases and the affected muscles show clear-cut degenerative changes on histological examination. The triceps muscle is often most strikingly weakened and wasted in such cases. It is a curious fact that the tendon reflexes usually remain brisk even in true myasthenia, while in the myasthenic syndrome accompanying bronchial carcinoma they are usually lost; in the latter condition, too, it is often found that the initial fatigability of an affected muscle during exercise is followed by an actual increase in strength (post-tetanic potentiation).

The prognosis is extremely variable; in the ocular cases the disease is benign, but acute generalised cases sometimes occur which despite treatment are fatal within a few months. In the cases of moderate severity, maintenance therapy with prostigmine and its analogues usually achieves for the patient considerable control of the muscular weakness and allows a reasonably active existence. Spontaneous remission, which can be heralded by reduced prostigmine requirements, is not uncommon and may last for months or years. In relatively acute myasthenia occurring in young women, and in other selected cases which show a poor response to drug therapy, surgical removal of the thymus gland may have a dramatic effect. The gland is enlarged in many individuals and some are found to have a thymoma, which always requires radiotherapy prior to surgery; however, no myasthenia-producing hormone secreted by this gland has yet been isolated and its exact role remains unclear. A history of variable ptosis, diplopia, dysphagia, jaw weakness or weakness of the limbs should always bring the possibility of myasthenia to mind and a diagnostic intramuscular injection of prostigmine (1·25 mg + 0·6 mg atropine sulph.) or an intravenous injection of 10 mg of the quick-acting edrophonium, a drug with a very transient effect, should be tried to see if the weakness is influenced thereby. In giving such an injection of edrophonium it is wise to inject 2 mg initially and to await side-effects, before proceeding to give the entire 10 mg.

MYOTONIA

The phenomenon of myotonia is in some respects the converse of myasthenia, for it results in an apparent delay in relaxation of skeletal muscle, accompanied by a peristent electrical 'after-discharge', even when voluntary innervation of the muscle has ceased. The nature of the abnormality in such cases is also in doubt, although the muscle fibre membrane is believed to be at fault. A characteristic feature of myotonia is that the patient, on taking a firm grasp of an object, is unable to let go, and typically a gradual uncurling of the clenched fingers, beginning in the index and middle fingers, is observed; the total period required for relaxation may be several seconds. The phenomenon can also be demonstrated by a firm tap upon the surface of a muscle, seen best in the tongue or thenar eminence when a clear-cut 'dimple' or furrow appears and may persist for several seconds. The electromyogram (*see* Chap. 3) is diagnostic. Myotonia is invariably accentuated by cold, and it is usually reduced either by warmth or by repeated contraction of the affected muscles, which results in a 'wearing-off' of the phenomenon. It can be partially or completely relieved by drugs such as quinine, procaine amide, cortisone and its analogues, and to a lesser extent by potassium-binding ion-exchange resins.

There are two major clinical syndromes in which the phenomenon of myotonia is observed. Both are inherited and in both the pattern of inheritance is that attributable to an autosomal dominant gene. In the first, **myotonia congenita** or Thomsen's disease, myotonia is generalised throughout the skeletal musculature, and is present from birth. The principal symptom is stiffness of the muscles, a difficulty in beginning muscular activity and in relaxing afterwards; these features are accentuated by cold and can be 'worked-off' by exercise. Generalised hypertrophy of the skeletal muscles usually develops during adolescence, but weakness and atrophy of muscles is not usually observed, except after many years, and most patients survive and remain active to a normal age. In **dystrophia myotonica** (myotonia atrophica), by contrast, myotonia is usually apparent only in the muscles of the hands and tongue, and may even be absent. The first symptoms of the disease usually develop in adolescence or adult life and in addition to myotonia affecting the grip there is progressive difficulty in walking. There are frontal baldness (in the male), impotence and testicular atrophy, cataracts, atrophy of the sterno-mastoids and of the facial and temporal muscles, and weakness and wasting of the peripheral muscles of the limbs; the latter are due to an associated muscular dystrophy which is an essential part of the disease process. Bilateral ptosis, and a typically long, lugubrious facies are usually seen. Many patients are of low intellect; the condition is progressive and eventually results in severe disability leading to a wheelchair existence, with death from cardiac failure (due to myocardial degeneration) or from respiratory infection, in middle-life. Whereas the myotonia in such cases can be relieved by drugs, the dystrophic process in the peripheral limb muscles, which is the principal cause of progressive disability, is uninfluenced by treatment.

Paramyotonia is an uncommon variant of myotonia congenita. In this condition the myotonia occurs only on exposure to cold and is then associated with attacks of generalised muscular weakness resembling closely those observed in cases of familial periodic paralysis but usually accompanied by a rise, rather than a fall, in the serum potassium (*vide infra*). **Myotonia paradoxia** is a term given to cases in which the myotonia is accentuated and not improved by exertion. Many such cases constitute merely an unusual form of myotonia congenita, but some in whom muscular pain and stiffness increase after exertion are suffering from a rare myopathy, due to a defect in muscle glycogen breakdown in muscles which are congenitally deficient in the enzyme phosphorylase (McArdle's syndrome); certain others are suffering from myxoedema, a disorder which can occasionally present with muscular symptoms (pseudomyotonia).

PROGRESSIVE MUSCULAR DYSTROPHY

This condition, in which progressive weakness and wasting of certain skeletal muscles occurs, has been defined as genetically-determined primary degenerative myopathy. The pathological changes in the diseased muscles, which are characteristic, clearly indicate a primary disorder of the muscle fibres themselves and there is no evidence of disease in the central or peripheral nervous system. One rare variety of muscular dystrophy, **ocular myopathy,** gives rise to progressive bilateral ptosis and eventually complete ophthalmoplegia and weakness of the orbicularis oculi, while another, **distal myopathy,** which is also extremely rare, except in Sweden, begins in the small muscles of the hands and feet and later spreads proximally in the limb muscles.

However, the commonly occurring varieties of muscular dystrophy fall into three principal groups which are clinically and genetically distinct. All are progressive, and uninfluenced by any form of treatment. The first, the **Duchenne or pseudohypertrophic type,** affects almost exclusively young boys, being inherited usually via a sex-linked recessive mechanism; often several boys in a sibship develop the condition; very occasionally affected girls are discovered and in these families the disease, which is somewhat more benign, is inherited as an autosomal recessive character. The onset is usually within the first three to five years of life; the child, who walked at the normal age, begins to be clumsy in walking, has difficulty in climbing stairs, falls frequently and rises by 'climbing up his legs'. He walks with his abdomen protruding (accentuated lumbar lordosis) and with a typical waddle. There is progressive weakness of the proximal muscles of the upper and lower limbs; often firm rubbery enlargement (pseudohypertrophy, due to fatty infiltration) of the calves, and sometimes of other muscles, is seen. The progress of the disease is inexorable. Often the child is unable to walk by the time he is 8 to 12 years old and later progressive contractures of the weakened muscles develop with secondary skeletal deformity, to give a tragic terminal state, from which the child is carried off by a series of respiratory infections or by acute cardiac failure often before the age of 20; a few isolated cases survive much longer.

The **limb-girdle variety** (Erb–Leyden–Möbuis) occurs equally in the two sexes and may begin at any age though it usually does so in adolescence or early adult life; it is usually inherited via an autosomal recessive gene. The disease may begin either in the pelvic girdle, giving difficulty in climbing stairs and a typical waddling gait, or in the shoulder girdle, resulting in an inability to lift the arms above the shoulders. Sometimes the muscular involvement remains confined to the shoulders or to the pelvic girdle for a great many years, but later spreads to the other. In the shoulder girdles the trapezii, serrati, pectorals, biceps and brachioradialis are commonly involved and the deltoids are spared, to give a characteristic clinical picture. Pseudohypertrophy of muscles is occasionally seen in this form of muscular dystrophy. The prognosis in this group of cases is much less grave than in the Duchenne variety, but nevertheless the disease is progressive, though sometimes intermittently so; most patients are severely disabled, as a rule in middle-life, and few survive to a normal age.

The **facioscapulohumeral form** (Landouzy–Dejerine) is the most benign. It, too, may begin at any age (usually in adolescence or early adult life) and in either sex, but it is generally inherited as an autosomal dominant character. The facial muscles are first affected, resulting in inability to close the eyes completely, a typical 'pout' of the lips and a 'transverse' smile. The shoulder girdle muscles are also involved, selectively as in certain of the limb-girdle cases, and the disease may not spread to the pelvic girdle for many years. Indeed in a small proportion of cases only a few muscles around the shoulders are involved and the disorder is then arrested (abortive cases). Whereas the muscular weakness may progress unusually quickly in a few affected individuals, the rapidity of advance of the disease is very slow in the majority, and some remain active, though with increasing disability, to a normal age.

The diagnosis of muscular dystrophy, in an established case, is rarely difficult, but in the early stages, particularly in a young child, the history of clumsiness in walking or of inability to run as quickly as other children of comparable age is often attributed to flat feet or to laziness, unless this diagnosis is borne in mind. Although the urinary output of creatine in such cases is increased, as is the serum aldolase, these are not diagnostic tests. However, estimation of the creatine kinase in the serum, which may be raised three-hundredfold in affected young boys, is virtually diagnostic of the Duchenne type of the disease but is less abnormal in the other varieties. This test can be used to identify the disease in its pre-clinical stage in the young male sibs of affected boys and is also useful in the diagnosis of the carrier state in their mothers and sisters. In cases of doubt, electromyography and muscle biopsy may be necessary. These procedures are also of value in distinguishing muscular dystrophy from poly-myositis (*vide infra*) with which the condition can sometimes be confused. In the absence of any effective treatment, all that can be done is to keep the patients active for as long as possible. Inactivity and bed rest have a deleterious effect; every effort should be made to delay the development of contractures for as long as possible by passively stretching tendons which are shortening, but surgical lengthening of such tendons is not indicated.

POLYMYOSITIS

This name has been given to a clinical syndrome produced by combined degenerative and inflammatory changes in skeletal muscle. It does not include suppurative and infective varieties of myositis which are rare, save for virus myositis (epidemic myalgia), which will be discussed below. In some instances the skin and mucous mem-branes are also involved, in which case the condition is known as dermatomyositis, but often the main brunt of the disease process falls upon the skeletal muscles. Although the syndrome may embrace several diseases of varying aetiology, it is clear that in most instances the pathological process responsible for the condition falls into the category of so-called 'collagen' disease. The syndrome has been observed in patients of all ages and in both sexes. Acute forms of polymyositis and dermatomyositis most often occur in adults and are characterised by the development of generalised muscular pains and weakness of comparatively rapid progression, associated often with a widespread erythematous rash on the face, limbs and trunk. The proximal limb muscles are more severely affected than the distal ones. The affected muscles are tender and the patients are ill and febrile; the respiratory muscles may be involved and the illness sometimes ends fatally within a few weeks or months. Subacute forms of polymyositis are much more common. In such cases muscular pain and tenderness and symptoms of constitutional upset are often absent, and the presenting features are those of progressive weakness and moderate atrophy of the muscles of the shoulder and pelvic girdles. In such a case the clinical picture can resemble closely that of muscular dystrophy, save for the fact that in polymyositis all the proximal limb muscles are weakened, and the deltoid, for instance, is not spared; furthermore the neck muscles are generally weak, dysphagia and a Raynaud phenomenon in the hands are common, and the muscular weakness is often greater than the degree of atrophy would suggest. This form of subacute polymyositis is particularly common in middle- and late-life and has been called by some 'menopausal muscular dystrophy'. When it occurs in child

M*

hood or adolescence there are commonly minor skin changes on the skin of the face and of the hands and fingers, resembling in many respects those of early scleroderma or acrosclerosis. In some cases, the skin lesions resemble those of lupus erythematosus, while in others, there may be associated evidence of another 'collagen' disease such as rheumatoid arthritis. Subcutaneous and intramuscular calcification (calcinosis universalis) is a not uncommon sequel of polymyositis. Another important point is that a significant proportion of cases of polymyositis and particularly of dermatomyositis in middle- and late-life develop in association with malignant disease in the lung or in some other organ.

The prognosis of polymyositis and dermatomyositis is variable. About half the acute cases are eventually fatal, despite modern methods of treatment. A proportion of the subacute cases in childhood remit spontaneously and many recover completely; others enter a chronic stage with the development of fibrous contractures in the muscles and severe deformity (chronic myositis fibrosa). Most of the subacute cases occurring in adult life are progressive if untreated but some become arrested. A considerable proportion of cases remit completely or partially when treated with cortisone and analogous remedies, but maintenance therapy may have to be continued for many months or years.

In the diagnosis of polymyositis, a raised E.S.R., which is found in up to two-thirds of cases, is important, and often the B.M.R. is also raised despite a normal radioactive iodine uptake. The serum aldolase, transaminases, creatine kinase and *Y*-globulin are also raised, but in most cases final diagnosis depends upon a combination of the clinical findings on the one hand with the results of electromyography and muscle biopsy on the other.

EPIDEMIC MYALGIA (*Bornholm Disease*)

This is the name given to a virus myositis, resulting generally from infection with one of the Coxsackie group of viruses. It gives rise to an acute febrile illness with severe pain in the upper abdomen and lower chest wall. Pain on breathing and coughing (pleurodynia) is a striking feature and the illness may simulate pleurisy or in some cases an acute abdominal emergency. The condition is self-limiting, occurs in localised epidemics, and usually clears up without residual symptoms in three to five days.

PAROXYSMAL MYOGLOBINURIA

Myoglobin may appear in the urine in any condition which produces sudden destruction of muscle, and if the quantity released into the blood stream is large, death may result from renal failure due to blockage of multiple renal tubules. Causes of myoglobinuria include massive crush injuries of muscle (crush syndrome), necrosis of the anterior tibial muscles in their tight fascial compartment after prolonged marching or similar exertion (the anterior tibial syndrome), acute polymyositis, and paroxysmal myoglobinuria. In the latter, a condition of unknown aetiology, patients experience intermittent febrile episodes, each lasting a few days, during which they complain of generalised muscular pain and pass dark brown urine containing myoglobin. The condition is uninfluenced by treatment, but even after repeated attacks, recovery is often complete, though death in an attack is a rare event. The disorder usually appears first in childhood and after repeated attacks some degree of permanent muscular weakness and wasting may be found.

FAMILIAL PERIODIC PARALYSIS

This is an uncommon condition of dominant inheritance which affects patients of either sex, usually from birth. Sufferers from this disorder experience attacks of generalised muscular weakness which vary in severity but may be sufficiently severe to paralyse them completely. A common story is that the patient wakens from sleep to find that he is unable to move. Although weakness of the skeletal musculature in such a case can be remarkably widespread and profound, swallowing is only occasionally disturbed, and respiratory muscle weakness is never sufficient to be of danger to life. The attacks vary in duration from one or two hours to as long as forty-eight hours. Commonly after a few minutes of total paralysis the patient is able to move but does so weakly and clumsily and may not be completely normal for two or three days. There are occasional cases in which the weakness is consistently localised to only a few muscle groups. It is well-recognised that the episodes are particularly likely to develop while the patient is resting after unusually heavy exertion, or after a heavy carbohydrate meal. Often they can be induced by the administration of insulin and glucose. In the majority of cases it is found that the serum potassium is low during the attacks and the weakness can be rapidly reversed by the administration of 2-4 g of potassium chloride by mouth. Maintenance therapy with 4-5 g of potassium chloride daily and sometimes aldosterone antagonists are useful prophylactically. Similar episodes can occur in patients whose serum potassium is lowered as a result of other causes, as in cases of potassium-losing nephritis, renal tubular acidosis, or aldosteronism.

It has recently become apparent that in some cases and families, attacks which are characteristic of the syndrome described above occur in association with a high, and not a low, serum potassium, This syndrome has been given the title of **adynamia episodica hereditaria.** The attacks in this form of the disorder are often less severe and of shorter duration than in the hypokalaemic type and may follow immediately after exertion, while some patients also have myotonia. The paralysis in this type of case is accentuated by the giving of potassium but can be terminated by the use of diuretics such as chlorothiazide or acetazoleamide which promote potassium excretion. Yet a third variety of periodic paralysis in which the serum potassium remains normal in the attacks and in which weakness is controlled by the administration of sodium, has been described. Clearly therefore it is essential in any individual who experiences attacks of this nature to estimate the serum potassium during an attack of weakness, so that appropriate treatment may be given.

ENDOCRINE MYOPATHIES

This group of disorders will be described in Chapter 19.

THE AMYOTONIA CONGENITA SYNDROME

To determine the nature of the pathological changes responsible for the production of widespread weakness and hypotonia of the skeletal muscles in infancy is a matter of the greatest difficulty. In most cases which present with these manifestations in severe form the disease process is one of infantile progressive spinal atrophy (Werdnig–Hoffman disease), whether the illness begins at birth or during the first year of life. In a considerable number of cases, however, the child's hypotonia may be a symptom of a variety of infective, metabolic and neurological disorders which are not primarily affecting the lower motor neurone or muscles. Thus muscular weakness and hypotonia of some degree is common in infants recovering from acute infection, in cases of intestinal malabsorption, malnutrition, hypocalcaemia, mental defect, and even in some of cerebral diplegia of the flaccid type. There exists, however, a third group of cases in which the weakness and hypotonia is benign, though of unknown aetiology, and in which considerable improvement and sometimes complete recovery may be expected. This latter condition was first described by Oppenheim under the title of myatonia congenita or amyotonia congenita, but this diagnosis has been widely utilised to include all infants which show severe generalised hypotonia soon after birth. As many of these have proved to be suffering from progressive spinal atrophy, this title has become discredited, and the term **benign congenital hypotonia** is now preferred by many for the group of cases which carry a good prognosis. These children, though weak and 'limp' or 'floppy' from birth, are never as severely paralysed as those with Werdnig–Hoffman disease and show gradual improvement. They sit up late and often do not stand or walk until late in the second or in the third year of life. Many recover completely but others, who are more severely affected in early life, improve up to a point, but no further, and have small, weak muscles throughout life. The latter condition has also been entitled 'congenital universal muscular hypoplasia' or 'congenital non-progressive myopathy'. In some cases of infantile hypotonia who are subsequently found to have generalised weakness and hypoplasia of muscles a curious defect of the centre of many muscle fibres can be demonstrated ('central-core' disease) while in yet others rod-shaped bodies of unknown composition are found to be collected beneath the sarcolemma of many fibres ('nemaline myopathy'). A similar hypoplasia of the skeletal muscles is seen in some individuals with long spidery fingers and a high arched palate (arachnodactyly).

One final condition requires to be mentioned, namely **arthrogryphosis multiplex congenita.** This is a condition of multiple contractures of skeletal muscle, combined with deformity of the limbs, which is present from birth. In some cases it appears to be due to a spinal muscular atrophy beginning in foetal life, in some to a myopathic process developing before birth, and in others, in which there is no evidence of disease in the motor nerves or muscles themselves, to excessive intra-uterine pressure, with abnormal posturing of the limbs.

REFERENCES

BRAIN, W. R., *Diseases of the Nervous System*, 6th ed., Chapters 18 and 19 (London, Oxford University Press, 1962).

BRANDT, S., *Werdnig-Hoffman's Infantile Progressive Muscular Atrophy* (Copenhagen, Munksgaard, 1950).

FORD, F. R., *Diseases of the Nervous System in Infancy, Childhood and Adolescence*, 4th ed. (Springfield, Ill., Thomas, 1959).

NATTRASS, F. J., 'Primary diseases of muscles', in *Modern Trends in Neurology*, Ed. Williams, D., 2nd series, Chapter 15 (London, Butterworth, 1957).

OSSERMANN, K. E., *Myasthenia Gravis* (New York, Grune and Stratton, 1958).

PERLO, V. and ADAMS R. D., 'Disease of the peripheral nerves', in *Principles of Internal Medicine*, Ed. Harrison, T. R., 4th ed., Chapter 291 (New York, McGraw-Hill, 1962).

THOMASEN, E., *Myotonia* (Copenhagen, Munksgaard, 1948).

TYLER, F. H. and ADAMS, R. D., 'Diseases of striated muscle', in *Principles of Internal Medicine*, Ed. Harrison, T. R., 4th ed., Chapters 83-87 (New York, McGraw-Hill, 1962).

WALTON, J. N., 'Genetic aspects of muscular and neuromuscular diseases', in *The Structure and Function of Voluntary Muscle*, Ed. Bourne, G. H., Chapter 34 (New York, Academic Press, 1960).

WALTON, J. N., (Ed.), *Disorders of Voluntary Muscle*, (London, Churchill, 1964).

WALTON, J. N. and ADAMS, R. D., *Polymyositis* (Edinburgh, Livingstone, 1958).

CHAPTER 19

METABOLIC DISORDERS AND THE
NERVOUS SYSTEM

INCREASING interest has been taken in recent years in the group of diseases or symptom-complexes in which symptoms depend not so much upon recognisable structural changes occurring in the parts of the body, but upon alterations in the chemical composition and metabolic activity of the tissues. In many of these disorders physical changes in the affected organs eventually develop, but this is not always so, and the primary change is a biochemical one. Under this heading it is usual to consider the so-called deficiency disorders which result either from an inadequate intake of certain foods, and particularly of vitamins, or from impaired absorption of these substances. Several of these deficiency disorders can have a profound effect upon the functioning of the nervous system, as may abnormalities in the endocrine glands and certain specific inborn errors of metabolism. The more common and important of these conditions will be described in this chapter. It will also be necessary to consider the effect of poisons upon the nervous system as well as the influence of various forms of physical injury, even though the latter type of insult is not a metabolic abnormality in the strictest sense of the term.

DEFICIENCY DISORDERS

Although many specific syndromes occurring in man have been ascribed to an insufficient dietary intake of certain vitamins, it is important to realise that these syndromes are not solely dependent upon vitamin deficiency. Thus total starvation does not as a rule result in the development of symptoms of scurvy, pellagra or beri-beri, while symptoms and signs of thiamine deficiency are greatly enhanced if the diet contains large amounts of carbohydrate. It seems therefore that some food must be taken before characteristic clinical evidence of vitamin deficiency can develop. Even so, the resultant clinical syndrome varies greatly in the individual cases; it is not, for instance, clear why thiamine (vitamin B_1) deficiency will produce Wernicke's encephalopathy in some cases, beri-beri in others, and optic neuritis or perhaps even 'burning feet' in yet others. It is, however, apparent that conditions such as pregnancy, or infective illnesses, which enhance the body's demands for vitamins,

347

may accentuate symptoms attributable to deficiency which were previously minimal. It is the vitamins of the B group, and particularly thiamine, nicotinic acid, pyridoxine and vitamin B_{12}, which are of greatest importance in relation to the nervous system. Clinical syndromes resulting from vitamin C deficiency (scurvy) and from deficiencies of the fat-soluble vitamins (A, D and K) are not as a rule attended by symptoms of nervous disease. The commoner manifestations of vitamin B_1 deficiency are Wernicke's encephalopathy and beri-beri, while nutritional amblyopia and the 'burning feet' syndrome are probably related, although the exact aetiology of these disorders has not yet been fully worked out. The clinical syndrome resulting from nicotinic acid deficiency is pellagra, while pyridoxine lack is attended by convulsions in infancy and by polyneuropathy in later life. The usual neurological effect of vitamin B_{12} deficiency is, of course, subacute combined degeneration of the spinal cord, though disturbances of cerebral function and optic atrophy are also occasionally seen.

Wernicke's Encephalopathy

Wernicke's encephalopathy is a clinical syndrome characterised by mental disturbance, disorders of eye movement and ataxia, and results from thiamine deficiency. It is most commonly observed in chronic alcoholic patients in whom alcoholic beverages have gradually replaced other forms of food, and gastrointestinal irritation has contributed by producing anorexia. However, the condition can develop as a result of thiamine deficiency arising from any cause. There is often an associated polyneuropathy. The principal pathological features are focal areas of haemorrhage and neuronal degeneration in the corpora mammilaria and upper mid-brain. Although in severe cases there is often a profound disturbance of consciousness, the characteristic mental symptoms are first, transient delirium and hallucinatory experiences, occurring particularly in alcoholic patients and resulting from alcohol withdrawal; secondly, apathy, listlessness and variable confusion; and thirdly, most characteristic of all, the Korsakoff syndrome (*see* Chap. 6). The principal abnormality in the Korsakoff syndrome is a memory defect resulting in an inability to record new impressions, from which spring disorientation in time and place and confabulation; events from the patient's remote past are described elaborately as if they had just happened. The principal neurological abnormalities which accompany these mental changes are coarse nystagmus, present in all directions of gaze, and ophthalmoplegia, which may consist merely of paralysis of both lateral recti or more often of disorders of conjugate ocular movement leading in some cases to immobility of the eyes. A profound truncal ataxia is also present as a rule, even though signs of cerebellar inco-ordination in the limbs can be singularly inconspicuous on formal testing. A characteristic feature of Wernicke's disease is that the neurological abnormalities generally remit promptly when the patient is treated with thiamine, although the mental disturbances, and particularly those of the Korsakoff syndrome, may take weeks or months before they resolve completely.

Beri-beri

Although thiamine deficiency is clearly an important factor in the aetiology of beri-beri, some additional factor is probably necessary in view of the rarity of the fully-developed syndrome in European or American chronic alcoholics and in view of the fact that it rarely occurs in its entirety except in populations who have fed upon milled rice. Polyneuropathy due to B-vitamin deficiency is, however, quite common in Western countries, not only in alcoholics, but in patients with prolonged anorexia due to mental disease and in elderly people who live alone.

The principal clinical features of beri-beri are due to polyneuropathy (*see* Chap. 18). Apart from the distal muscular atrophy and sensory loss which is common to all varieties of peripheral neuropathy, a characteristic feature of this form is that the patients often complain of intense burning and tingling feelings in the extremities and especially in the feet; touching the skin is sometimes particularly unpleasant, so that walking becomes impossible, not as a result of muscular weakness, but because of sensory disturbance. In some individuals, these are the only clinical manifestations ('dry' or 'neuritic' beri-beri) but generally there is also peripheral oedema, breathlessness, tachycardia and cardiac enlargement, indicating myocardial involvement. In this condition, the administration of thiamine in large doses is usually attended by gradual improvement and by eventual complete recovery.

The 'Burning Feet' Syndrome

A syndrome which was commonly observed in prisoner-of-war camps during World War II was one in which pain and intense burning developed in the feet, but signs of a motor neuropathy were absent, and often sensory changes were inconspicuous even on careful examination. Usually there was associated intense itching of the scrotum with occasional ulceration. Clearly the syndrome was nutritional in origin and it responded to treatment with vitamins of the B group in high dosage; very probably it was a form of nutritional polyneuropathy but the exact aetiology of the syndrome has never been clearly established.

Nutritional Amblyopia

In some individuals existing on diets which are low in vitamin B content, a progressive blurring of vision develops and the visual fields show central or paracentral scotomas, at first for coloured objects and later for white. Clinical evidence of optic disk swelling is not a feature but if the condition is left untreated, optic atrophy follows. The condition is clearly similar clinically and perhaps aetiologically, to the forms of amblyopia which have been attributed to alcohol and tobacco. It has been attributed to a deficiency of riboflavine and certainly responds to treatment with mixed vitamins of the B group given in high dosage, but recent work suggests that a deficiency of vitamin B_{12} is the principal factor. Hence the condition resembles the optic atrophy which occasionally complicates subacute combined degeneration of the spinal cord.

Tobacco Amblyopia

This condition occurs particularly in heavy pipe-smokers who customarily smoke thick dark tobacco; slow visual deterioration occurs and paracentral or centrocaecal scotomas are usually found. There is some evidence that in these cases B_{12} metabolism may be involved, but the visual symptoms usually recover completely if the individual gives up smoking or changes to a more innocuous tobacco. Possibly some toxic substance in the tobacco or some form of sensitivity causes an impairment of the utilisation of Vitamin B_{12}.

Pyridoxine Deficiency

It has become apparent in recent years that pyridoxine (vitamin B_6) deficiency in early infancy can be responsible for repeated convulsions. Recurrent epileptiform seizures developed in a large number of infants in the United States who were fed upon artificial milk which, through an accident of manufacture, was deficient in pyridoxine. It has also been discovered that pyridoxine deficiency can cause a form of polyneuropathy and it now appears that polyneuropathy following isoniazid administration is due to metabolic antagonism of pyridoxine and may be corrected by giving high dosage of this vitamin.

Pellagra

The syndrome of pellagra is generally attributed to a dietary deficiency of nicotinic acid, but a secondary factor is often a defective protein intake, as the amino acid tryptophane is a chemical precursor of nicotinic acid. Hence it occurs in individuals who are existing on a predominantly vegetable or cereal diet which is deficient in animal protein; thus it is not uncommon in vegans who refuse all foods derived from animal sources. Commonly the skin lesions of pellagra, which consist initially of erythema on the face, hands and other exposed surfaces, and later give rise to vesiculation, pigmentation and thickening of the skin, are produced by exposure to sunlight. The symptoms of nervous system involvement, which almost invariably develop in such cases, are predominantly mental. Sometimes the clinical picture is that of a severe confusional state, while in other cases there is impairment of memory, apathy, fatigue, depression and insomnia. Evidence of polyneuropathy is commonly found, but this is probably due to an associated deficiency of other B-vitamins. However, in some cases of apparently uncomplicated pellagra there are symptoms and signs of spinal cord involvement, with spastic paresis of the lower limbs and with variable evidence of disease in the posterior columns.

Vitamin B12 Deficiency

Although a primary dietary deficiency of vitamin B_{12} has been observed in vegans, the clinical effects of vitamin B_{12} deficiency upon the nervous system are generally seen only in patients with pernicious anaemia, in whom the dietary intake of the vitamin is adequate but its absorption is prevented by the absence of the necessary intrinsic factor in the gastric juice. Histamine-fast achlorhydria is invariable in such cases and usually there are changes in the blood or in the bone-marrow to indicate a diagnosis of pernicious anaemia. Rarely, however, neurological symptoms and signs antedate any recognisable change in the blood and even in the bone-marrow. Although the principal neurological symptoms and signs indicate disease of the spinal cord, there are occasional cases in which **cerebral symptoms** are predominant, at least initially. These symptoms include defects of intellect, of memory and of concentration or episodes of confusion or paranoia; it may at first be difficult to distinguish these cerebral manifestations of vitamin B_{12} deficiency from the clinical features of early presenile dementia or from those resulting from any organic confusional state. Occasionally, too, there is progressive bilateral visual loss with central scotomas in the visual fields and **optic atrophy** is observed on physical examination.

Subacute Combined Degeneration of the Spinal Cord

Symptoms and signs indicating involvement of the nervous system occur in about 80 per cent of cases of pernicious anaemia. The principal sites of pathological change, in which initial loss of myelin with subsequent axonal degeneration occur, are the posterior columns and the pyramidal tracts. There is some evidence that the disease process occasionally involves the posterior roots and even the peripheral nerves, giving clinical features suggestive of a polyneuro-pathy, but this suggestion is not yet fully substantiated.

The clinical features of the illness depend upon which tracts of the spinal cord are principally affected by the disease process. Since the lesions in the posterior columns are usually predominant, the principal initial symptoms are generally paraesthesiae, tingling, numbness and pins and needles in the extremities. It is common for patients to describe sensations as if a tight band of constriction were present around one toe, around a limb or about the waist; feelings suggesting that cold water is trickling down the legs are also frequent. Physical signs may be minimal but usually vibration sense is impaired early in the disease, Romberg's sign is positive, the appreciation of position in the toes and fingers is defective and the threshold for two-point discrimination is raised. As evidence of posterior column involvement becomes more severe, so the patient develops an ataxia of sensory type, in which locomotion or maintenance of the upright posture are particularly difficult in the dark or when the eyes are closed. Impairment of the appreciation of light touch in the periphery of the limbs is sometimes seen, together with tenderness of the calves, and it is these features, along with depression or absence of the tendon reflexes, which have led to the suggestion that the peripheral nerves or posterior nerve roots are sometimes involved. Very rarely, pain and temperature sensation are impaired, due to pathological changes in the spinothalamic tracts, and there may even be a sensory 'level' on the trunk.

Disturbances of motor function result from a disturbance of function in the pyramidal tracts. This gives rise to the characteristic stiffness and slowness of the gait which develops in a case of spastic paraparesis of whatever cause. The abdominal reflexes are lost, and the lower limb reflexes may be exaggerated, with clonus, unless the lesions in the sensory pathways have interrupted the reflex arc; the plantar responses are extensor. The condition is, however, very variable in presentation. Usually sensory symptoms are predominant but there is a significant proportion of cases in which spasticity of the lower limbs is striking and signs of posterior column involvement, though present, are relatively slight. Hence this diagnosis should be seriously considered in any case of spastic paraplegia which develops subacutely in adult life; even if examination of the peripheral blood and bone-marrow reveals no abnormality it is usually essential to examine the gastric juice for the presence of free hydrochloric acid. If histamine-fast achlorhydria is discovered, estimation of the level of vitamin B_{12} in the serum may then be an essential investigation. It should also be remembered that even when gastric acidity is normal,

B_{12} deficiency can result from intestinal malabsorption or from a small bowel 'blind-loop' syndrome. It is of the greatest importance to recognise this condition as early as possible, as the neurological manifestations can resolve completely following treatment with parenteral vitamin B_{12}. Sensory symptoms and signs are usually the first to improve and may be completely relieved, but if there is a spastic paraplegia of moderate severity before treatment is begun, there is usually some persistent residual disability.

NERVOUS DISORDERS DUE TO PHYSICAL AGENTS

There are a number of physical agents which, though influencing the metabolic behaviour of many of the tissues of the body, have a particular tendency to impair profoundly the functioning of the central and peripheral nervous system. Among the aetiological agents which are important in this connexion are oxygen lack (anoxia, hypoxia), electricity, decompression sickness, excessive heat, and excessive cold. Radiation injury, due either to excessive exposure to X-rays or to atomic explosions, has comparatively little effect upon the nervous system when compared with the severe damage which may be caused to the haematopoietic system. However, therapeutic irradiation of the neck or mediastinum is sometimes followed within six to twelve months by the development of a slowly progressive spastic paraparesis with sensory impairment in the lower limbs (**post-radiation myelopathy**).

Anoxia

The commonest varieties of anoxia met with in clinical practice are those in which there is deficient oxygenation of the arterial blood due either to a failure of adequate quantities of oxygen to reach the lungs (high altitudes, drowning); or to diminished oxygenation resulting from pulmonary disease (emphysema); or anaemic anoxia in which there is a deficiency in circulating haemoglobin or a chemical alteration in the haemoglobin which prevents it from carrying oxygen. Local anoxia of the tissues can of course be due to arterial disease producing ischaemia. Oxygen lack may have a profound effect upon the brain, but the spinal cord and peripheral nerves seem capable of resisting degrees of anoxia which produce irreversible cerebral damage. Common causes of severe cerebral anoxia include carbon monoxide poisoning and cardiac arrest during anaesthesia. When the oxygen supply to the brain is moderately reduced over a long period, the most frequent symptoms are fatigue, drowsiness, apathy and failure of attention, followed later by impairment of judgement and of memory, ataxia and inco-ordination. Sudden profound anoxia produces almost instantanous loss of the senses, and normally the brain cannot withstand more than three minutes of total anoxia, after cardiac arrest. If the period of anoxia is considerably more prolonged, respiration ceases and death rapidly ensues. After a period of from five to fifteen minutes of cardiac arrest, even if the circulation is re-established, the patient may survive for a time in a semicomatose decerebrate state but full intellectual function is never restored. Even after less prolonged periods of anoxia the patient may regain full control of his limbs, and consciousness is restored after several hours or days, but there is commonly some degree of permanent intellectual deficit; epileptic seizures of temporal-lobe type are a frequent sequel, resulting from the pathological changes which anoxia commonly produces in Ammon's horn and in contiguous areas of the hippocampus. In some cases of carbon monoxide poisoning the patient is initially unconscious but then may regain his senses at least to some extent after twenty-four or forty-eight hours. A relatively lucid interval may then be followed by progressively deepening coma and death (post-anoxic encephalopathy). In other cases a surprising degree of recovery may occur after prolonged unconsciousness so that the prognosis is difficult to predict in any single case.

Electrical Injuries

Electrocution, occurring either as a result of accidental contact with an electrical supply or from being struck by lightning, can be immediately fatal due to cardiac arrest. In such cases there are extensive pathological changes in the brain, muscles and peripheral nerves as well as in other tissues. Less severe and more localised injuries commonly produce extensive burning or electrical necrosis of the tissues. It is not uncommon in such cases for a temporary flaccid paralysis of the lower limbs to occur, with sensory loss; this usually passes off in twenty-four hours and is believed to be due to profound vasoconstriction in the arteries of the spinal cord. A variety of other syndromes resulting from focal injury to the brain, spinal cord or peripheral nerves may occur in other cases.

Decompression Sickness

This condition, which is commonest in divers and in tunnel workers who work in an atmosphere of compressed air, is due to the release of bubbles of nitrogen into the blood stream during the process of decompression. A variety of neurological symptoms, including hemiplegia, paraplegia, scotomas in the visual fields, vertigo and diplopia can occur in such cases, presumably as a result of gas embolism of the arteries of the brain or spinal cord. The development of symptoms of this type in a compressed-air worker is an indication for immediate recompression in a compressed-air chamber, a measure which will almost invariably relieve the symptoms; subsequently decompression must be repeated much more slowly. Non-neurological symptoms include chest pain, dyspnoea, cough, aching in the limbs and infarction of the bones, with subsequent arthropathy, particularly of the hip joints.

Heat Stroke

In an individual who has been exposed to a consistently high environmental temperature, the typical manifestations of heat stroke are a rapidly mounting temperature and a hot dry skin with total absence of sweating. The patient is at first apathetic, later stuporose or comatose, and convulsions are common. Circulatory collapse will soon follow if rapid cooling is not instituted. Variable degrees of cerebral damage may persist even in those patients who recover; variable confusion, slurring dysarthria, and ataxia are common during the phase of recovery. Indeed, the Purkinje cells of the cerebellum are particularly sensitive to heat injury and a severe cerebellar ataxia may persist as a permanent sequel.

Hypothermia

Accidental hypothermia is usually a result of prolonged exposure or immersion in cold water. Hypothermic coma is, however, an occasional complication of myxoedema and can occur without obvious physical cause in elderly people living in unheated rooms in cold weather. Induced hypothermia is nowadays commonly used as an adjunct to anaesthesia; this too may have important complications and sequelae. Unduly prolonged hypothermia can lead to convulsions, irreversible coma, cardiac arrest and death, while hypothermia which has been excessive but less prolonged can lead to sequelae similar to those of cerebral anoxia. Semicoma, confusion and a curious alternating rigidity of the limbs with coarse myoclonic jerking are sometimes seen during recovery. Immersion foot is a syndrome of local hypothermia involving the lower limbs; it occurs particularly in shipwreck survivors and in soldiers living in trenches whose feet have been cold for a prolonged period. In this condition there are extensive pathological changes in peripheral nerves, muscles and blood vessels and the neurological symptoms and signs are those of a severe peripheral neuropathy which may or may not be associated with gangrene. In frost-bite, by contrast, the principal pathological changes are in the blood vessels, and symptoms and signs of peripheral nerve injury are unobtrusive.

DISORDERS DUE TO DRUGS AND OTHER CHEMICAL AGENTS

Whereas a great many drugs may, if taken to excess, produce manifestations of disordered nervous activity, those most commonly encountered in clinical practice as a cause of poisoning or intoxication are alcohol, either ethyl or methyl, barbiturates, opiates, amphetamine and its derivatives, and heavy metals. Intoxication may result from excessive indulgence in the drug over a prolonged period or it may be acute, as in a suicidal attempt. In the case of heavy metals, it is usually due to accidental ingestion, often in the course of the patient's occupation. Not only are the symptoms induced by some of these drugs themselves of considerable importance and interest, but a characteristic clinical syndrome may follow their sudden withdrawal.

Alcoholism

Chronic alcoholism due to an excessive intake of ethyl alcohol is a form of drug addiction like any other and as a rule has potent psychological causes. It can develop insidiously in an individual who is at first merely a social drinker. Gradually his or her consumption of alcohol steadily increases so that any excuse or opportunity, however trivial, is regarded as a reason for having a drink, or another drink. It is when the patient begins to drink alone, when alcoholic beverages take the place of his meals, and when he has a compulsive and irresistible urge to drink, no matter the time of day, that he becomes an alcoholic. The individual who indulges in occasional episodes of excessive drinking with intervals of abstinence is not strictly an alcoholic, though he may become so if the intervals between the episodes shorten progressively, or if his debauches last for days rather than hours (a 'lost weekend'). Only occasionally does alcoholism develop quickly as a result of acute emotional stress and then it usually implies a basically insecure personality. Even small quantities of alcohol impair significantly the performance of skilled motor activity as well as mental functions. Although the individual who has taken one or two drinks may be elated and may feel himself to be in a state of heightened perception, his reaction time is increased and his senses are dulled. Alcohol also increases water and electrolyte excretion by the kidneys and this has a diuretic effect. Dehydration and gastrointestinal irritation are largely responsible for so-called 'hangover' symptoms, including headache.

The symptoms of alcoholism are first gastrointestinal, and secondly nervous. The principal **gastrointestinal symptoms** are nausea, anorexia and diarrhoea, due to chronic gastritis and enteritis; these frequently contribute to malnutrition which in turn results in **polyneuropathy** and/or **Wernicke's encephalopathy** (*vide supra*). So-called alcoholic cirrhosis of the liver, generally a sequel of long-continued alcoholism, is probably a result of associated nutritional deficiency combined with the toxic effects of alcohol. The **nervous symptoms** can be divided into those resulting from acute intoxication and those which follow alcohol withdrawal. The symptoms and signs of acute alcoholic intoxication are well-known. The speech is slurred, the gait unsteady and the patient is either jocular and inattentive, noisy and aggressive, or dulled, confused and retarded. More severe degrees of intoxication result in stupor or coma; the diagnosis must be made not only upon the flushed face and alcohol-laden breath, but upon the absence of signs of other diseases of the nervous system; it must always be remembered that subarachnoid haemorrhage, for instance, can occur during an alcoholic debauch. Pure alcoholic coma, however, is rarely deep or prolonged, and focal neurological signs are not discovered. It is important to realise that although an estimation of blood-alcohol level may indicate the amount of alcohol that the individual has consumed, it is unsafe to regard this level as signifying the degree of clinical intoxication, as individual tolerance varies widely and depends to some extent upon habituation.

A wide variety of symptoms and physical signs may be provoked by the **withdrawal of alcohol** after prolonged intoxication or after several days of particularly heavy drinking. The commonest feature of this state is a state of nervousness or **intense tremulousness** ('the shakes'), which is relieved by a further intake of alcohol, but returns more severely when once again the patient abstains. He is alert, jumpy and easily startled, and has a marked tremor of the limbs. Sometimes these symptoms settle within a few days but occasionally there is a superadded **hallucinosis** which can take the form of vivid visual experiences, or less commonly auditory hallucinations, in the form of voices, motor cars, radios and the like. Occasionally, too, a series of convulsions ('rum fits') occur during this stage. The most severe of all the symptoms of alcoholic withdrawal is **delirium tremens.** It commonly develops two to four days after the last drink and usually does so in individuals who have been excessive drinkers for several years. Often it is seen when the patient develops an intercurrent illness such as pneumonia or is admitted to hospital for an operation, or following an accident. The patient is typically restless, voluble and sleepless, living in a state of intense physical and mental activity both day and night. At the same time there are tremor of the limbs, intermittent muscular twitching, confusion and, as a rule, hallucinations. A fatal outcome, resulting from circulatory failure or even, in certain cases, from exhaustion despite sedation, is not uncommon. In most instances the illness last for three to four days, and the patient at last goes into a calm sleep and awakens lucid but amnesic, having no recollection of the period of his illness.

Among the much less common syndromes which result from alcoholism are **alcoholic cerebellar degeneration,** which gives a progressive, symmetrical cerebellar ataxia of subacute type, and **degeneration of the corpus callosum** (Marchiafava–Bignami disease), a syndrome of progressive dementia with fits and eventual spastic paralysis, which develops almost exclusively in Italian wine-drinking males. Even less common is **central pontine myelinolysis** which gives rise to pseudobulbar palsy and quadriparesis. Alcoholic polyneuropathy has been considered in Chapter 18.

The syndrome produced by the ingestion of **methyl alcohol,** which occurs in methylated-spirit drinkers and in others who consume home-made liquor containing wood alcohol, is characterised by an acute acidosis and by nausea, vomiting, visual loss, muscle pains and impairment of consciousness. If large quantities have been taken, death in coma is not infrequent. If recovery takes place, permanent visual loss due to optic nerve damage is common; some patients remain blind, while others show bilateral central scotomas.

Barbiturate Intoxication

Drugs of the barbiturate group are nowadays prescribed so extensively by the medical profession that they are being used very frequently for suicidal attempts by the depressed patient. Accidental excessive dosage is also seen, when a patient awakens during the night, and being in a bemused state as a result of a tablet taken on retiring, proceeds to take several more. In this connexion it is important to remember that alcohol can greatly potentiate the action of barbiturates. There are also a number of individuals to whom these drugs have been given for purposes of sedation who gradually increase their habitual dose and thus develop a syndrome of chronic barbiturate intoxication.

Symptoms of **acute barbiturate poisoning** depend upon the dose taken. Mild intoxication results from taking about two or three times the maximum recommended dose; the patient is drowsy, but easily awakened and often there are nystagmus, dysarthria and ataxia. When the dose is five to ten times the normal, the patient is semicomatose and can only be awakened by the most vigorous stimulation, when he may mutter a few words and will then lapse again into unconsciousness. The patient who has taken from fifteen to twenty times the usual dose or more is deeply comatose with shallow respiration, absent reflexes and extensor plantar responses; sometimes blisters develop on the feet and legs. When the patient is in this condition, which can be fatal, treatment is imperative (*see* Chapter 20).

The clinical features of **chronic barbiturate intoxication** and those of withdrawal are very similar to those of alcoholism. Increasing tolerance can be considerable, so that the patient who is habituated is able to take many times the recommended dose of the drug with comparatively little clinical effect. Characteristically the barbiturate addict is slow in his mental reactions, his perception is dulled and he is slovenly in his dress and habits. The physical signs are those of nystagmus, dysarthria and cerebellar ataxia. Withdrawal of the drug is followed by a few hours of temporary improvement but later by tremulousness, nervousness, weakness and confusion. There may be a phase of delirium with hallucinations and delusions, and major convulsions are particularly common following barbiturate withdrawal.

Amphetamine Intoxication

Amphetamine drugs and related compounds (benzedrine, dexedrine, preludin) have been increasingly used in recent years not only for their stimulant and antidepressive effects, but also in order to reduce appetite in patients who are attempting to lose weight. It is not uncommon in such individuals for the dose to be steadily increased up to a point where symptoms of intoxication or of chronic addiction appear. The principal symptoms of overdosage are restlessness and overactivity, dryness of the mouth, tremor, palpitations and tachycardia, hallucinations, irritability and profound insomnia. Very heavy dosage can produce fits, hypertension and fatal ventricular arrhythmia. The withdrawal of amphetamines is followed by an acute delirious state with severe hallucinations and sometimes by a delusional psychosis which may last for days or weeks.

Opiates

The drugs of the opiate group which are occasionally a cause of symptoms indicating intoxication are opium itself and its tincture (laudanum), morphine, heroin (diacetylmorphine), dilaudid (dihydromorphine) and codeine (methylmorphine.) Synthetic analgesics such as pethidine (demerol), methadone and dromoran are similar pharmacologically and can also give rise to addiction; so they are conveniently considered together with the true opiates.

Acute poisoning with drugs in this category is relatively uncommon except as a result of accidental ingestion or mistakes in dispensing, as the issue of these remedies is carefully controlled by law. The usual clinical features are stupor or coma, pin-point pupils, shallow respiration and bradycardia.

Chronic **opiate intoxication or addiction** is characterised by an initial phase of tolerance in which increasing doses of the drug are required to produce the desired effect, whether it be the pleasurable feeling of detachment which first encourages the eventual addict to use these drugs, or the relief of symptoms for which the drug was initially prescribed. Prolonged therapeutic use of these drugs in illness is a potent cause of addiction, particularly in doctors and nurses. The phase of tolerance is followed by one of drug dependence, in which attempted withdrawal results in the development of a series of characteristic symptoms. Some twelve hours or so after the last dose the patient begins to yawn repeatedly and there is lacrimation and running of the nose. This is followed by restlessness, insomnia, muscular twitching, generalised aching and shivering, and then by nausea, vomiting and diarrhoea. Commonly, these acute symptoms last for two or three days, but insomnia and weakness can persist for several days or even for weeks. Even when the stage of withdrawal and physical dependence has passed, emotional dependence or habituation remains and is an important cause of relapse. Physical, mental and moral dilapidation is an invariable sequel in the established addict, and the majority of addicts will resort to any measure involving lying, feigning illness and a variety of other subterfuges in order to obtain supplies of the drug.

Heavy Metals

Whereas poisoning with a considerable number of heavy metals is accompanied by symptoms indicating involvement of the nervous system, the most important in clinical practice are arsenic, lead and mercury.

ARSENICAL POISONING

The principal symptoms of acute arsenical poisoning are gastro-intestinal, namely vomiting, diarrhoea and acute abdominal pain, though convulsions may occur. In chronic arsenical poisoning, however, whether resulting from criminal intent, from the excessive use of therapeutic arsenical preparations, or from contamination of food with arsenical insecticides, the main symptoms are neurological though hyperkeratosis, pigmentation and desquamation of the skin are also common. The nervous symptoms include headache, drowsiness, confusion and a symmetrical polyneuropathy which gives burning paraesthesiae in the extremities followed by muscular weakness and atrophy, distal sensory loss and absence of the tendon reflexes.

LEAD POISONING

In children, the principal symptom of lead poisoning, which has sometimes resulted from chewing painted objects covered with lead paint, is an encephalopathy giving rise to somnolence, convulsions and coma. In adults, and particularly in painters using paint which contains lead, agonising colicky abdominal pain and anaemia are often the most frequent presenting symptoms. A peripheral neuropathy is also common, but is rarely symmetrical, and more often affects one limb. Thus it is not infrequent for a worker who is making batteries or accumulators to develop a unilateral wrist drop in the arm most often used, and the presence of a blue line on the gums and of punctate basophilia in the red blood cells will confirm that this is due to lead.

MERCURY POISONING

Acute mercurial poisoning gives severe vomiting and diarrhoea followed by anuria and uraemia due to renal tubular necrosis. In infants, however, chronic mercurial poisoning due to excessive use of calomel teething powders is probably the cause of most cases of pink disease (acrodynia). A syndrome of chronic mercurial poisoning in adults has been described, due either to the inhalation of mercury vapour or in police officers working with mercurial finger-print powders. In some instances this has produced a cerebellar ataxia, but more often a syndrome characterised by excessive salivation, tremulousness, vertigo, irritability and depression or erethism (childish over-emotionalism) occurs.

An attempt has been made above to outline the symptoms of nervous dysfunction which can result from a variety of drugs and other poisons. There are many other poisons which give rise to neurological symptoms, but these are much less commonly encountered in clinical practice. Thus atropine and related drugs in excess produce a clinical picture of nervous excitation and confusion which may progress to mania; bromism, which is rarely observed nowadays, is characterised by drowsiness, lethargy, dysarthria and sometimes by psychosis. Chloral hydrate has an effect similar to alcohol, and antihistamine drugs too may produce lethargy or coma and sometimes convulsions in children. For a full description of the effects of these and of the many other drugs which affect the nervous system if taken to excess, the reader is referred to textbooks of medicine and toxicology.

NEUROLOGICAL COMPLICATIONS OF ENDOCRINE DISEASE

It is becoming increasingly recognised that neurological symptoms and signs are sometimes produced by hormonal abnormalities resulting from disease of the ductless glands. Thus in **hypopituitarism,** leaving aside the local effects of the pituitary tumours (chromophobe adenomas) which sometimes produce this syndrome, it is not uncommon for widespread muscular weakness and atrophy to develop. These improve when the hypopituitarism is treated. In **Cushing's syndrome,** which is due as a rule to hyperadrenalism, and much less commonly to a basophil adenoma of the pituitary (a tumour which is never large enough to produce local symptoms), mental symptoms, including depression, paranoid ideas and confusional episodes are not uncommon, while occasionally there is clinical evidence of increased intracranial pressure, with headache and papilloedema. A myopathy, often painful, and usually affecting thigh muscles predominantly to give weakness, atrophy and histological changes, has also been observed in some patients with Cushing's syndrome, and resembles the so-called steroid myopathy seen in some patients who are being treated for long periods with steroid drugs (particularly triamcinolone). The exact pathogenesis of **exophthalmic ophthalmoplegia** remains in doubt, but this syndrome is still believed by many to result from an excessive output of pituitary thyrotropic hormone. Histologically there is striking oedema of the orbital muscles and of other tissues. The first symptom is usually severe pain in one eye followed by unilateral exophthalmos and diplopia. Often the superior rectus or superior oblique is the first muscle to become paretic. Although exophthalmos may be predominantly unilateral for some time, the other eye is eventually affected, and paresis of several extrinsic ocular muscles becomes apparent. Occasionally the degree of exophthalmos is sufficiently severe for orbital decompression to be imperative but in less severe cases it can be reduced by radiotherapy. The syndrome sometimes develops acutely after thyroidectomy. Usually there are few if any symptoms of thyrotoxicosis.

Thyrotoxicosis (primary Graves' disease) is occasionally sufficiently acute to produce a severe confusional state, but this is uncommon. It is sometimes associated with myasthenia gravis and a rare syndrome of thyrotoxic periodic paralysis, which clears up when the thyrotoxicosis is relieved by surgery or drugs, has been described. A more common complication is a myopathy of girdle and proximal limb muscles (thyrotoxic myopathy). This condition improves, and generally recovers completely, when the thyrotoxicosis is adequately treated. In severe **myxoedema,** hypothermic coma is an occasional complication due to lowering of the body temperature, while acute psychiatric episodes (myxoedematous madness) and even a reversible syndrome of depression and mild dementia may occur. More often there is muscular pain and aching, accentuated by exertion, with overall slowness of muscular contraction and relaxation (pseudomyotonia). These symptoms respond to treatment with thyroid hormone.

In **diabetes mellitus,** polyneuropathy is a well-recognised complication (*see* Chap. 18). It has been suggested that lesions in the spinal cord (diabetic myelopathy) also occur, but this is not yet fully substantiated. Isolated cranial nerve palsies of the third and sixth cranial nerves are also a common complication, but usually clear up spontaneously within a few weeks or months. An important complication, not of diabetes itself, but of its treatment, is **hypoglycaemia,** resulting from excessive insulin administration. Excessively low blood-sugar readings are also seen in some cases of hypopituitarism, in patients with hyperinsulinism due to an adenoma of the islets of Langerhans, and sometimes in insulin coma when used as a form of treatment for schizophrenia. The first symptom of hypoglycaemia is commonly profuse sweating and light-headedness followed by confusion and sometimes abnormal behaviour. Vertigo, diplopia and a variety of other nervous symptoms occasionally occur. Gradually the patient lapses into coma and is found, sweating profusely, with flaccid limbs and extensor plantar responses. If the coma is severe, generalised epileptiform convulsions may develop. A deep hypoglycaemic coma which lasts more than a few hours can produce permanent cerebral damage, with clinical after-effects and histopathological changes resembling those of anoxia. Even after several hours of unconsciousness, however, complete recovery is still possible, but often takes several days. A rare complication of hyperinsulinism is a peripheral neuropathy of motor type.

Lassitude and asthenia are salient clinical features of **Addison's disease,** which results from hypoadrenalism, but in addition, progressive muscular weakness and wasting (Addisonian myopathy) occur in some cases, while papilloedema due to cerebral oedema has also been described. A myopathy, responsible for symptoms of generalised muscular weakness, is also an occasional feature of **hypoparathyroidism,** while paradoxically, muscular weakness, lassitude and polyuria can also be prominent in cases of hyperparathyroidism due to a parathyroid adenoma. In hypoparathyroidism following accidental operative removal of the parathyroid glands, or in **hypocalcaemia** due to any cause, there is excessive neuromuscular irritability, giving rise to tetany and a positive Cvostek's sign. Idiopathic hypoparathyroidism is much less common, but in this condition, mental defect, recurrent major fits and calcification of the basal ganglia are constant features. The severity and frequency of the attacks of epilepsy are greatly reduced by treatment with calciferol or dihydrotachysterol.

PORPHYRIA

The term porphyria embraces a group of diseases which have in common the excretion of excessive amounts of uroporphyrin and coproporphyrin and of porphyrin precursors (porphobilinogen) in the urine.

Congenital porphyria is a rare inherited disorder in which there is excessive photosensitivity from birth. Any exposure to sunlight results in blistering of the skin, and porphyrins are laid down in the affected area to give pigmentation; eventually extensive scarring takes place. When a similar disorder develops in adult life it is known as **porphyria cutanea tarda.**

It is, however, in **acute idiopathic porphyria,** which is also the result of an inborn error of metabolism, that neurological manifestations occur. Attacks of this condition can be produced by the administration of drugs, particularly barbiturates and sulphonamides. They occur usually in early adult life and in either sex. The cardinal manifestations are attacks of abdominal pain which are often diagnosed initially as acute surgical emergencies, episodes of mental confusion, and the development of a polyneuropathy. Bulbar paralysis occasionally occurs. During latent periods between attacks there is generally excessive porphobilinogen in the urine, but in the acute episodes, which can be provoked by drugs, the urine is port-wine coloured and contains large quantities of porphyrins. Remissions invariably occur and can last weeks, months or years, but many patients are seriously disabled by the polyneuropathy, even though this, too, may remit.

HEPATIC COMA (PORTAL-SYSTEMIC ENCEPHALOPATHY)

In patients with liver disease, either acute hepatic necrosis or chronic cirrhosis, a number of characteristic neurological symptoms and signs can result from the fact that blood from the bowel, containing large amounts of nitrogenous substances, by-passes the liver through anastomoses between the portal and systemic arterial systems, and enters the systemic circulation. These nitrogenous substances, of which the level of blood ammonia is a useful index, can have a profound effect upon the brain. The early symptoms of 'hepatic coma' are confusion, apathy, difficulty in concentration and inappropriate behaviour. Gradually the patient may lapse into coma. In certain cases the patients enter a chronic phase which is characterised by episodic confusion and abnormal behaviour; this may last for several weeks or months and is sometimes wrongly attributed to cerebral atherosclerosis or to presenile dementia, if clinical evidence of liver disease is unobtrusive. Although exaggeration of tendon reflexes is commonly discovered, the most important neurological sign, which is almost pathognomonic, is a flapping tremor of the outstretched hands, a movement which is reminiscent of the flapping of a bird's wings. The electroencephalogram in such cases reveals diffuse slow activity.

Clearly the mechanism by which this condition is produced is enhanced by surgical procedures which create artificial anastomoses between the portal and systemic circulations. Episodes of encephalopathy can follow a high-protein meal, or a gastrointestinal haemorrhage (due to absorption of blood products). Treatment consists of a low-protein diet and the regular administration of intestinal antibiotics (e.g. neomycin) which destroy bacterial flora and so reduce the absorption of protein derivatives.

HEPATOLENTICULAR DEGENERATION (*Wilson's Disease*)

Hepatolenticular degeneration was first clearly defined by Kinnier Wilson in 1912, although similar cases had previously been described by Westphal and Strumpell under the title of pseudosclerosis. This condition, which affects either sex, is familial, being due to an autosomal recessive gene, so that it can affect several members of a sibship, but there is generally no history of the disease having affected members of the family in previous generations. It usually begins during the first two decades and is characterised first by the appearance of symptoms indicating progressive degeneration of the basal ganglia, secondly by the development of cirrhosis of the liver, and thirdly by the presence of a ring of brown pigment around the margin of the cornea, the Kayser–Fleischer ring. It is now apparent that the primary defect is one of copper metabolism and copper is deposited in the brain and liver as well as in the periphery of the cornea. Characteristic biochemical features include amino-aciduria, an excessive output of copper in the urine (normal upper limit 70 μg/24 hr), and a reduction of the serum copper level (normal range 75-100 μg/100 ml); the serum copper oxidase is also reduced. The primary defect appears to be a congenital deficiency of caeruloplasmin, the copper-binding fraction of the serum proteins; as there is too little of this substance available to absorb ingested copper, the latter is either deposited in the tissues or excreted in the urine.

The principal clinical manifestations are usually neurological although occasionally symptoms of liver disease (jaundice, ascites, splenomegaly) predominate. The neurological manifestations, which generally begin in adolescence, include facial grimacing, tremor, dysarthria, ataxia and personality change. The tremor is usually of

N

the action type, but is sometimes present at rest, as in Parkinson's disease, or accentuated towards the end of movement, as in cerebellar ataxia. Sometimes there is a flapping or wing-beating movement of the outstretched hands, as in patients with hepatic coma, and occasionally choreiform or athetoid posturing of the limbs, or plastic rigidity, are observed. Speech is invariably slurred, and facile euphoria or intellectual deterioration are frequent in the later stages. There are as a rule no changes in the reflexes or in sensation and the plantar responses are flexor. Often there is little clinical evidence of hepatic dysfunction, but spider naevi on the skin, 'liver palms', and splenomegaly are not infrequent, while gastrointestinal bleeding from oesophageal varices is an important complication, and liver function tests usually gives results which are grossly abnormal.

If untreated, the disease is usually fatal in five to fifteen years from the onset; neurological disability is progressive, leading to immobility, emaciation and dementia, and death is usually due to intercurrent infection, gastrointestinal haemorrhage, or hepatic failure. There is considerable evidence, however, that treatment with BAL (dimercaprol) or with calcium EDTA (versene) may modify the course of the disease, as these agents promote copper excretion. However, these agents have now been superseded by penicillamine (dimethylcysteine) which should be given continuously in a dosage of 1-1·5 g daily. If treated early enough the disease is completely controlled and affected individuals become virtually normal, both mentally and physically, and remain so.

Potassium sulphide in a dosage of 20 mg three times daily diminishes the absorption of copper and is a useful adjuvant.

REFERENCES

CARTWRIGHT, G. E., 'Hepatolenticular degeneration' and 'Disorders of porphyrin metabolism', in *Principles of Internal Medicine*, Ed. Harrison, T. R., 4th ed., Chapters 91 and 93 (New York, McGraw-Hill, 1962).

CUMINGS, J. N., *Heavy Metals and the Brain* (Oxford, Blackwell, 1959).

CUMINGS, J. N. and KREMER, M. (Eds.), *Biochemical Aspects of Neurological Disorders*, 1st and 2nd series (Oxford, Blackwell, 1959 and 1965).

KENNEDY, A., 'Alcoholism', in *Early Diagnosis*, Ed. Miller, H. G. (Edinburgh, Livingstone, 1959).

SPILLANE, J. D., *Nutritional Disorders of the Nervous System* (Edinburgh, Livingstone, 1947).

VICTOR, M. and ADAMS, R. D., 'Alcohol', 'Barbiturates' and 'Nutritional disorders of the nervous system', in *Principles of Internal Medicine*, Ed. Harrison, T. R., 4th ed., Chapters 99, 101 and 288 (New York, McGraw-Hill, 1962).

WALSHE, J. M., 'Neurological complications of liver disease and hepato-lenticular degeneration', in *Diseases of the Nervous System*, Ed. Walshe, F. M. R., 11th ed., Chapters 12 and 13 (Edinburgh, Livingstone, 1958).

CHAPTER 20

TREATMENT IN NEUROLOGY — AN OUTLINE

WHEREAS the preceding chapters have been concerned with the foundations of neurological diagnosis and with descriptions of specific syndromes in which the functioning of the nervous system is disordered, it must be remembered that it is the treatment of the patient's disease and not diagnosis itself which is, or should be, the ultimate aim. While accurate diagnosis of the nature of the illness may be an essential first step before appropriate therapeutic measures can be recommended, this is not always the case and there are certain patients suffering from nervous disease in whom the correct management is clearly apparent even though diagnosis remains obscure. In a case of progressive dementia arising in the presenium, for instance, there may be no certain means of deciding whether the illness is the result of cerebral degeneration or of atherosclerosis. Provided, however, that treatable conditions such as general paresis, vitamin B_{12} deficiency and frontal meningioma have been excluded, management then depends upon the patient's behaviour and social circumstances. If he is placid and manageable, despite his dementia and associated incontinence, and if he has a capable wife or other female relatives, the situation should be explained to his relatives and he should be nursed at home with suitable sedative drugs and nursing assistance. But if, on the other hand, he is violent or severely disturbed in his behaviour, if he lives alone, or if his relatives are frail or incompetent, there will generally be no alternative to arranging for the patient's admission to a mental hospital.

Treatment, it must be remembered, is not merely a matter of prescribing drugs, and of seeing that they are properly administered (a problem which is sometimes much more difficult than the simple act of writing a prescription). It also involves management of the individual and of his relatives. When should the patient be treated and nursed at home and when in hospital? How far should special investigations be pursued, particularly if they are unpleasant or potentially dangerous? Are they to be carried out because of possible benefit to the patient, or merely to satisfy the doctor's curiosity? How much should the patient be told of the nature and prognosis of his illness, and how much information should be given to his family? When is it necessary to ask for a second opinion? These are questions which arise every day in clinical practice and unfortunately they cannot easily be answered in the pages of a textbook. The ability to solve these problems with tact, patience and understanding stems not only from a knowledge of disease, but also from experience of patients as individuals and of their personalities, emotional reactions and family background. So diverse may be the personal and domestic circumstances of two patients suffering from identical illnesses, that although the correct treatment in a pharmacological sense is similar in the two cases, the appropriate management when considered in more general terms may be totally different. The first and most important lesson that the student must learn is that his value as a doctor in the community does not depend merely upon his ability to diagnose illness and to prescribe appropriate drugs, but also upon the way in which he manages sick people and their relatives.

When one comes to consider specific disorders of the nervous system, it is now apparent that an increasing number of conditions can be cured or benefited by pharmacological or surgical methods of treatment. Even in the large number of neurological disorders in which the basic pathological process is relatively uninfluenced by any form of treatment which is at present available, substantial improvement in the patient's symptoms or in his own attitude to his disease can be achieved by means of drugs or with physical methods of treatment. Often it is of the greatest value to the patient if the doctor can do no more than give an accurate forecast of the natural history and eventual outcome of the illness. In the case of inherited conditions, it is also important to be able to give appropriate advice concerning the prospects which exist of other members of the family being affected, if this information is sought, and particularly if the parents of an ill child are considering adding to their family. If, on the other hand, they already have other children, if may be wise to conceal the possibility that they may be affected until the parents become aware of the possibility themselves. It is also preferable in cases of progressively crippling illness, to keep a glimmer of hope alive by referring to research work which is being done in many parts of the world upon the chronic neurological diseases and by saying that these are not incurable conditions, but rather diseases for which the cure has not yet been found. It is, however, equally important to be sure in such a case that the hopes of the patient and his relatives should not be too lavishly encouraged, only to be shattered by the subsequent course of events.

Although treatment of individual syndromes was touched upon briefly when they were described in many of the preceding chapters, it is now proposed to give in outline some of the principal methods of treatment of neurological diseases and also methods which can be employed for the relief of important symptoms of disordered nervous function.

N*

THE RELIEF OF PAIN

As mentioned in Chapter 4, pain is a common symptom of nervous disease, and the doctor is frequently called upon to choose an appropriate remedy for its relief. Much depends upon its severity, its situation and its cause. Musculoskeletal pain which is relatively mild and not due to serious organic disease can be relieved by the local application of heat, or by immobilisation, while the most appropriate remedy for headaches which result from muscular tension is not analgesic drugs but sedatives (*vide infra*) designed to relieve emotional stress. When the cause of the pain cannot immediately be eliminated, however, analgesic remedies are commonly indicated in order to produce symptomatic relief. Of these the one most commonly prescribed is aspirin (acetylsalicylic acid) in various forms, usually in a dosage of 10-15 gr (600-900 mg) in adults. Children may require a dosage of 1-10 gr depending upon their age. The irritative effect of this drug upon the gastrointestinal system, and the dangers of gastric haemorrhage, are reduced to some extent by utilising neutral soluble aspirin ('disprin', 'solprin', 'paynocil'). Another mild and useful remedy is paracetamol (500-1000 mg every four hours). When the relief obtained from aspirin is inadequate, owing to the severity of the pain, it is often sufficient to utilise compound tablets containing a combination of aspirin, phenacetin and codeine. The usual dosage of tab. codeine co. in adults is two tablets, in children from five to ten years of age, one tablet, and this dose can be repeated every four to six hours if necessary. Often headache, and pain of nerve or nerve-root compression of moderate severity is substantially relieved by the use of these tablets. More severe and continuous pain may, however, require more powerful remedies; one such is dihydrocodeine (30-60 mg) and yet another is propoxyphene (65 mg). It should always be remembered that all of the more powerful analgesics are drugs of addiction which should therefore be used sparingly. These powerful remedies are nevertheless appropriate when pain is the result of a self-limiting illness in which analgesics will only be required for a few days or at the most for a few weeks. When the duration of the illness is likely to be measured in months, it is generally unwise to begin treatment with these remedies, unless the patient's expectation of life is short, either because of the nature of the disease, or on account of his age. In younger patients suffering from chronic pain, it is important to persist with the less powerful analgesics or to employ physical or surgical methods for its relief, for the patient may very readily become addicted to the more powerful remedies. Of these powerful drugs, morphine and its derivatives remain the most satisfactory, except in patients with increased intracranial pressure or intrathoracic disease, in whom the depressant effect of these remedies upon respiratory function can be dangerous. The average adult dose of morphine sulphate is 16 mg by injection, but for a maximum analgesic effect, up to 32 mg can be given, except in elderly patients. Dihydromorphone (dilaudid) is a similar preparation, of which the dose is 2 mg. The newer drug levorphanol tartrate (dromoran) is more powerful than morphine but is similar in its side-effects and in its tendency to produce addiction. It is given in an oral dose of 1·5-3 mg or 2 mg by subcutaneous or intramuscular injection. Each of these drugs may be given every four hours if necessary. Very large doses of morphine (up to 120 mg) can often be tolerated if given in combination with daptazole (12·5-15 mg), as the latter drug counteracts the soporific and respiratory depressant effects of morphine.

There are several synthetic analgesics which are comparable with morphine in their analgesic effect, but which are less severe respiratory depressants. Of these, the most commonly employed is pethidine hydrochloride (Demerol) which is given by mouth or by intramuscular injection in a dosage of 25-100 mg. This drug is commonly used for the relief of intense headache resulting from subarachnoid haemorrhage or cerebral tumour; if there is associated vomiting, it is useful to give in addition chlorpromazine 25-50 mg every four to six hours, as this remedy may not only potentiate the action of pethidine but will also assist by reducing the frequency and severity of vomiting. Pethidine is also very useful in the control of severe pain resulting from inflammation or compression of nerve roots. Pethilorfan, a combination of pethidine, 100 mg, with 1·25 mg of levorphan, is a valuable and powerful remedy for very severe pain. A less commonly-employed analgesic which has a similar effect is amidone (physeptone, methadone) which is given in tablet form or by injection in a dosage of 10 mg. Also to be regarded as dangerous drugs which can be habit-forming but which are comparable to morphine in their effects are dipipanone (10 mg) and dextromoramide (5 mg) which can be given in tablet form. Another remedy which is occasionally employed with some success in patients suffering from pain of nerve-root origin, particularly when this is due to chronic degenerative changes in multiple intervertebral disks, is phenylbutazone (butazolidine) in a dosage of 100 mg three or four times daily, but this drug, which has important toxic effects upon the haematopoietic system and upon the kidneys in some cases, is more often utilised in cases of painful arthropathy. Less effective but less toxic and of value in musculoskeletal pain are carisoprodol (175-350 mg) and ethoheptazine (75 mg). These and many other drugs are available commercially in a bewildering variety of combined tablets which may make the choice of remedy in any single case a matter of considerable difficulty, but in general it is wise to begin with simple remedies and only to employ those which are more powerful in resistant cases.

It should also be remembered that the pain (headache) which is produced by increased intracranial pressure can be relieved by measures designed to reduce this pressure. Lumbar puncture is not as a rule indicated under such circumstances because of the danger of tentorial or cerebellar herniation, but detensifying therapy (dehydration) is occasionally successful, at least temporarily. Remedies usually employed to produce this effect are intravenous sucrose (100 ml of a 50 per cent solution every twelve hours) or rectal hypertonic magnesium sulphate (8 oz of a 25 per cent solution every six hours). There is recent evidence that an intravenous infusion of a 30 per cent solution of urea in a dosage of 1·0-1·5 g per kg body weight may be even more effective but this remedy has a temporary effect only and is best utilised for its immediate effect during a surgical operation. Steroid drugs (prednisone, dexamethasone) are of considerable value in reducing cerebral oedema due to the presence of a brain tumour or to some other cause, while the new and powerful diuretic frusemide (40-120 mg) is also useful in this connexion.

Whereas the pain of self-limiting or treatable diseases can be successfully relieved by means of the therapeutic agents described above, **intractable pain** which is resistant to the milder analgesics presents a much more difficult problem of management. In certain cases, local physical measures are effective. Thus in a patient with a painful phantom limb following amputation, repeated percussion of a neuroma in the stump several times daily with a rubber mallet or some other appropriate instrument may be helpful. Pain referred to a specific skin area is also relieved on occasion by repeated subcutaneous infiltration around the painful area either with procaine hydrochloride or even with saline. This method occasionally works in cases of persistent postherpetic neuralgia, a syndrome which follows herpes zoster and is particularly troublesome and long-lasting in the elderly. The pain of this condition and many other varieties of intractable cutaneous pain are also relieved in some cases by the application, several times a day, of an electrical vibrator or of an ethyl chloride spray to the affected area of skin.

If local measures of this nature are ineffective, it is often necessary to resort to *surgical methods* of pain relief. First, however, it is wise to try the effect of chlorpromazine in gradually increasing dosage, up to 600 mg daily, if tolerated, as this drug reduces the patient's emotional reaction to his pain, and can almost be considered to produce a pharmacological leucotomy. There are, nevertheless, certain varieties of pain which regularly require surgical treatment. Causalgia, for instance, following peripheral nerve injury, can only be relieved in the majority of cases by sympathectomy, interrupting the autonomic innervation of the affected member. In tic douloureux, if the pain is strictly limited topographically, it is occasionally relieved by operative section of the appropriate peripheral nerve (supraorbital, infraorbital). As a rule, these measures are ineffective, and until recently it has been necessary in most cases to divide the sensory pathway more centrally, either by alcohol injection of the Gasserian ganglion, or by surgical division of the sensory root of the trigeminus. Now, however, the new drug carbamazepine ('tegretol'), given in a dosage of 200 mg three, four or even five times daily has proved to be remarkably successful in relieving pain in the majority of cases, though it may have to be continued for many months until a spontaneous remission occurs. Only patients who are unable to take this drug owing to side-effects or in whom pain relief is inadequate now require injection or surgical treatment. Alcohol or aqueous phenol injection has usually only a temporary effect, giving relief for one to two years in most cases, and is therefore the appropriate method to use in the elderly, but in patients under the age of sixty, surgical division is more suitable. It is important to explain to all patients undergoing these procedures that the affected side of the face will be rendered permanently numb, and one must always be certain that the pain is sufficiently severe for this after-effect to be tolerated. Some patients in whom the pain was not particularly severe or disabling have been known to complain that the cure was worse than the disease. It is also important that these procedures should only be carried out in patients suffering from true tic douloureux, as the pain of atypical facial neuralgia, which is often of emotional origin, is not relieved thereby.

When intractable pain is more extensive, measures which can be utilised, when other methods have failed, include intrathecal injections of phenol in glycerine around appropriate nerve roots, surgical division of the spinothalamic tract in the spinal cord (anterolateral cordotomy), surgical destruction of appropriate thalamic nuclei, utilising stereotaxis, and, as a last resort, prefrontal leucotomy. Leucotomy, which usually must be performed bilaterally, with destruction or sectioning of the white matter in both frontal lobes, does not relieve pain, but by altering the patient's emotional responses, renders it more bearable. However, the selection of appropriate cases of intractable pain in which these skilled techniques are indicated, and the choice of the appropriate method, are matters which are the concern of specialist neurologists and neurosurgeons.

SEDATION

Sedative and hypnotic drugs are required in patients with nervous disease not only in order to control agitation or violent and disturbed behaviour, but also in order to achieve restful sleep in patients whose illness produces sleeplessness. If pain is contributing to the patient's insomnia it is often necessary to give an analgesic as well as a sedative or hypnotic remedy. Drugs which fall into this category are also of value in the relief of anxiety and emotional tension, but the tranquillising remedies will be considered below when the treatment of mental disease is considered.

In restless, disturbed or confused patients suffering from brain disease, the most valuable drug of all is paraldehyde, given in an oral dose of from four to six drams (15-20 ml). Usually, in circumstances where this drug is needed, the patient is insufficiently co-operative for this route to be employed, and while it can be given rectally, it is generally more satisfactory to give 5-10 ml of the drug by deep intramuscular injection. In small children, 1-2 ml may be sufficient, and the dose can be repeated in four to six hours if necessary. This drug is very safe and often remarkably effective. When mental disturbance is less severe, another safe remedy, chloral hydrate, may be employed in an average dose of 1·3-2·0 g. It is often given in the form of a syrup of which the usual dose is half a fluid ounce (15 ml). Correspondingly lower doses are utilised in children, in whom this is a particularly useful hypnotic.

The commonest sedative and hypnotic drugs in use nowadays are those of the barbiturate group. Long-acting barbiturates such as phenobarbitone (dosage 30-120 mg) are slow to have an effect; this remedy is of little value in promoting sleep but is useful for long-continued mild sedation. When a rapid effect is desired, then drugs which act rapidly, such as quinalbarbitone (seconal, 50-200 mg) or cyclobarbitone (phanodorm, 200-400 mg) are more appropriate. However, since the effect of these remedies wears off in about four hours, those drugs which have an activity of medium duration are usually employed to give a more prolonged sleep. In this category are butobarbitone (soneryl, 100-200 mg), pentobarbitone (nembutal, 100-200 mg) and amylobarbitone (sodium amytal, 65-200 mg). There are a great many commercial preparations in which short and medium-acting barbiturates are combined to give a rapid action and a prolonged effect. If a barbiturate must be given parenterally, the drugs usually employed are sodium gardenal (soluble phenobarbitone, 200 mg) or somnifaine (aprobarbital and barbitone, 2-4 ml).

There are numerous other non-barbiturate remedies which also have a mild sedative effect. Among those in common use are carbromal, 300-1,000 mg, which is a derivative of urea, and glutethimide (doriden, 250-500 mg). A useful combined tablet, particularly in elderly confused patients, is carbrital, which contains 250 mg of carbromal and 100 mg pentobarbitone. Because of their side-effects and comparative inefficacy, bromide preparations are now rarely used for the purpose of sedation.

<h2 style="text-align:center">THE MANAGEMENT OF EPILEPSY</h2>

There are now a great many drugs available for the treatment of epilepsy. But the doctor's responsibility does not end when he prescribes appropriate remedies for the control of seizures. There are also social and educational problems in which his help and advice are needed. Since the answer to many of these questions must depend upon the degree to which the attacks can be controlled by medication, and since the medication appropriate to the individual case depends upon the nature of the seizures, it is first important to consider some important points which arise in the investigation of patients who present with recurrent seizures. It is true that brief 'blank spells' occurring in childhood are usually correctly diagnosed as being the result of 'petit mal' epilepsy, a condition which generally responds to drugs of the troxidone (tridione) group. On the other hand, attacks of major epilepsy and those of temporal lobe epilepsy are more appropriately treated by phenobarbitone and the hydantoinates or similar remedies. Phenobarbitone has little effect upon true petit mal, while troxidone sometimes makes major attacks more severe and frequent. When clinical diagnosis is accurate, treatment is often comparatively straightforward, but there are a great many varieties of minor epileptic seizures which are difficult to classify according to clinical criteria, so that the correct choice of drug is not always easy. It is in this respect that the EEG can be of great value. Unfortunately this investigation gives negative findings all too often, despite the utilisation of all available techniques of activation, and under such circumstances, treatment must be based upon clinical evidence alone. Probably, however, an EEG should where practicable, be carried out in the great majority of patients who present for the first time with seizures which are presumed to be epileptic, as it sometimes gives findings which are of great value in deciding upon appropriate treatment.

In a child who is suffering from **petit mal** attacks alone, who has never had a major seizure and whose EEG reveals symmetrical generalised spike-and-wave activity, it is reasonable to begin treatment with troxidone (tridione) in an initial dosage of 0·15-0·3 g twice daily, depending upon age. In a child over the age of three years, the dosage of this drug can be increased if necessary up to the maximum adult dose of 0·3 g four times daily. It is true that some cases of agranulocytosis have been described following the use of this drug, but routine white blood counts are of little or no value in anticipating this complication and it is preferable to warn the parents that the patient should stop the tablets and report to his doctor immediately if he develops a sore throat or a high temperature. Other side-effects, including an acneiform rash and a sensation of 'glare', which is particularly troublesome in bright sunlight, rarely necessitate any reduction in the dose of this drug. Should the patient who is being treated with this drug develop major seizures, then phenobarbitone, or one of the hydantoinates, or a similar remedy, should be added to the troxidone. In patients who experience both petit mal and grand mal from the beginning, treatment should be started with troxidone, phenytoin sodium (epanutin) and phenobarbitone in combination. If troxidone fails to control the minor attacks, then paramethadione (paradione) may be added, in a dosage of up to 0·3 g four times daily, in addition to troxidone, or alternatively phensuximide (milontin) can be given in a dosage of 0·5 g three or four times daily, or acetazolamide (diamox) (250-500 mg each morning) can be tried. Perhaps the most effective of all is the comparatively new remedy ethosuximide ('zarontin') which is given in a dosage of 250 mg, three to six capsules daily. Of these remedies, troxidone, ethosuximide and paramethadione, either alone or combined, seem to be the most effective in petit mal; for very young children, these drugs are available in dulcet or elixir form. Occasionally, combinations of as many as three or four drugs must be tried before maximum effect is obtained. Very occasionally dextroamphetamine sulphate (5-10 mg each morning) appears to have a beneficial effect in minor epilepsy and so does chlortetracycline (aureomycin) 250 mg three times daily, but there are a small number of cases of petit mal which show virtually no response to any form of treatment, and in these individuals it is sometimes preferable to withdraw all medication.

It should always be remembered that in some cases of major or focal epilepsy, including the temporal lobe variety and particularly when the epileptic seizures begin in middle- or late-life, epilepsy is symptomatic of intracranial disease. It is often difficult to be sure how far investigations should be pursued in any case of epilepsy of late onset. It is true that a proportion of such cases eventually prove to be harbouring intracranial neoplasms, but there are a much greater number in which this is not the case. In some of the latter the lesion responsible is a scar in one or other temporal lobe, resulting from birth injury; in others it may be a cortical scar in some other situation resulting from previous head injury or even from asymptomatic infarction. Again in cases of this type, the EEG is of value, as it may demonstate a focus of spike or sharp-wave discharge, or of paroxysmal slow activity either in one or other temporal lobe or in some other situation, indicating that the patient's epilepsy is the result of a localised cerebral lesion. Or occasionally it will show focal slow activity of a type suggesting the presence of a cerebral tumour. In the latter circumstance it will then be wise to proceed to specialised radiological and other studies such as echo-encephalography, gamma-encephalography, angiography or air encephalography. Furthermore, in a small proportion of cases in which a focus of spike discharge has been demonstrated in the EEG and in which anticonvulsant therapy using all available drugs has failed, surgical excision of the epileptogenic lesion, should it be accessible, is indicated. Usually, however, if the EEG is negative, or if it shows focal or generalised spike discharges, and if there are no other symptoms or physical signs indicating brain disease, it is wise to give anticonvulsant drugs and not to carry out air studies routinely, no matter the age of the patient. Should headache, papilloedema or localising neurological signs develop subsequently, specialised radiological studies will then be indicated, but little will usually have been lost during the waiting period.

In the treatment of cases of **major** or **focal (including temporal lobe)** epilepsy in adult life it is usual to begin treatment with 30-60 mg of phenobarbitone twice daily and with phenytoin sodium (epanutin, dilantin) 100 mg twice daily. Children are given proportionately lower doses. An average dose in a child aged five years would be 30 mg of phenobarbitone and 50 mg phenytoin, each twice daily. Maximum doses for adults are usually 200 mg of phenobarbitone and 400 mg of phenytoin a day. Side-effects of phenobarbitone are skin rashes, drowsiness and ataxia, and hyperkinesis in childhood; these can often be avoided by substituting methylphenobarbitone (phemitone) in doses of up to 600 mg daily. Phenytoin in excessive dosage gives rise to sponginess and swelling of the gums, which must often be tolerated if the drug is effective in controlling the patient's seizures; more troublesome are drowsiness, nystagmus and severe ataxia, symptoms which necessitate a reduction in dosage but not necessarily withdrawal, as the level of dosage producing toxic symptoms in the individual is often finely balanced. If phenobarbitone and phenytoin alone are insufficient to control the patient's attacks it should be remembered that in those individuals whose seizures are major in type but in whom the EEG reveals generalised spike-and-wave activity, troxidone is occasionally effective, and this drug may be cautiously added in an initial dosage of 0·3 g twice daily, increasing if necessary. More often, however, and particularly when

N**

the EEG has shown generalised spike discharges or temporal-lobe spikes, it is preferable to substitute primidone (mysoline) for pheno-barbitone, while continuing with phenytoin. The initial dose of this drug is 0·25 g twice daily, increasing if necessary up to a maximum of 0·5 g four times daily, but few patients can tolerate this level of dosage. Many patients are intolerant of this drug and suffer from vomiting, severe drowsiness, dysarthria and ataxia, and these symptoms often necessitate its withdrawal or a substantial reduction in dosage to a level which is insufficient to control the seizures. Under these circumstances, another remedy which can be tried is methoin (mesontoin), which though chemically similar to epanutin can be given in combination with the latter drug in a dosage of up to 100 mg four times daily. Cases of agranulocytosis and aplastic anaemia have, however, been reported as a result of this remedy. It should always be remembered that megaloblastic anaemia has resulted from prolonged medication with phenytoin and with mysoline, but responds to treatment with folic acid. Another effective anticonvulsant which is unfortunately even more toxic than the drugs previously mentioned is phenacetylurea (phenurone, dose 0·5 g up to four times daily), which seems to be particularly useful in myoclonic epilepsy. The latter remedy is now being supplanted by phenylethylacetylurea (benuride) of which the dosage is 200 mg three times daily; it is equally as effective and less toxic. Almost completely non-toxic, but relatively ineffective as an anticonvulsant, and also very expensive, is beclamide (nydrane, hibicon), given in a dosage of 500 mg three to six times daily. A recent addition to the range of hydantoinates is peganone (500 mg and 100 mg tablets; 1-5 g daily). Another most important drug which has been intro-duced within the last few years is sulthiame (ospolot) which can be given in a dosage of 200 mg three or four times daily along with full doses of phenobarbitone and phenytoin, and has proved to be remarkably effective in many resistant cases.

The treatment of **status epilepticus** (recurrent major convulsions occurring without recovery between attacks) is a matter of consider-able difficulty and the condition has a significant mortality. Sodium gardenal (200 mg every six hours) and phenytoin (100 mg six-hourly) should be given intramuscularly but are rarely sufficient. Paral-dehyde (10 ml intramuscularly every four to six hours) will control the attacks in most cases but must sometimes be given by intravenous drip. If these measures fail, intermittent positive pressure respiration with curarisation of the patient may be required for several days in addition to anticonvulsant therapy.

There are also a considerable number of commercial preparations containing several of the anticonvulsant drugs in various combinations, but these are mentioned only to be condemned, as in the majority of cases it is important to be able to adjust the dosage of the various remedies independently. There can be no condition which is more rewarding to treat than epilepsy, since with patience and repeated trial and error, provided the principles mentioned above are taken into account, a very large proportion of epileptics can have their fits controlled by anticonvulsant medication. Some patients require three or four such drugs in combination and patient trial and error of different combinations is often required before success is achieved. Most epileptic children can attend ordinary schools and many lose their attacks (particularly if these have been only petit mal) after puberty. Only a small proportion whose attacks are impossible to control require prolonged institutional care or education in special epileptic schools or colonies. Restrictions to be imposed upon the activity of the child epileptic are largely dictated by common-sense and depend to some extent upon the frequency and severity of his attacks. Thus it is reasonable to forbid cycling on the highway, climbing, and swimming except in company, but other restrictions are as a rule unnecessary and an over-protective attitude upon the part of the parents must be avoided.

In adult life, too, most epileptics can play a useful part in society, though there are a small number with mental defect, frequent fits or behaviour changes resulting from temporal lobe epilepsy, who require institutional care, usually in a mental hospital. The latter is generally also true of some patients who have degenerative cerebral disease, of which epilepsy is merely a symptom. In other individuals, the guiding principle with regard to employment must be that the individual should not be placed in any situation in which he might injure himself or others if he had a fit. Thus he should not work at heights, with moving machines, and must not drive a mechanically-propelled vehicle. The law with regard to driving is perfectly clear. No patient who has had an epileptic fit can hold a driving licence. Exceptionally, on medical advice, the licensing authority may restore a licence to an epileptic patient who has been free from fits, usually without medication, for three or four years. But this is a purely individual matter, and there is no legal obligation to restore the licence. Equally, while it is the doctor's duty to impress upon the patient the danger to himself and others which may ensue if he continues to drive, he has at present no obligation to report to the authorities the epileptic who continues to drive a car.

MANAGEMENT OF THE PARAPLEGIC PATIENT

The nursing and medical care of the patient who has paralysis of the lower limbs or of all four limbs can be considered under three principal headings. First it is essential that proper care be taken of the skin to prevent the development of pressure sores (bedsores); secondly, particular attention should be paid to the functioning of the bladder and bowels; and thirdly, contractures and deformities must be prevented as far as possible and physiotherapeutic measures must be utilised in order to make the best possible use of the voluntary activity, if any, which remains or returns in the weakened limbs. Pressure sores are due to prolonged pressure upon an area of skin which is at first reddened and then, as a result of ischaemia, it either becomes gangrenous or breaks down to form an ulcer. Loss of cutaneous sensibility and urinary or faecal incontinence leading to frequent wet or soiled beds are important contributory factors. The prevention of sores must depend first upon the posturing of the patient, with the assistance of special mattresses or foam-rubber cushions, secondly upon frequent turning, with a change of position every half-hour, and thirdly upon strict cleanliness of bed-linen with frequent washing and massaging of vulnerable skin areas. Various forms of skin protectives, such as barrier creams, may be helpful. Susceptible areas include the elbows, the skin over the scapulae, the sacrum and buttocks, the lateral aspect of the hips and the heels.

The patient with a flaccid paraplegia of whatever cause almost invariably develops retention of urine, though sometimes from the beginning there is retention with a dribbling overflow. Catheterisation is then essential. Authorities differ as to whether intermittent catheterisation with a strictly sterile 'no-touch' technique, or an indwelling catheter is preferable. If an in-dwelling catheter (always of rubber or polythene and not of gum-elastic) is used, it should be changed every two or three days, and the technique of tidal drainage can usefully be employed in such a case. Almost invariably some degree of urinary infection supervenes, and it is important to examine the urine microscopically for the presence of pus cells every day. When infection develops, the urine should be cultured and appropriate therapy with alkalies (potassium citrate), with mandelic acid, with sulphonamides or with antibiotics is given depending upon the infecting organism and its sensitivity to these drugs as revealed by bacteriological tests. Every few days, the catheter should be removed, or intermittent catheterisation delayed, to see whether satisfactory evacuation of the bladder can be achieved either by voluntary effort, with the aid of manual compression above the pubis, or following the intramuscular injection of 0·25 mg of carbamylcholine (carbachol). If a single injection of this drug has no effect, it can be repeated half an hour later, but if there is still no evacuation of urine, the catheter should be reinserted and the procedure attempted again a few days later. Eventually, in the majority of cases of spastic paraplegia, automatic bladder action becomes established, even if the paraplegia remains complete, within a few weeks or months and the bladder is then evacuated automatically every few hours, whenever the intravesical pressure reaches a certain level. In some cases, surgical resection of the bladder neck becomes necessary to facilitate this process, as the internal urethral sphincter becomes greatly hypertrophied. Once automatic bladder action is established, the male patient can be helped by the use of disposable urinals made of plastic which prevent inadvertent wetting of his garments. Incontinence pads may be used in the female but are much less satisfactory. Following lesions of the cauda equina, the bladder remains permanently atonic and in many such cases evacuation is only achieved by means of abdominal contraction or manual compression. In some such cases permanent catheter drainage is necessary.

Care of the bowels does not as a rule give rise to as many problems as care of the bladder. Retention of faeces is usual in the initial stages and enemas are generally required every two or three days. Subsequently as a rule the patient regains some voluntary control over the act of defaecation, unless the nerve roots of the cauda equina are damaged, when regular enemas may be needed indefinitely.

The posture of the patient is all-important in the prevention of muscular contractures and consequent skeletal deformity. Thus a cage is usually required to take the weight of the bedclothes which would otherwise cause foot drop. Splinting of the legs is also required in some cases in order to prevent contractures of the hamstrings. When flexor spasms at the hips and knee develop, mephenesin or mephenesin carbamate (tablets 0·5 g, dosage up to 6 g daily) or diazepam 2-5 mg four times daily are sometimes of value. If these spasms are severe, surgical division of the obturator nerves or intrathecal injections of phenol in glycerin are sometimes necessary for their relief.

MANAGEMENT OF THE COMATOSE PATIENT

As in the paraplegic, so in the comatose patient, appropriate nursing care is essential if life is to be saved and undue disability avoided. The first essential is maintenance of an adequate airway. This is usually first achieved by turning the patient on to his side so that the tongue cannot fall back down the throat. Secretions and vomit, if present, should then be removed from the mouth, pharynx and upper respiratory passages, using suction if possible. If the period of unconsciousness is at all prolonged it is wise to pass a nasal tube into the stomach and to aspirate the gastric contents so that the danger of inhalation of vomit can be avoided. If difficulty is encountered in keeping the respiratory pathways free from secretions, a tracheotomy should be performed. Despite these precautions, comatose patients are particularly liable to develop pulmonary collapse and/or consolidation. It is therefore usual to give prophylactic antibiotic therapy, usually with penicillin, half a mega unit every six hours, and the chest should be examined frequently. Care of the skin is equally as important as in paraplegic patients, and if there is retention of urine, catheterisation will be required. The urine should also be examined at frequent intervals, because of the danger of urinary infection. If faecal incontinence is troublesome it is often preferable to give daily enemas. It is also important to maintain an adequate intake of fluid and of food if unconsciousness is likely to be prolonged. No particular steps are necessary in this connexion as a rule if the patient is unconscious for twenty-four to forty-eight hours or less. Intravenous fluid may be necessary, but is best avoided initially because of the danger of pulmonary oedema. Subcutaneous infusions of fluid using hyaluronidase are useful in such cases, but the serum electrolytes should be estimated daily and may indicate the need for intravenous therapy. Subsequently, if there is no vomiting, an adequate fluid and food intake can be achieved by intragastric tube feeding, which can be continued indefinitely until the patient is capable of taking adequate nourishment by mouth. Milk and various protein hydrolysate preparations are the basis of most meals given by tube, but care should be taken to see that vitamin supplements and adequate quantities of sodium and potassium are added.

MANAGEMENT OF RESPIRATORY PARALYSIS

There are numerous disorders of the nervous system in which paralysis of the muscles of respiration can develop, with fatal results if some form of assisted respiration is not employed. It is most important that these methods of treatment should be instituted early, when the patient is showing symptoms merely of restlessness, anxiety, irritability and sleeplessness and before cyanosis or impairment of consciousness have resulted from respiratory insufficiency. The commonest conditions in which this is necessary are acute anterior poliomyelitis, postinfective polyradiculopathy (the Guillain–Barré syndrome), transverse myelitis, myasthenia gravis and polymyositis or dermatomyositis, but there are many others in which respiration may cease while the heart continues to beat strongly. As a general rule, techniques of assisted respiration should only be used if the illness from which the patient is suffering is one in which some degree of recovery may be expected, for once a respirator has been started it is rarely justifiable to stop. It is, for instance, usually a waste of medical and nursing skill to utilise assisted respiration in a patient who has stopped breathing as a result of a massive intracerebral haemorrhage, unless surgical evacuation of clot is proposed.

Two principal methods of artificial respiration are available. The first method, which utilises intermittent external pressure upon the thorax, is employed in the tank (iron lung) and cuirass respirators, and is applicable in cases in which the muscles of respiration are paralysed but those of swallowing are unaffected. When, however, the pharyngeal muscles are also paralysed, so that the patient is unable to swallow food or secretions, intermittent positive-pressure respiration, in which the lungs are mechanically inflated and deflated through a cuffed tracheotomy tube, is needed. Each of these methods requires a team of doctors and of nurses to give the patient constant supervision and to check continually that ventilation is adequate and that the patient is not developing evidence of anoxia or of carbon-dioxide retention. Many other nursing problems arise in connexion with care of the patient's skin, bladder and bowels, quite apart from the physiotherapeutic and other treatment he requires for the primary condition which was responsible for the respiratory paralysis.

PHYSIOTHERAPY AND REHABILITATION

Physiotherapy has a most important part to play in the treatment of many neurological disorders. Thus when disease results in a partial or complete paralysis of a limb, or of more than one limb, appropriate physiotherapeutic treatment must be instituted as soon as possible. The purpose of this treatment is to help the patient to make the best possible use of the available power in the affected limb if the paralysis is partial, and to prevent muscular contractures, stiffening and deformity if it is complete. When paralysis is almost complete, whether it be flaccid (a lower motor neurone lesion, or an upper motor neurone lesion during the stage of spinal shock) or spastic (upper motor neurone lesion), the first essential is that passive movements of the affected muscles should be carried out repeatedly through a maximum range at all affected joints. This action will maintain the elasticity of the muscles, will prevent the development of contractures and may, if spasticity is present, help in modifying the increased muscular tone. Later, once voluntary power begins to return, active movements are encouraged, first with support or positioning of the limb to nullify the effect of gravity and later against resistance. In a patient with a hemiplegia following cerebral thrombosis, for instance, this process is sometimes very slow, requiring great patience and continual encouragement on the part of the physiotherapist and nurse, and confidence and persistence on the part of the patient. Nearly all hemiplegic patients can eventually be helped to walk, although in many, little useful function in the paralysed fingers is regained. The help of a skilled physiotherapist is also essential in patients with respiratory paralysis, as skilful positioning will not only help the patient to expectorate secretion which might otherwise obstruct the bronchi, but will also help him to make the best possible use of the ventilatory capacity which he regains.

Rehabilitation is important not only in restoring to useful activity those patients who are recovering from an illness resulting in paralysis, but may also be of inestimable value in individuals suffering from certain chronic neurological diseases. Thus in patients with ataxia resulting from cerebellar disease, Fraenkel's walking exercises, in which the patient learns to walk along a line or to follow foot-prints drawn on the floor, may be very beneficial. Similar exercises, if utilised with enthusiasm and persistence, and combined with vigorous passive movements, are also of great value in the rehabilitation of the paraplegic, and in the education of children with cerebral palsy. They may even produce considerable improvement in patients with diseases such as disseminated sclerosis and Parkinsonism, in whom there is hope of remission or arrest. On the other hand, physiotherapeutic treatment of this type is not indicated in other remorselessly progressive disorders such as motor neurone disease; it is disappointing to the patient and frustrating for the physiotherapist, as the disease progresses sufficiently rapidly to nullify any temporary benefit which may result from the treatment. Much the same is true in cases of muscular dystrophy, although it is sometimes of benefit in such cases to demonstrate to the parents of affected children the passive movements (dorsiflexion of the ankle, extension of the knees) which they can employ to delay the onset of contractures for as long as possible.

There are many appliances which can be utilised to compensate for disability and to aid the physiotherapist in her efforts. Thus in the patient who is beginning to walk following a disabling illness, walking machines, walking tripods, crutches, calipers and walking-sticks, may all be required at some stage to give the patient the support and confidence which he needs. Night splints applied to a spastic or paralysed limb are often a useful means of preventing contractures, while in a patient with foot drop, a toe-spring fitted to his shoe to prevent the toe from dragging will improve his walking considerably. Similarly, a 'cock-up' forearm splint will be required in a patient with wrist drop. In obtaining for his disabled patients appropriate appliances and invalid aids, the neurologist is dependent upon the advice of his colleagues in physical medicine and upon the help of skilled physiotherapists.

Closely related to physiotherapy and rehabilitation are techniques of **manipulation** and **immobilisation.** Manipulation of muscles and joints is often required to overcome stiffness, or the adhesions and contractures which sometimes follow paralysis. An example is the painful 'frozen shoulder' which not uncommonly develops in the hemiplegic patient and which is often benefited also by an injection of 1 ml of 'intra-articular' hydrocortisone into the capsule of the shoulder joint. The place of manipulation in spinal disorders and particularly in the treatment of intervertebral disk prolapse is a much more controversial matter, and one upon which there is singular lack of agreement amongst neurologists, physicians in physical medicine, orthopaedic surgeons and neurosurgeons. In a case of acute disk prolapse, whether lumbar or cervical, most neurologists would favour an initial period of bed rest for two to three weeks, with the aid (in cervical disk prolapse) of a collar made of soft 'gamgee' tissue. In some cases of lumbar disk disease continuous traction applied through a suitable belt applied over the lower abdomen and attached to weights (15-30 lb) which are suspended over a pulley at the bottom of the bed relieves pain which is not relieved by bed rest alone. Continuous or intermittent traction of the neck is also helpful sometimes in cervical disk prolapse. If symptoms persist at the end of this period, then immobilisation in a plastic-moulded collar or in a plaster jacket or firm lumbar support (in lumbar disk disease) is then advised, usually with success. Should these measures fail, then manipulation in skilled hands has a place, although the risks of paraplegia following cervical manipulation or of a cauda equina lesion after lumbar manipulation must be borne in mind. Surgical exploration is only as a rule indicated in relatively young patients in whom other measures tried over an adequate period have failed to relieve pain or when there are physical signs (paraparesis, lower motor neurone paralysis, sensory loss) indicating persisting compression of the spinal cord or of one or more spinal roots. Impairment of sphincter control, a 'cauda equina syndrome' or even foot-drop resulting from acute lumbar disk prolapse, are always indications for laminectomy, but minimal neurological signs (an absent ankle jerk or a small patch of sensory loss) may resolve with conservative treatment. In cases of chronic cervical sponylosis with spinal cord compression, immobilisation of the neck in a collar is rarely of benefit save for the relief of pain. Nevertheless it is often utilised *faute de mieux,* as the results of surgical decompression of the cervical spinal cord are singularly unimpressive except in patients who are showing rapid deterioration and in whom there is myelographic evidence of severe compression of the spinal cord by one (or at the most two) intervertebral disks.

OCCUPATIONAL THERAPY

The value of the occupational therapist in helping patients suffering
from chronic neurological diseases, or in those who are recovering
slowly from disabling disorders of the nervous system (including head
injury) cannot be denied. As days and weeks of comparative mono-
tony slip by, with improvement which may at first be imperceptible,
particularly to the patient, it is essential that he or she should be kept
occupied and interested. Not only does he require constant encouragement, but time spent in basket- or rug-making is not only an
antidote for despondency, but will also help to improve the power
and co-ordination of his limbs. Occupational therapy is of particular
value to the disabled housewife in assisting her to adjust to or
compensate for her disability in the performance of domestic tasks,
but is also invaluable in the rehabilitation of the wage-earner as well
as in the management of the seriously disabled. Television and
organised sports (such as archery for the paraplegic) are also excellent
for morale in appropriate long-stay hospitals. Even greater ingenuity
may be demanded of the doctor who is supervising the slow recovery
of a patient who has been ill in his own home.

SPEECH THERAPY

The speech therapist is another invaluable member of the team of
individuals who are concerned in the treatment and rehabilitation of
neurological cases. The greater part of her time is spent in the pains-
taking education of children who are born with defective speech or
who begin to speak in an abnormal way. Two important categories
are the deaf child and the child with severe cerebral palsy. While
considerable improvement may be expected in these children with
patient training, complete recovery can be achieved within a few
years in children with dyslalia. But speech therapy is also useful in
patients suffering from dysarthria and more particularly aphasia as
a result of disease of the brain (as after cerebral vascular accidents).
With the aid of patient re-education, recovery can be accelerated
and is in the end much more complete, provided the patient is capable
of enthusiastic co-operation.

THE TREATMENT OF INFECTIONS

Whereas no specific therapy is available for most of the virus infections of the nervous system, bacterial infections of the brain and
meninges, as elsewhere, are favourably influenced by chemotherapy
and by antibiotics and it is important that treatment should be
given in adequate dosage and by the most effective route.

Meningitis

PYOGENIC MENINGITIS

The prognosis of meningococcal meningitis, the commonest variety of pyogenic meningitis, has been transformed since the introduction of the sulphonamides and the antibiotics. The most satisfactory combination of drugs for treatment of this condition is intramuscular penicillin with sulphadiazine given by mouth. Although very little penicillin normally penetrates the blood-brain barrier, substantial amounts of this drug will cross the inflamed arachnoid to enter the subarachnoid space, so that intrathecal therapy is rarely necessary in this condition. The usual adult dose is one or two mega units of penicillin given intramuscularly every six hours, and sulphadiazine, 4 g as an initial dose and thereafter 1 g every four hours. Treatment should be continued for at least five to seven days and sometimes longer, depending upon the clinical response.

The treatment of **other varieties of pyogenic meningitis** is similar, provided bacteriological tests reveal that the organism is penicillin-sensitive. However, in pneumococcal, streptococcal and staphylococcal meningitis, intrathecal penicillin therapy is usually essential, at least for the first few days. As penicillin is irritative when injected into the subarachnoid space, the maximum dosage which can safely be given is 10,000 units of crystalline penicillin, well diluted in 10 ml of sterile normal saline, and this should be repeated not more often than every twelve hours until a satisfactory reduction in the number of cells in the cerebrospinal fluid is achieved and cultures become sterile. Often systemic penicillin and sulphadiazine must be continued for two or three weeks. If the organism, on culture, is found to be penicillin-resistant, then other antibiotics such as streptomycin, chloramphenicol, one of the tetracyclines, or erythromycin will be required, again depending upon sensitivity. The tetracyclines in common use are tetracycline itself (achromycin), chlortetracycline (aureomycin) and oxytetracycline (terramycin); the standard dose of each is 250 mg, six-hourly. These drugs are reserved for penicillin-resistant Gram-positive infections. Erythromycin, of which the dose is 250-500 mg, six-hourly, is best reserved for staphylococcal infections which resist penicillin, while chloramphenicol (250 mg, six-hourly) is also useful as a wide-range antibiotic, and particularly in influenzal meningitis, but should only be used for relatively short periods as it is liable to produce blood dyscrasias. In influenzal meningitis, streptomycin, 1 g daily intramuscularly, may also be effective, as is sulphadiazine; streptomycin is also required in the rare cases of *B. coli* meningitis. Antibiotic and sulphonamide therapy may have to be continued for many weeks in influenzal meningitis before the spinal fluid returns to normal.

Systemic penicillin is also required, or other antibiotics depending upon the sensitivity of the infecting organism, if known, in cases of **extradural, subdural or cerebral abscess.** In each of these conditions, however, the most essential part of treatment is surgical drainage of the abscess, or sometimes, in cases of cerebral abscess, its total excision. Surgical drainage at an early stage is particularly imperative in cases of spinal extradural abscess.

TUBERCULOUS MENINGITIS

The essential drugs in the treatment of tuberculous meningitis are streptomycin (1 g intramuscularly daily), sodium aminosalicylate (PAS, in cachets, 16-20 g daily) and isoniazid (200-300 mg daily). There is much controversy as to whether intramuscular streptomycin therapy in combination with PAS and isoniazid is sufficient, as many workers believe, or whether intrathecal streptomycin is also required. Some workers still favour the administration of 0·1 g streptomycin intrathecally, daily for six or seven days and thereafter twice weekly for three or four weeks, in adults. In children, a proportionately lower dose (25-50 mg) is given by intrathecal injection. However, in general it is now believed that systemic treatment alone is sufficient in most cases and fewer and fewer patients are receiving intrathecal medication. It is now usual to give 100-150 mg of cortisone or 20-30 mg of prednisone daily in addition, as it appears that this drug prevents the development of adhesions in the subarachnoid space. In cases in which multiple subarachnoid adhesions and spinal block have developed despite treatment, it is sometimes necessary to give intrathecal streptomycin via cisternal puncture or even through burr holes into the lateral ventricles. There is also some evidence that in cases of this type, in which the prognosis seems poor, intrathecal tuberculin may be of value, but this method of treatment must be used with the greatest caution and is only rarely applicable.

Other Bacterial Infections

Leprosy is a disease which can now be treated effectively with drugs of the sulphone group, of which the most effective is dapsone, which is given in a dosage of 25-50 mg twice weekly, increasing to a maximum of 400 mg twice weekly. The treatment of **tetanus** is complicated and difficult, particularly in the severe generalised cases and always requires skilled nursing in hospital. The first essential is to neutralise free circulating antitoxin; this is done by giving 60,000 to 100,000 units of antitoxin, half intravenously and half intramuscularly. As the tetanus bacillus is penicillin-sensitive, penicillin should be given in a total dosage of two mega units daily, preferably by six-hourly intramuscular injection, but this treatment does not modify the effects of the antitoxin. The next essential is, if possible, to remove the source of exotoxin by excising the wound in which the bacteria are growing. It is also important to maintain adequate hydration, electrolyte balance and nutrition, and this must be achieved by appropriate tube-feeding and/or intravenous therapy. Most important and difficult of all, however, is the control of the tetanic spasms. The patient should be nursed in a dark room, insulated as far as possible from noise. Many forms of treatment have been advised, including sedation with paraldehyde, avertin or other barbiturates, high dosage of chlorpromazine, or intravenous infusions of mephenesin. It now seems probable that the most effective treatment in severe cases is to perform a tracheotomy and to institute intermittent positive-pressure respiration, while keeping the patient's muscles continuously relaxed with tubocurarine, succinylcholine, or other relaxant drugs. The danger of hyperpyrexia may have to be averted by means of tepid sponging or other techniques of generalised cooling.

In cases of **botulism,** the only really effective treatment is to give 5,000 units of botulinus antitoxin after the tainted food has been ingested but before symptoms have developed. When symptoms have developed, the appropriate dose is 20,000 units given intravenously, and a daily dose should be given intramuscularly for several days thereafter.

Virus Infections

Although some few of the larger viruses, such as that which causes primary atypical pneumonia, appear to be sensitive to the tetracycline group of drugs, unfortunately none of the dangerous neurotropic viruses appear to be influenced significantly by antibiotic therapy. Thus treatment depends essentially upon the provision of adequate fluid and nourishment, the administration of sedatives or analgesics as required, careful nursing including the institution of artificial respiration in appropriate cases (as in some patients with poliomyelitis), and the application of methods of physiotherapy and rehabilitation once the acute illness has subsided. In the acute stage of anterior poliomyelitis, physical exertion should be avoided as much as possible as this may increase the severity of the paralysis.

Spirochaetal Infections

Although there is some evidence that the leptospirae of **Weil's disease** and **canicola fever** may be moderately sensitive to penicillin, and this antibiotic should certainly be given to such cases in appropriate dosage, it does not appear to have much influence upon the course of the illness in clinical cases, and treatment depends upon general principles of dietary and nursing care.

Penicillin is, however, the sheet-anchor of treatment for **neuro-syphilis,** and is in the view of many neurologists the only drug required for cases of meningovascular syphilis, of general paresis, and of tabes dorsalis. This view is, however, contested by many venereologists. Despite this difference of opinion there is no doubt that penicillin is effective in each of these conditions. An average course of treatment is one mega unit of procaine penicillin given intramuscularly each day for twenty-one days. Often the course of treatment must be repeated at three-monthly intervals, on two or possibly three occasions until the cerebrospinal fluid cell count and protein content reverts to normal and the Wassermann and Kahn reactions become negative. It is not nowadays considered necessary to begin treatment with small doses of penicillin as Herxheimer reactions (exacerbation of symptoms at the commencement of treatment) are extremely rare. Penicillin is almost invariably curative in meningovascular syphilis, but in general paresis particularly, and in tabes dorsalis to a lesser extent there is a body of opinion which favours the administration of fever therapy, generally by infecting the patient with blood containing the plasmodia of benign tertian malaria, or by utilising a heating cabinet designed to produce hyperthermia. Patients treated with malaria are generally allowed to have seven to ten febrile episodes before antimalarial drugs are given. The use of bismuth and arsenical drugs in cases of syphilis has now been virtually abandoned, but there is some evidence that a short course of iodides in cases of tabes dorsalis may partially relieve residual 'lightning pains' when penicillin has failed to do so.

Parasitic and Fungal Diseases

A long discussion of methods of treatment of parasitic and fungal disorders would be inappropriate in a textbook of neurology; many of those which affect the nervous system are relatively uninfluenced by treatment but torulosis, it now appears, can be effectively treated with the new antibiotic amphotericin B, while actinomycosis is sensitive to large doses of penicillin given in association with sulphadiazine. Malaria, alone among the protozoa, can be effectively treated by means of a wide variety of agents, including quinine, chloroquine and primaquine.

SYDENHAM'S CHOREA

No single drug is effective in the treatment of rheumatic chorea. Some physicians still give salicylates in adequate dosage (sodium salicylate or aspirin 2 g, four-hourly at first, reducing to a maintenance dosage of 1·3 g six-hourly) but there is no convincing evidence that this treatment affects the course of the disease and cortisone and other steroid drugs appear to be of no benefit. Rest, quiet surroundings and sedation, with either phenobarbitone 30 mg eight-hourly or amylobarbitone 60 mg eight-hourly, are the most important measures.

ALLERGIC DISORDERS

There is now increasing evidence to suggest that many of the nervous diseases which appear to result from hypersensitivity, and particularly postinfective encephalomyelitis and the Guillain–Barré syndrome, are favourably influenced by treatment with cortisone and related drugs of the steroid group (*vide infra*).

THE TREATMENT OF MENTAL DISORDERS

A detailed review of the innumerable methods of treatment for mental disease which are now available would be inappropriate in a volume devoted to neurology, but an outline will be given of some of the more important methods which are available for the relief of symptoms of disorders of the mind. In cases of anxiety state or reactive depression, a willingness to listen to a description of the patient's symptoms and to his explanation of their probable cause, and an attitude of patience and understanding on the part of the doctor may be of more benefit than drugs. Indeed some individuals are cured by simple psychotherapy, particularly if the basic cause of their anxiety can be revealed and eradicated. Psychotherapy of this type often requires little more than wise counselling and humanity and does not involve the more complex and time-consuming techniques of psychoanalysis. Often, however, the judicious use of drugs is of great benefit, though drug therapy without understanding, and without confidence of the patient in the doctor, will achieve little. Anxiety and tension can be substantially relieved by the administration of amylobarbitone 60 mg or of quinalbarbitone 50 mg three times daily. When insomnia is also a feature of the illness, a larger dose of an appropriate hypnotic will be required before retiring. Should these measures be ineffective, then a variety of other tranquillising drugs are available, of which the most useful are chlorpromazine (25-50 mg three times a day), promazine (50 mg three times daily) meprobamate (200-400 mg three or four times a day), trifluoperazine (2-6 mg daily), chlordiazepoxide (5-10 mg three times daily), thioridazine (25-50 mg three times daily)and diazepam (2-5 mg three times daily). If there is considerable weight loss and anorexia, as in cases of anorexia nervosa, 10-20 units of subcutaneous insulin and

50 g of glucose given before each meal are often useful for promoting appetite. If reactive depression is superimposed upon anxiety, a tablet combining dextroamphetamine sulphate (5 mg) with amylobarbitone (50 mg), such as drinamyl, is sometimes effective, and should be given at 8 a.m. and 12 noon. These drugs are also available in 'spansule' (long-acting) form. This type of combined tablet should, however, be used with great caution as patients may become dependent upon amphetamine preparations and this type of remedy is now being largely supplanted by other drugs which carry less risk of habituation. Similar forms of treatment are sometimes of benefit in cases of hysteria, but hysterical symptoms are often much more intractable unless their cause can be removed, and may require more sophisticated methods of treatment such as hypnosis or abreaction during light pentothal anaesthesia.

Many drugs are now available for the treatment of depression. Reactive depression or anxiety-depression often responds best to a combination of phenelzine (15 mg three times daily) and trifluoperazine (1 mg three times daily). For severe endogenous depression, however, the drugs of choice are imipramine (25 mg three times daily increasing up to 75 mg three times daily), amitriptyline (25-50 mg three times daily) and nortriptyline (25-50 mg three times daily). Maintenance treatment may have to be continued for many months or even for years in some cases. The dangers of liver damage in patients receiving chlorpromazine and phenelzine or other amineoxidase inhibitors or of toxic reactions due to the ingestion of cheese in those receiving the latter group of drugs should be borne in mind. Nevertheless these drugs have transformed the treatment of depressive illness. Cases of severe depression which fail to respond to drugs require electroconvulsion therapy (ECT) and may be cured by six to eight treatments given at intervals of two or three days.

The control of mania is essentially a problem of sedation, and paraldehyde, 10 ml intramuscularly, is the most valuable drug. Remarkable benefit can be obtained in some cases of schizophrenia with reserpine in an initial dosage of 0·25 mg three times daily, increasing up to 1 mg or more three or four times a day, but this drug occasionally produces severe depression. It is also particularly valuable in senile psychoses. Trifluoperazine, too, given in a dosage of up to 5 mg three times a day is often useful in cases of paranoid psychosis or other delusional states. Chlorpromazine and its derivatives can be of great benefit in some severely disturbed schizophrenic patients and may have to be given in a dosage of 200-300 mg three or four times daily. In many cases of this disease, however, the maximum therapeutic response may be obtained from electroconvulsion therapy given repeatedly over a long period.

POISONING, ADDICTION AND DRUG WITHDRAWAL

In all cases of accidental or suicidal poisoning it is first important whenever possible to determine the nature of the poisonous agent, in order that appropriate treatment may be given. For instance, in cases of carbon-monoxide poisoning, oxygen, and artificial respiration if need be, should be given. In cases of poisoning by drugs, unless the substance ingested has a strong corrosive effect, the stomach should be washed out immediately, and if, for instance, the patient has taken a strongly acid substance, an appropriate bland alkali (magnesium carbonate or sodium bicarbonate) should be given, while if the poison was a powerful alkali, vinegar in water is a suitable antidote. The commonest drugs which are utilised for suicidal attempts nowadays are sedatives, particularly the barbiturates. In such a case the first essential is to maintain adequate ventilation, by preservation of the airway and using artificial respiration if need be. Whereas many analeptic drugs have been utilised in such cases, including metrazol, picrotoxin and amphetamine, it is now apparent that the most effective remedies in such cases are bemegride (megimide) and amiphenazole (daptazole). Unless it is clear that the dose taken was small enough for the patient to recover spontaneously, these drugs should usually be administered; certainly they should be given to any patient who is comatose (showing no response even to painful stimuli). Their administration is greatly facilitated if an intravenous infusion of saline or glucose saline is set up; 1 ml of a 1·5 per cent solution of amiphenazole and 10 ml of a 0·5 per cent solution of bemegride are then given intravenously every three to five minutes until the tendon reflexes are obtainable and usually until there is some sign of returning consciousness. In severe cases, intermittent positive pressure respiration is needed and there is evidence that a powerful diuretic such as frusemide (40-120 mg) may promote excretion of the drug via the kidneys. In occasional cases, if these methods of treatment fail, dialysis with the aid of an artificial kidney is successful in removing barbiturate from the body. Similar methods of treatment can be used not only in barbiturate intoxication, but in poisoning with narcotic drugs.

The treatment of **heavy metal poisoning** (arsenic, lead, copper), if acute, is similar to that of any form of acute poisoning. In chronic intoxication with heavy metals, the appropriate remedies are dimercaprol (BAL) or chelating agents such as calcium EDTA (versene). BAL is given by deep intramuscular injection in a 5 per cent solution; the dosage is 2 ml, four times on the first day, three times on the second, twice on the third and then daily for four days. Several courses of treatment may be required at intervals of a few weeks. The dosage of calcium EDTA is 0·5 mg given intravenously in 200 ml of saline over two hours; this should be repeated every eight to twelve hours for five days and another course may be required a few days later.

Drug addiction, whether to opiates, barbiturates, amphetamine or alcohol is extremely difficult to treat. There is hope of success if the underlying psychiatric disorder which caused the addiction can be treated effectively, but more often there are basic defects in personality in the addict which are immutable. Some addicts, and particularly alcoholics, are salvaged through the interest and support they obtain from organisations such as Alcoholics Anonymous, whose members often attain a zeal for reform which has almost a religious intensity. In the addict who genuinely desires a cure, the process, though often painful and long-lasting, is worth-while, but many addicts undergo prolonged and distressing courses of treatment, only to relapse immediately when once more they enter society. The cure of addiction almost always requires treatment in an appropriate hospital. The complicated series of steps required to treat the opiate addict are beyond the scope of this volume. In chronic barbiturate intoxication, withdrawal must be gradual in order to prevent psychosis and convulsions. Usually the patient is given 200-400 mg of pentobarbitone or a similar barbiturate three or four times daily, and the dosage is reduced by 100 mg daily. If severe withdrawal symptoms appear, a higher dosage can be recommenced for two or three days and then the process is begun again until complete withdrawal is achieved.

In cases of chronic alcoholism, a similar regimen of gradual withdrawal is often effective, using progressively lower amounts of whisky or brandy. Sudden withdrawal may result in delirium tremens; in this condition, intramuscular paraldehyde is often required to control excitement and/or convulsions, and intravenous fluid may be needed in order to correct dehydration and electrolyte imbalance. There is some evidence that corticotrophin (ACTH), 100 units daily by intramuscular injection on the first two or three days, is beneficial, as some of the symptoms of delirium tremens are believed to be due to adrenal exhaustion. Vitamins of the B group should also be given in heavy dosage parenterally and are conveniently administered in the form of 'parentrovite'. Insulin (fifteen units) and glucose (50 g) three times daily are also of value, and can usefully be continued after the acute stage in order to promote appetite. Residual tremulousness is often relieved by meprobamate, chlordiazepoxide or chlorpromazine, although the danger of jaundice following administration of the latter drug should be remembered. Vitamins in high dosage, including thiamine 200 mg or more should be given daily over a prolonged period, particularly if there is any evidence of polyneuropathy. Once withdrawal has been achieved, prolonged abstinence can be helped by the use of disulfiram (antabuse). This drug is given in a dosage of from half to one tablet (0·25-0·5 g) daily. When a patient who is taking this drug regularly takes alcohol, acetaldehyde is released into the circulation and gives rise to headache, palpitations, nausea and vomiting. Great care must be exercised in the use of antabuse, as fatal reactions have been described following a large intake of alcohol; it is usually wise to begin its administration in hospital and to give the patient a small glass of an alcoholic beverage during his stay, so that he may know what to expect if he drinks while receiving the drug. If he has no real desire to be cured, he has only to stop taking the tablets on leaving hospital; but antabuse is nevertheless of considerable value in strengthening the resolve of those who wish to overcome their addiction, and certainly helps them to resist temptation.

MIGRAINE AND RELATED DISORDERS

Although migraine is a constitutional disorder which cannot be cured completely, it can be relieved considerably in the majority of cases. The frequency and severity of attacks is unquestionably increased by stress, fatigue and/or anxiety; adequate rest, relaxation, avoidance of stress, and the use of tranquillisers to relieve tension and anxiety are thus of benefit in some cases. In the patient who is suffering frequent severe attacks, their incidence and intensity can often be reduced significantly by the continued use, for several months, of the old-fashioned Gowers' mixture: liq. trinitrini, m. 1, tinct. nux. vom., m. 15, tinct. gelsemii, m. 10, phenazone, gr. 5, sod. brom., gr. 5, aq. chlorof. to $\frac{1}{2}$ oz, three times daily. Sometimes tablets of ergotamine tartrate, if taken regularly for short periods, have a prophylactic effect but prolonged treatment is dangerous because of the risk of ergotism. An increased frequency of migrainous attacks in women at about the time of the menopause is commonly due to an associated depressive illness which can usually be relieved by treatment with phenelzine or amitriptyline (*vide supra*) with dramatic improvement in the attacks of migraine. However, the greatest advance in the prophylaxis of migraine has been the introduction of methysergide (1-3 mg three times daily) which often reduces dramatically the frequency and severity of attacks and may have to be continued in diminishing dosage for several months. The actual attack, if it is mild, will often be greatly relieved by aspirin or by two tablets of tab. codeine co. For more severe attacks, tablets containing ergotamine tartrate, and an antihistamine drug to combat nausea and vomiting, are often very effective, provided they are taken during the aura or the moment the attack begins. Examples of useful proprietary preparations are cafergot (ergotamine tartrate 2 mg, caffeine 100 mg, belladonna alkaloids 0·25 mg, *iso*butylallyl-barbituric acid 100 mg) and migril (ergotamine tartrate 2 mg, caffeine 100 mg, cyclizine hydrochloride 50 mg); one or two tablets is the appropriate dose for a single attack. If these oral remedies prove ineffective, then ergotamine tartrate in suppository form or inhaled as a fine powder should be tried, or else the more intelligent patients can be taught to give themselves a subcutaneous injection of ergotamine tartrate (0·5 mg) at the beginning of the aura. If the patient is then able to lie down for approximately thirty minutes, the attack may be aborted.

Ergotamine tartrate is also the most appropriate drug for the treatment of **migrainous neuralgia.** Oral therapy should first be tried when a 'bout' begins; a tablet of cafergot or migril or of some similar preparation should be given two or three times daily. If effective, this treatment should be continued for several weeks, depending upon the duration of previous 'bouts', and repeated attempts to withdraw the tablets are then made until withdrawal is accomplished without the return of pain. Should these remedies be ineffective, then dimethysergide (1-2 mg three times daily) should be given according to a similar programme. If oral therapy is ineffective injections of ergotamine tartrate, 0·5 mg subcutaneously, may be required once or twice daily during a bout. Treatment should not be continued indefinitely because of the danger of ergotism.

NARCOLEPSY AND RELATED DISORDERS

The drug of choice in the treatment of narcolepsy and other conditions causing prolonged somnolence is amphetamine sulphate, or dextro-amphetamine which are given in an initial dosage of 5 mg at 8 a.m. and 12 noon, and the dose is then increased if necessary depending upon the requirements of the individual patient. Some patients require as much as 40 mg daily to keep them awake, but this is exceptional.

EPISODIC VERTIGO

Episodic vertigo of labyrinthine origin (e.g. Menière's syndrome) can be very difficult to control. Phenobarbitone in a dosage of 30 mg two or three times daily has been used for many years, but is of comparatively little value, and diuretics which have also been widely employed are disappointing, despite the fact that the essential pathological change in Menière's syndrome is a hydrops of the membranous labyrinth. Somewhat more effective are dimenhydrinate (dramamine) 50 mg three times daily, promethazine (avomine) 25 mg three times daily, prochlorperazine (stemetil) 5 mg three times daily and thiethylperazine (torecan) 10 mg also three times daily. These remedies appear to reduce the severity of the attacks but not necessarily their frequency. They are also of great value in motion sickness and in vestibular neuronitis (epidemic vertigo) and have fewer side-effects than 0·5 mg hyoscine which is equally if not more effective. In a small proportion of cases of Menière's disease involving only one ear, if the attacks of vertigo are frequent and severe, labyrinthectomy is justifiable, despite the fact that the ear is rendered permanently deaf by this operation. In elderly patients, the ataxia which normally follows this operation, but is usually brief, can be very persistent and difficult to overcome. Some neurosurgeons still practise section of the labyrinthine division of the eighth nerve, but this must be done intracranially with all the risks of a posterior fossa exploration. The most satisfactory method, which is likely to be used increasingly in the future, is destruction of the membranous labyrinth by means of ultrasonic waves; this method is effective, carries little risk and leaves hearing intact.

SPASTICITY

Although numerous drugs have been advised for the relief of spasticity, none produce any dramatic improvement in the mobility of spastic limbs. Chlorpromazine in doses of up to 100 mg three times daily, or zoxazolamine 0·5 g four times daily are occasionally of some benefit, if combined with physiotherapeutic measures. Mephenesin carbamate (tolseram) which is given in an initial dose of 0·5 g four times daily, increasing gradually if tolerated up to 3-4 g four times a day, is occasionally beneficial, but is very costly and rarely produces sufficient clinical improvement to justify the expense of prolonged use. Meprobamate, 400 mg three or four times daily, is sometimes helpful, but chlordiazepoxide (10-20 mg three or four times daily) and diazepam (5 mg three times daily) seem to be more effective and are probably now the drugs of choice. Occasionally, however, they so reduce extensor tone that the patient's lower limbs become almost flaccid so that he is unable to walk and hence treatment may have to be discontinued. When severe adductor spasms develop in the thighs, obturator neurectomy is occasionally necessary, while painful flexor spasms may be relieved in a proportion of cases by means of intrathecal injections of phenol in myodil or glycerine (described earlier for treatment of intractable pain) around the L1 and L2 roots. Rarely the pain of flexor spasms is sufficiently severe to justify intrathecal injections of alcohol, despite the certainty of producing bladder paralysis, or alternatively spinothalamic tractotomy may be considered. In most cases nowadays, however, the judicious use of phenol injections is the most effective method and a surprising degree of voluntary power in the affected limbs may be preserved.

PARKINSONISM

A great many drugs are available for the partial relief of muscular rigidity in Parkinsonism and related conditions, and striking improvement can be produced in a considerable proportion of cases when the optimum combination and dosage of drugs is achieved. This is an individual matter; drug tolerance varies widely from case to case; some patients respond to one drug, others to another, and sometimes if a particular drug appears to be losing its effect, substitution of a different though similar remedy is remarkably successful. Although tremor is relieved much less by drugs than is rigidity, it too can be reduced in amplitude and severity. The traditional remedies, tinct. stramonii, 15-30 m three times daily, atropine and hyoscine, 0·5-1 mg three or four times daily, have largely been abandoned, despite their effectiveness, in favour of more modern proprietary preparations, because of their troublesome side-effects (severe dryness of the mouth and blurring of vision). The most popular and effective remedies are: benzhexol hydrochloride (artane), 2 mg three times a day initially, increasing up to 20 mg or more per day, orphenadrine hydrochloride (disipal), 50 mg tablets, three to eight daily, ethopropazine hydrochloride (lysivane), 50 mg tablets, four to ten daily, procyclidine hydrochloride (kemadrin), 5-20 mg three times daily, benztropine methanesulphonate (cogentin), 2 mg tablets taken at night or twice daily and phenglutarimide (aturbane) 5 mg tablets, four to ten daily. Promethazine hydrochloride (phenergan) and other anti-histamine drugs are also of value in occasional cases, while methixene hydrochloride (tremonil) 5 mg tabs, 3-12 daily, is a useful adjuvant and is believed to have a selectively beneficial effect upon tremor. It is always wise to begin treatment of the condition with a small dose of any remedy and to increase the dosage gradually. Useful combinations are to give artane and cogentin or disipal and cogentin together, in the maximum dosage which can be tolerated. Side-effects of all of these drugs include blurred vision (due to disordered accommodation), dryness of the mouth, nausea, dizziness, mental confusion and urinary retention, and may be sufficiently severe to demand a reduction in dosage or trial of another remedy.

Side-effects of this type, and confusion in particular, are often most troublesome in atherosclerotic Parkinsonism and patients with this form of the disease are occasionally unable to tolerate any of these remedies. Patient trial of many remedies in different combinations is, however, well worth while in most cases of this condition, and can usefully be combined with physiotherapy. Oculogyric crises are influenced comparatively little by means of drugs, but are occasionally helped by means of amphetamine sulphate, 5-10 mg given at 8 a.m. and 12 noon. The place of surgical treatment will be mentioned below.

MYASTHENIA GRAVIS

Although edrophonium chloride (tensilon) is useful in the diagnosis of myasthenia, its transient effect means that it is not an effective method of treatment and the most important therapeutic agent is still neostigmine (prostigmine). Whereas in occasional severe cases, intramuscular injections of this drug, 2·5-5 mg or even larger doses, are required every three or four hours, symptoms can be adequately relieved in most instances by means of oral treatment. Tablets of neostigmine bromide, each containing 15 mg, are used, in an initial dosage of one or two, four times daily. These are increased depending upon the adequacy of the therapeutic response, and the presence or absence of side-effects, up to as many as fifty or sixty tablets a day in occasional cases. An average dose is two to four tablets, five or six times daily. Tablets should be taken every 2 or 3 hours depending upon the needs of the individual patient. Atropine sulphate, 0·5 mg should also be given two or three times a day to counteract the colicky abdominal pain and other muscarinic side-effects of the drug which are otherwise troublesome. Another useful remedy is pyridostigmine (mestinon, 60 mg tablets) which has a more long-lasting effect than prostigmine and can therefore be given usefully in the morning and at night before retiring. Some authorities prefer to treat all cases with pyridostigmine tablets four-hourly but most patients seem to do best on a combination of pyridostigmine and neostigmine as the latter drug gives a quicker 'boost' effect. Ephedrine, ½ gr (32 mg) three times daily is a useful adjuvant in some cases. A number of newer remedies such as ambenonium have been introduced but have not yet found a permanent place in treatment, although in some cases spironolactone (25 mg four times daily) appears to be helpful. Patients with this disease generally become skilled in adjusting the level and timing of their medication to suit their individual needs. It should be remembered that excessive dosage of prostigmine may produce an increase in weakness (cholinergic crisis). If doubt exists as to whether weakness is due to under- or overdosage, an intravenous injection of tensilon will usually resolve the difficulty, since it will increase weakness in the patient suffering from overdosage, but will improve the patient who requires more neostigmine. Unfortunately there are some cases in which different muscles respond differently and a dose of neostigmine adequate to improve strength in limb muscles may paralyse the diaphragm. Management in such cases may be a matter of considerable difficulty. Cases of the myasthenic-myopathic syndrome complicating lung carcinoma are often extremely sensitive to neostigmine and readily pass into cholinergic crisis.

In very occasional cases of myasthenia gravis, severe respiratory weakness develops despite treatment and artificial respiration is needed. The place of thymectomy remains controversial. Although it should be considered in all severe cases of the disease, it is most effective in young women who have suffered from the condition in a relatively severe form for a short period of time. If X-rays reveal the presence of a thymic tumour, this should be treated first by radiotherapy and later the thymus should be removed. In some few cases of myasthenia, particularly those in which the external eye muscles are primarily affected, the muscular weakness eventually becomes unresponsive to treatment and permanent structural changes develop in the muscles. Once this has happened, the condition cannot be significantly influenced by any form of treatment. In other cases, however, spontaneous remissions occur from time to time and are usually heralded by decreasing neostigmine requirements.

METABOLIC AND DEFICIENCY DISORDERS

The appropriate treatment of **deficiency disorders** is clearly to correct the deficiency. In cases of alcoholic polyneuropathy, Wernicke's disease and other varieties of vitamin B_1 deficiency, thiamine 100 mg three times daily should be given, while pellagra is treated with nicotinamide 200 mg three times daily. Since most vitamin deficiencies are multiple, it is often more satisfactory to give multiple vitamin therapy, provided it is adequate. A useful preparation is 'parentrovite', which contains thiamine, nicotinamide, riboflavine, pyridoxine and ascorbic acid and which can be given intravenously or intramuscularly. It is normal to begin treatment with one of each of the high-potency ampoules, given twice daily for the first two or three days, and then to give one of each of the 'maintenance' ampoules daily. After a week it is generally possible to change over to oral treatment, say, with one or two tablets of 'orovite' (50 mg thiamine, 5 mg riboflavine, 200 mg nicotinamide, 5 mg pyridoxine) or a similar combined tablet, three times daily.

In patients with vitamin B_{12} deficiency, the anaemia is satisfactorily corrected as a rule by means of intramuscular injections of cyanocobalamin (vitamin B_{12}), 100-250 μg given daily or on alternate days at first and thereafter weekly or twice weekly. When neurological symptoms or signs are prominent, however (as in cases of subacute combined degeneration of the spinal cord), a substantially higher dosage is required and it is usual to begin treatment with 1,000 μg daily, reducing later to 500 μg twice weekly or weekly. When maximum benefit has been obtained (usually within three to six months) the maintenance dose can often be reduced to 250 μg every two weeks.

Neurological complications of endocrine disease are treated by controlling the primary endocrine disorder, and the detailed treatment of diseases of the ductless glands is beyond the scope of this volume. Cases of hypopituitarism usually require about 12·5 mg of cortisone daily and often thyroxin and testosterone as well, while Cushing's syndrome resulting from adrenal hyperactivity may necessitate bilateral adrenalectomy followed by steroid maintenance therapy. The nervous complications of diabetes mellitus are improved when the diabetes is satisfactorily controlled with diet and insulin, and cases of hypoglycaemia due to an adenoma or to hyperplasia of the islets of Langerhans usually demand surgical removal of the tumour or subtotal pancreatectomy. Hypoglycaemia following gastric operations is best treated by glucose, while reactive hypoglycaemia paradoxically responds best to a high-protein, low-carbohydrate diet. Similarly, the neurological complications of Addison's disease improve when the hypoadrenal syndrome is treated with appropriate steroids, while thyrotoxic myopathy is also improved when the thyrotoxicosis is treated with carbimazole, radioactive iodine or by surgery. The myopathy and the mental disturbances which occasionally complicate myxoedema can be corrected immediately by the administration of tri-iodothyronine, followed by maintenance therapy with thyroxin. The treatment of exophthalmic ophthalmoplegia is often very difficult. Mild cases are sometimes improved by the administration of l-thyroxine 0·1 mg once or twice daily combined with a thiouracil preparation or carbimazole if there are signs of associated thyroid over-activity. Cortisone and related steroids are probably contra-indicated, and if the condition is progressive and severe, deep X-ray therapy to the orbit or surgical decompression may be required. In cases of idiopathic hypoparathyroidism, the associated epileptic seizures require anticonvulsant therapy, but additional benefit is also obtained from the use of dihydrotachysterol (AT10), 4-10 mg (3-8 ml) daily. When symptoms and signs of hypoparathyroidism follow thyroidectomy, symptoms can usually be controlled by the regular administration of calcium in the form of lactate or gluconate.

The most important measure in the control of symptoms of **hepatic coma** (portal-systemic encephalopathy) is restriction of the amount of protein in the diet. The absorption of protein derivatives can also be reduced significantly by the prolonged oral administration of neomycin, 4-10 g daily.

In cases of **hepatolenticular degeneration** (Wilson's disease), treatment with potassium sulphide, 20 mg three times daily, is useful as a long-term measure, as this preparation reduces the absorption of copper. Repeated courses of BAL or calcium EDTA (*vide supra* under 'heavy metal poisoning') promote excretion of copper and often produce clinical improvement. The most effective agent, however, appears to be penicillamine (dimethylcysteine) which is nontoxic and can be given continuously in a dosage of 0·5-1·5 g daily; it is, however, very expensive.

CORTISONE AND RELATED HORMONES IN NEUROLOGY

The principal neurological disorders in which cortisone is of value are acute postinfective encephalomyelitis and its variants, postinfective radiculopathy (the Guillain-Barré syndrome), polymyositis and dermatomyositis, temporal arteritis, and the neurological complications of 'collagen' or 'connective-tissue' disease. There is also some evidence that prolonged administration of these remedies may possibly reduce the frequency and severity of relapse in disseminated sclerosis, but this question is still in doubt. Cortisone will also reduce or abolish myotonia, but is probably inferior in this respect to procaine amide, while injections of 'intra-articular' hydrocortisone beneath the carpal ligament will relieve symptoms in a proportion of cases of median nerve compression in the carpal tunnel. Steroid drugs are also useful in preventing or delaying the development of adhesions in the subarachnoid space in cases of tuberculous meningitis.

Cortisone itself has now been largely supplanted by the newer steroid remedies which produce less salt and fluid retention and less reduction in the serum potassium. There is no convincing evidence that corticotrophin (ACTH), which must be given by injection, is superior to oral treatment with cortisone or related hormones, though fifty to a hundred units of ACTH should be given daily for two to three days when cortisone therapy is being withdrawn, in order to re-establish spontaneous adrenal function. There is, however, a suggestion from clinical trials that ACTH is preferable to cortisone in cases of multiple sclerosis and an initial course of 80 units daily may be followed by 80 units every other day and later twice weekly for several months. The usual initial dose of cortisone is 300 mg and the long-term maintenance dose is 50-100 mg, depending upon clinical response. Of the newer related steroids the most useful in clinical practice are still prednisone and prednisolone, of which the initial dosage is 60 mg daily, and the maintenance dose 10-20 mg daily. Methyl-prednisolone and triamcinolone, of which 4 mg are approximately equal in their effects to 5 mg of prednisone, are also effective remedies, but triamcinolone given over a prolonged period sometimes produces widespread muscular weakness and wasting. Similar objections apply to betamethasone (1 mg three times daily at first, later reducing to 0·5-1 mg daily) and to dexamethasone (4·5 mg daily reducing to 1-1·5 mg daily) but in some cases these drugs are apparently superior to prednisone or appear to be effective when the latter seems to be losing its effect. It is impossible to define an appropriate course of treatment applicable to each of the neurological conditions mentioned above, as the dosage of treatment must be varied in individual cases, depending upon clinical response, but it is usual to give 60 mg prednisone daily for two or three days, 40 mg daily for one or two weeks, 30 mg daily for another two weeks or more, and the dose should then be progressively reduced to 20, 10 or even 5 mg daily provided the patient's disease is kept under control. In cases of encephalomyelitis, treatment can be discontinued within two to three months, but in patients with the Guillain–Barré syndrome, temporal arteritis and polymyositis, maintenance therapy may need to be continued for six months to one year or even longer. Sometimes potassium supplements are necessary and it is wise to give calcium, in order to prevent osteoporosis, to patients receiving these drugs over long periods. Apart from the systemic side-effects (moon-face, fluid retention, hirsutes) of these remedies, peptic ulceration is an occasional troublesome complication and is occasionally overcome by the use of enteric-coated capsules of prednisone. Steroid-induced diabetes may be permanent and requires the standard treatment for diabetes.

ANTICOAGULANT THERAPY

The value of anticoagulant therapy in cases of cerebral vascular disease has yet to be finally determined. One serious difficulty is that differential diagnosis between cerebral infarction on the one hand and cerebral haemorrhage on the other cannot yet be established with certainty by any method, whether clinical or investigative. The evidence which has been collected to date, however, suggests that this method of treatment is of no real value in cases of established cerebral 'thrombosis', particularly if the resultant hemiplegia is complete. It is, however, probable that in patients suffering from cerebral embolism, particularly when there is a known source of emboli, long-term anticoagulant therapy reduces strikingly the frequency and severity of subsequent episodes. There is also some evidence to suggest that in cases of carotid or basilar insufficiency, particularly when recurrent ischaemic attacks are occurring, these episodes can be abolished by this form of treatment, which should probably be continued for a year or more. Anticoagulants are probably of no real value in patients with a slowly-evolving 'stroke' due to cerebral infarction, or in those in whom weakness is increasing in an episodic manner; nevertheless in some such cases, certain authorities continue to advise a course of treatment lasting for four to six weeks. The usual regimen of treatment is to begin with intra-venous heparin, 10,000 units every eight hours for thirty-six to forty-eight hours and with phenindione (dindevan) 200 mg on the first day, 150 mg on the second day, and a dosage which thereafter is varied according to the plasma prothrombin level, which should be estimated daily at first. The aim should be to reduce the prothrombin concen-tration to a consistent level of between 20 and 30 per cent of normal average. This can generally be done by a dosage of 25-75 mg of phenindione daily, but individual tolerance varies widely. After two weeks it is usually possible to find a level of maintenance dosage which produces adequate and consistent lowering of the prothrombin and it may then be possible to carry out the estimation twice weekly, once weekly and later even fortnightly. Many patients become skilled at assessing the dosage they require, depending upon the prothrombin level, in much the same way as the intelligent diabetic works out his own insulin requirements. Complications are few, but haemor-rhage from any site, unless scanty, generally necessitates immediate withdrawal of the drug and the administration of menaphthone (vitamin K).

With increasing experience of the use of this group of drugs in cases of cerebral vascular disease the indications for their use appear to be diminishing; certainly in patients with carotid insufficiency who are shown to be suffering from a stenosis of the internal carotid at its origin, surgical endarterectomy is a preferable method of treatment provided the patient is fit for operation.

SURGICAL TREATMENT

A detailed discussion of the indications for and techniques of neuro-surgical treatment would be inappropriate in this volume, and the brief commentary given below is included in order to draw attention to some of those neurological disorders in which judicious surgical treatment may be of benefit.

Head Injury

In cases of concussion and cerebral contusion, the essential aims of treatment are; to maintain an airway and to ensure that ventilation of the lungs is adequate; to sedate the noisy or disturbed patient; and to give adequate fluid and nutrition while partial or complete restoration of cerebral function is gradually being achieved through natural reparative processes. In occasional cases, particularly those of severe brain-stem injury, tracheotomy is required, and if hyperpyrexia develops it may be necessary to reduce the body temperature, either by surface cooling, or by the administration of chlorpromazine and pethidine, 25-50 mg of each every four to six hours. Routine antibiotic therapy, generally with penicillin, should be given in all severe cases because of the danger of respiratory infection. An associated linear skull fracture does not as a rule necessitate any immediate surgical treatment, but if there has been bleeding or leakage of cerebrospinal fluid from the ears or nose, subsequent operation is often required to close the tear in the dura, since there is a serious risk of meningitis developing as a result of the spread of infection from the middle ear or paranasal sinuses. If the fracture is not linear, but there is actual depression of skull fragments, early operative treatment is generally indicated in order to raise or excise the depressed portions of bone, and subsequently it may be necessary to close the skull defect with a tantalum plate or some similar prosthesis. The most imperative indications for surgical treatment in cases of head injury are, however, **extradural haemorrhage** and **subdural haematoma.** In cases of extradural haematoma the haemorrhage must be evacuated and the middle meningeal artery is plugged or coagulated. A subdural haematoma can usually be evacuated satisfactorily through one or more burr holes. Only rarely in longstanding cases is it necessary to excise the membrane which has formed as a lining of the subdural space.

Cerebral and Spinal Abscess

The appropriate surgical treatment for an extradural intracranial abscess is systemic treatment with the appropriate antibiotics, and drainage of the abscess, either through the ear, if it is otogenic, or through a burr hole. A subdural empyema can also be evacuated successfully through a burr hole in many cases and it is often necessary then to irrigate the subdural space with a weak antibiotic solution. Occasionally a wider exposure is needed and a bone flap

o

must be turned in order to achieve complete evacuation of the sub-dural space. Early surgical drainage of the spinal extradural space is imperative in cases of spinal extradural abscess and the laminae of two or three adjacent vertebrae must sometimes be removed to allow adequate exposure and drainage, although occasionally drainage is satisfactory without laminectomy. A cerebral or cerebellar abscess should not be approached surgically until it seems likely that the infection has become reasonably confined as a result of systemic antibiotic therapy. However, all such cases should be under neuro-surgical observation in case a sudden rise in intracranial pressure should result in tentorial or cerebellar haematoma with consequent brain-stem compression, when urgent decompression may be required. Certain abscesses in 'silent' areas of the brain can be excised completely, including the capsule. More often it is necessary to aspirate the abscess and to instil antibiotic with a radio-opaque substance such as thorotrast and thereafter to aspirate and inject antibiotic daily until the cavity is seen to shrink.

Intracranial Tumour

In cases of presumed intracranial tumour in which there are localising signs indicating that the lesion lies within one cerebral hemisphere, carotid arteriography is often a diagnostic measure, as the vascular pattern may not only localise the neoplasm but will also give some indication of its nature. However, when there are symptoms and signs of raised intracranial pressure, without localising neurological signs, ventriculography is more appropriate, since in many such cases the neoplasm lies in the posterior fossa. A considerable proportion of meningiomas can be excised completely, except for some of those in the cerebellopontine angle or in the region of the sphenoidal ridge; these often envelop important structures such as cranial nerves and major cerebral arteries. In some such cases the surgeon may have to be content with an incomplete removal. The same difficulty may arise in cases of acoustic neuroma, but many of these neoplasms, if diagnosed sufficiently early, can be removed completely, although there is generally a residual facial paralysis and some facial anaesthesia on the side of the lesion. It is virtually impossible to remove any glioma of the cerebral hemisphere com-pletely; if such a tumour is confined to one frontal lobe, say, it is sometimes advisable to carry out a frontal lobectomy in order to create an internal decompression which may prolong life. Generally it is essential to turn a bone flap and to take a biopsy from the tumour (sometimes this can be done via a burr hole) as its histological characteristics will be of value in assessing the prognosis, but radical surgery, and decompression achieved by removing areas of the skull vault, are generally contra-indicated in such cases as these measures merely prolong and accentuate suffering. The situation with regard to gliomas and particularly cystic astrocytomas of the cerebellar hemisphere is, however, quite different, as these can sometimes be completely excised, particularly in children, with excellent results and sometimes without recurrence. The same is true of haemangioblastomas of the cerebellum. Also benign and slow-growing, and occasionally completely removable, are oligodendrogliomas, particularly if lying in one frontal or temporal lobe. Gliomas of the brain stem and of the spinal cord are also comparatively benign in some cases and considerable and prolonged improvement may be achieved with radiotherapy. Cytotoxic drugs given systemically have been shown to have a markedly beneficial though temporary effect in some patients with gliomas but this work is still in the experimental stages.

Colloid cysts of the third ventricle can also be removed completely in many cases, though the technical approach is difficult, but medulloblastomas, ependymomas and craniopharyngiomas are often inoperable. However, the drainage of a cyst in cases of craniopharyngioma is sometimes of considerable, though temporary, benefit, while children with medulloblastomas can usually be greatly improved, again temporarily, by radiotherapy. Some ependymomas of the fourth ventricle can also be removed in their entirety. Radiotherapy is also a useful adjuvant in cases of pituitary adenoma, but in most cases, particularly when the tumour is a chromophobe adenoma, surgical removal is indicated. Sometimes when a relatively benign but inoperable neoplasm is present in the posterior fossa and is giving rise to internal hydrocephalus through blockage of the aqueduct, an appropriate palliative measure is to perform Torkildsen's operation or some similar procedure such as the insertion of a Spitz-Holzer valve by means of which cerebrospinal fluid from one lateral ventricle is allowed to drain through a tube into the basal cisterns of the subarachnoid space or into the venous circulation.

Finally it is important to mention the intracranial arteriovenous angioma; a small proportion of these malformations which are small and lie in relatively silent areas of the brain (e.g. the frontal lobe) can be excised completely, but there are many which are too large or are situated too close to important areas of cortex for this measure to be considered. Some few cases of this type are benefited temporarily by the ligation of major superficial vessels which enter the malformation.

Parkinsonism and other Involuntary Movements

Stereotaxic surgery, a technique through which, with radiological aid, an intrument can be inserted into individual nuclei in the depths of the brain with considerable accuracy, has transformed the surgical treatment of Parkinson's disease. It is true that in some patients with severe unilateral tremor, this can be abolished by dividing the crossed pyramidal tract in the cervical spinal cord, but destruction of the globus pallidus or more often of a part of the lateral thalamic nucleus, by the passage of a coagulating current, by injecting alcohol, or by the use of a freezing (cryogenic) probe, not only abolishes contralateral tremor in a considerable proportion of cases but also reduces rigidity. The operation should be considered in patients with Parkinson's disease who are physically fit, mentally alert, under the age of sixty-five, and who are considerably disabled by tremor and/or mainly unilateral rigidity. Sometimes the operation can be done in older patients and in those with bilateral signs, but the risks are greater when the operation must be done on both sides. Stereotaxic surgery has also been utilised for the abolition of involuntary movements in patients with hemiballismus, torsion spasm and Huntington's chorea, with some measure of success and is now being applied in the treatment of intractable pain. It is less successful in the treatment of athetosis. The procedure is time-consuming and carries certain risks so that the selection of appropriate cases for this form of treatment is a matter for the specialist.

Epilepsy

Surgical treatment can only be utilised in cases of epilepsy when clinical and electroencephalographic evidence indicates that the epileptic seizures are the result of focal epileptic discharge arising in a limited and relatively superficial area of the brain. It is only indicated when adequate treatment with anticonvulsant drugs has been given over a prolonged period and has failed to control the patient's seizures. The primary aim of the procedure is to localise by means of electrocorticography and then to excise the diseased area of the cerebral cortex and/or the subcortical structures in which the epileptic discharge is arising. Clearly, therefore, surgical treatment would not be appropriate if the focus is found to be in the primary motor or sensory area. Surgical treatment is particularly applicable in the treatment of intractable cases of temporal lobe epilepsy, in which excision of the anterior portion of the affected temporal lobe will sometimes cure the patient's attacks and will also improve his temperament and behaviour. In some cases of infantile hemiplegia in which epilepsy and behaviour disorders are intractable, surgical removal of the entire diseased cerebral hemisphere, with the exception of the basal ganglia (hemispherectomy) may result in an abrupt cessation of the attacks, without significant worsening of the hemiplegia; this operation is particularly appropriate in cases of the Sturge–Weber syndrome.

Cerebral Vascular Disease

Surgical treatment is being utilised to an increasing extent in cases of intracranial haemorrhage. Evacuation of a subdural haematoma is of course essential once the diagnosis is made, but it is now becoming apparent that a small proportion of relatively young patients who develop a primary cerebral haemorrhage due to hypertension or some other cause can be improved if the haemorrhage is localised by arteriography or ventriculography and then drained through a burr hole. Surgical methods of treatment are, however, even more appropriate in cases of subarachnoid haemorrhage resulting from rupture of an intracranial aneurysm or angioma. Everything depends upon the results of carotid arteriography, which should ideally be performed within the first few days after the haemorrhage. If it reveals an intracranial or subdural extension of the bleeding, this may require evacuation, but the essential problem is to deal with the primary cause. Some aneurysms can be excised, their parent arteries can sometimes be ligated, they can be trapped between ligatures, opened and packed with muscle, or coated with a layer of acrylic resin. The use of hypothermia as an aid to anaesthesia has greatly reduced the risks of operation. The appropriate technique to be utilised and the timing of the operation is a matter for the expert, but all cases of subarachnoid haemorrhage should now be considered as possible candidates for surgical treatment.

It is also becoming increasingly apparent that in some patients suffering recurrent cerebral ischaemic attacks, particularly in the distribution of one internal carotid artery, angiography will demonstrate a localised stenosis of the artery in the neck. In such cases and in certain others in whom aortic arch angiography demonstrates local stenosis of major vessels, thrombo-endarterectomy is curative and will prevent a major stroke.

Spinal Cord and Root Compression

In every case in which myelography gives appearances which could be the result of a benign intraspinal neoplasm, laminectomy should be performed, as the great majority of these neoplasms can be totally removed, with excellent results. Surgical treatment is not, however, indicated as a rule in cases of traumatic paraplegia due to fracture-dislocation of the spine, as damage to the spinal cord is generally at its maximum immediately after the injury. Laminectomy is, however, indicated in any other case in which there is evidence of localised spinal cord compression resulting in a progressive para-

plegia, unless there is evidence to indicate that the lesion responsible
is a metastasis or some other lesion of equally sinister prognosis.
Even if the lesion compressing the cord is known to be malignant (e.g.
metastasis or myeloma) laminectomy and decompression may be
needed to avoid total paralysis before radiotherapy or chemotherapy
can be effective. The place of surgery in the treatment of cases of
cervical spondylosis involving the spinal cord remains controversial.
Any attempt to remove the prolapsed intervertebral disks or the
bony ridges into which they have often been converted, is almost
certain to result in severe damage to the spinal cord. Simple laminectomy of two or three vertebrae with division of the denticulate
ligaments in order to produce a decompression, is indicated in those
cases in which neurological disability is advancing despite other forms
of treatment and in which myelography indicates the presence of
central disk protrusions at one, two or very rarely three levels. Surgical
treatment is also indicated sometimes when there are symptoms and
signs of long-standing compression of one or two spinal roots, either
in the cervical or in the lumbar region, and particularly if the myelogram shows that the root-sleeve or sleeves at the appropriate levels
fail to fill with contrast medium. Under these circumstances the root
canal should be opened and it may be necessary to divide fibrous
adhesions. It should also be remembered that occasionally a large
lumbar disk prolapse can compress multiple roots of the cauda
equina giving a clinical picture like that of a cauda equina tumour;
in such a case, too, surgical removal of the prolapsed portion of disk
should be carried out.

Peripheral Nerve Disorders

The surgical management of lesions of the peripheral nerves is
often regarded as being the province of the orthopaedic or general
surgeon rather than of the neurosurgeon. In this category one must
include operations such as removal of a cervical rib or fibrous band
which is compressing the inner cord of the brachial plexus, or
removal of a neurofibroma growing from the sheath of a peripheral
nerve such as the sciatic. Section of the carpal ligament to relieve
median nerve compression is an operation which is done by orthopaedic, general and neurological surgeons; the operation can be
done 'blind', using an instrument known as a retinaculotome which
is inserted through a small incision, or else an open exposure
of the carpal tunnel can be made. Both methods are successful. In
the surgical management of peripheral nerve injuries it is now generally agreed that if a nerve has been divided by an injury, the results
are usually better if secondary suture is performed some weeks after
the original injury, rather than immediately when the primary

laceration of the skin is sutured. The results of ulnar nerve suture are much better than those achieved after suture of the median nerve. If the results of peripheral nerve repair are unsatisfactory, it is often possible to carry out various operations involving muscle or tendon transplants to compensate for residual disability, but these do not require detailed discussion here. Transplantation of the ulnar nerve to lie in front of the elbow is, however, often required in patients who present with symptoms and signs of a progressive ulnar nerve lesion due to compression and irritation of the nerve trunk as it lies behind the medial epicondyle of the humerus.

THE MANAGEMENT OF THE 'INCURABLE' CASE

So many of the chronic neurological disorders are relatively un-influenced by any form of treatment that patients suffering from this group of conditions present particularly difficult problems in management. The specialist and more particularly the general practitioner will often need to mobilise all his reserves of patience, tact and human understanding in dealing with these problems. It is true, as already mentioned, that physiotherapy is often of temporary benefit in some such cases and that many appliances and invalid aids are available to assist patients in compensating for and adjusting to their disabilities. But when the patient, despite his efforts and those of his doctors, sees himself deteriorating it is not surprising that he often becomes despondent. To strike the right note of encouragement, of sympathy combined with firmness, to offer a glimmer of hope without unjustifiable optimism, and to think of something new to say to the patient and his relatives at each weekly visit; these are the problems which often strain the doctor's resources to the utmost. When to tell the patient the truth about his condition? When to encourage his desire for yet another opinion and when to dissuade him? What to tell his relatives and what to withhold? These are questions which cannot be answered in any text-book, as so much depends upon the patient's personality, his responsibilities and his domestic circumstances. The correct path to follow can only be chosen in the light of experience and there can be few circumstances in which the doctor's judgement is more important. Some patients demand and deserve to be told the truth and their resolve and resis-tance is strengthened by knowing the facts of the situation, however gloomy, while others prefer ignorance and seem to be curiously lacking in insight to the end. Some are helped by sedative or anti-depressive remedies when despair deepens, others regard their illness as a challenge, and triumph in every minor victory over disability. It is only to be expected that some patients will resort to unorthodox forms of treatment when orthodox medicine has failed. While it is the doctor's duty in such a case to advise his patients against accepting potentially dangerous or totally inappropriate remedial measures, particularly if this involves a financial outlay he can ill afford, the physician who regards this deviation upon the part of his patients as being a personal affront or evidence of loss of faith in his ability shows lack of understanding.

When it becomes clear that the illness is drawing towards its close, management must be guided by a number of simple principles. The most important are that pain and suffering should be relieved, and emotional distress alleviated by all available means, so that the patient can be made as comfortable as possible. The question as to whether he should be nursed at home or in hospital during this terminal period depends upon many variables, including the efficiency and devotion of his relatives and the nature of his illness. If there is no reason to suppose that the nursing and medical care which the patient would receive in hospital would be in any way superior to that he is obtaining at home, it is better that he should remain in familiar surroundings. But even in the best of circumstances there are occasions when, because of confused or irrational behaviour, incontinence and the like, admission to hospital cannot be avoided. Of the drugs which are available for the relief of pain and suffering in a terminal illness, morphine and its analogues are unquestionably the best, but sedatives such as paraldehyde, chloral or barbiturates are often required in addition, while chlorpromazine too is of considerable value, as it not only potentiates the action of many of these drugs but also helps to relieve the nausea and vomiting which are often troublesome features. If the patient dies peacefully in reasonable comfort, and his relatives have been well-informed and know that everything possible has been done, from both the medical and nursing standpoint, the doctor can be satisfied that his duty has been done.

REFERENCES

CONN, H. F., *Current Therapy* (Philadelphia and London, Saunders, 1965).

DUNLOP, D. M., DAVIDSON, S. and ALSTEAD, S., *Textbook of Medical Treatment*, 3rd. ed. (Edinburgh, Livingstone, 1963).

FORSTER, F. M., *Modern Therapy in Neurology* (London, Henry Kimpton, 1957).

GOODMAN, L. S. and GILMAN, A., *The Pharmacological Basis of Therapeutics*, 2nd ed. (New York, Macmillan, 1955).

MARSHALL, J., *Neurological Nursing* (Oxford, Blackwell, 1956).

MILLER, H. G. (Ed.), *Modern Medical Treatment* (Edinburgh, Livingstone, 1962).

O*

413

Index